Praise for *The Harvard Medical School Guide to Men's Health*

"Excellent. . . . Much like a very caring family doctor, Simon presents both sides of issues and lets the reader know what the evidence recommends as best practice. This comprehensive, informative, engagingly written guide is a standout among a slew of similar titles."

—*Library Journal*

"Men, and the women who love them, might actually read *The Harvard Medical School Guide to Men's Health*. . . . This extremely reader-friendly book is chock full of useful information, and with chapter titles like 'What Makes a Man?' and a whole section on 'What Keeps Men Healthy?' (yeah, yeah, the 'Sexuality and Reproduction' chapter is there, too), every guy should be able to find something of interest."

—*Arkansas Democrat-Gazette*

"[Simon] offers a number of ways to deal with every health issue raised and does it in a practical, straightforward manner that just may convince men that women needn't outlive them, on average, by more than five years."

—*Chicago Tribune*

"Dr. Simon's men's health guide reads like a novel. It is logical, it is scientific, and it poses all the questions men should ask or are asking. He combines science with humor and wit. It truly is about time for men. If we really are going to see increasing survival and life expectancy in men, following the recommendations in *The Harvard Medical School Guide to Men's Health* is the means to do it. The chapters dealing with reducing cancer risk and understanding prostate cancer couldn't be clearer. Every man needs to read this book."

—David S. Rosenthal, M.D., past President, American Cancer Society

"I have always called men 'ostriches' when it comes to their health care because they have their heads in the sand. Men need to take their heads out of the sand, put on their glasses, and read this informative book by Dr. Simon. The book not only gives an easily understandable description of the major diseases that men experience but it also discusses treatment and, more important, prevention. The book is easy to read, informative, and comprehensive."

—E. Darracott Vaughan, Jr., M.D., President, American Urological Association

"Cardiovascular disease is the number-one killer in our society, causing death in one of every two men in the United States. Just as important, through the development of problems like heart failure and stroke, it is also the number-one cause of disability as men age. Based on the newest and most up-to-date information, Dr. Simon explains these issues clearly and accurately. As a cardiologist, I'm particularly impressed by Dr. Simon's lucid program to prevent heart attacks and strokes. This guide can help men stay 'heart healthy.' I highly recommend it. If American men would adopt the straightforward suggestions made by Dr. Simon, we would truly be able to make progress in preventing the heart disease epidemic."

—Valentin Fuster, M.D., Ph.D., past President, American Heart Association

OTHER HARVARD MEDICAL SCHOOL BOOKS
PUBLISHED BY SIMON & SCHUSTER

Harvard Medical School Family Health Guide
by Harvard Medical School

Six Steps to Increased Fertility
by Robert L. Barbieri, M.D.; Alice D. Domar, Ph.D.,
and Kevin R. Loughlin, M.D.

The Arthritis Action Program
by Michael E. Weinblatt, M.D.

Healthy Women, Healthy Lives
by Susan E. Hankinson, Sc.D.; Graham A. Colditz, M.D.;
JoAnn E. Manson, M.D.; and Frank E. Speizer, M.D.

Eat, Drink, and Be Healthy
by Walter C. Willett, M.D.

The Aging Eye
by Harvard Medical School

The Sensitive Gut
by Harvard Medical School

The Harvard Medical School Guide to Taking Control of Asthma
by Christopher H. Fanta, M.D.; Lynda M. Cristiano, M.D.; and Kenan Haver, M.D.;
with Nancy Waring, Ph.D.

ALSO BY HARVEY B. SIMON, M.D.

Conquering Heart Disease: New Ways to Live Well Without Drugs or Surgery

Staying Well: Your Complete Guide to Disease Prevention

The Athlete Within: A Personal Guide to Total Fitness
(with Steven R. Levisohn, M.D.)

Tennis Medic
(with Steven R. Levisohn, M.D.)

THE HARVARD MEDICAL SCHOOL GUIDE TO

Men's Health

Lessons from the Harvard Men's Health Studies

Harvey B. Simon, M.D.

Illustrations by Harriet Greenfield
Editorial Review by Julie E. Buring, Sc.D.; I-Min Lee, Sc.D.; and Robert Krane, M.D.

FREE PRESS
NEW YORK • LONDON • TORONTO • SYDNEY

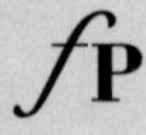

FREE PRESS
A Division of Simon & Schuster, Inc.
1230 Avenue of the Americas
New York, NY 10020

First Free Press trade paperback edition 2004

FREE PRESS and colophon are registered trademarks
of Simon & Schuster, Inc.

For information regarding special discounts for bulk purchases,
please contact Simon & Schuster Special Sales:
1-800-456-6798 or business@simonandschuster.com

DESIGNED BY LISA CHOVNICK

Manufactured in the United States of America

10 9 8 7 6 5 4 3 2

The Library of Congress has cataloged the hardcover edition as follows:
Simon, Harvey B. (Harvey Bruce), 1942–
The Harvard Medical School guide to men's health / Harvey B. Simon.
p. cm.
1. Men—Health and hygiene. 2. Self-care, Health. I. Harvard
Medical School. II. Title.
RA777.8 .S545 2002
613'.0423—dc21 2002021723

ISBN 0-684-87181-5
ISBN 0-684-87182-3 (Pbk)

Acknowledgments

LIKE ALL BOOKS OF AMBITIOUS SCOPE, *The Harvard Medical School Guide to Men's Health* has depended on the efforts of numerous individuals. While I am entirely responsible for the book's shortcomings, many people deserve credit for its possible virtues. At the considerable risk of omitting some valued contributors, I would like to express my gratitude to those who have helped. My heartfelt thanks are extended:

To the many researchers who have worked so hard and fruitfully on the Harvard Alumni Health Study, the U.S. Physicians' Health Study, and the Health Professionals Follow-up Study—and to the 96,000 men who volunteered to be subjects in these seminal investigations that continue to provide unique and important insights into men's health. Clinical studies such as these are the bedrock of modern scientific medicine. The researchers who participated in the three Harvard studies are identified along with their principal publications in the bibliography, which is available at www.health.harvard.edu/HMS_mens_health.

To the Harvard faculty members who reviewed portions of the manuscript and suggested many improvements. I am particularly indebted to Dr. Julie Elizabeth Buring and Dr. I-Min Lee, who have been major contributors to the Harvard men's health studies, and to Dr. Robert Krane, an eminent urologist. I am profoundly sad that Dr. Krane succumbed to cancer before he could see how the book turned out. Other expert reviewers who contributed important insights include Dr. Christopher M. Coley, Dr. William C. DeWolf, Dr. Greg L. Fricchione, Dr. James B. Meigs, and P. J. Skerrett.

To Ed Coburn, Joan Perry, and our other colleagues at Harvard Health Publications. My particular thanks to our Editor-in-Chief, Dr. Anthony L. Komaroff, who inspired this book and offered much sage advice. Thanks, too, to Mr. William Rosen at Simon & Schuster, who edited my manuscript with insight and care.

To my editorial assistant Kathleen Sweeny Laing and the Harvard Faculty members who serve on the Editorial Board at the Harvard Men's Health Watch for their ongoing partnership on behalf of men's health. They include Dr. Christopher M. Coley, Dr. Gilbert H. Daniels, Dr. William C. DeWolf, Dr.

Daniel A. Dyreck, Dr. Robert H. Fletcher, Dr. Greg L. Fricchione, Dr. Marc B. Garnick, Dr. Edward L. Giovannucci, Dr. Niall M. Heney, Dr. Fred H. Hochberg, Dr. Ashby C. Moncure, Dr. Patrick T. O'Gara, Dr. Russell S. Phillips, Dr. Gregory W. Randolph, Dr. Stanley J. Rosenberg, Dr. William U. Shipley, Dr. John M. Siliski, and Dr. Stephen E. Goldfinger, who convinced me to begin writing on men's health in 1996, when few thought we would find readers.

To my patients, who have granted me the privilege of serving them for more than thirty-five years. Also, to the physicians, nurses, and office staff who assist in that care and fill in for me so admirably when I put down my stethoscope to pick up my pencil.

Finally, my deepest thanks to my family for their loving support in this venture, as in all things.

—Harvey B. Simon, M.D.

For Rita
The guide to one man's health and happiness

Contents

Prologue: The Time Has Come

EVER SINCE THE DAWN OF SCIENCE, the profession has been dominated by men. It has been true of physics, chemistry, and biology, and it has occurred in every society in the world.

In America, as in other countries, medicine has been a predominantly male pursuit, both in basic research and clinical practice. Perhaps because of this, clinical research trials have historically included many more male than female subjects.

With more scientists, more studies, and more doctors, you might think men would be healthier than women—but we're not. In fact, every one of the ten leading causes of death in America is substantially more common in men than women. Which is why women are way ahead in the area that counts most, longevity. The average American woman will outlive her male counterpart by more than five years.

Over the past thirty years, the women's movement has changed the face of American medicine. Medical schools now admit nearly as many women as men. It is a change for the better, but more progress is needed, particularly in the basic sciences and in leadership positions.

The changes in clinical research have been just as profound. Large, well-funded studies are now focusing on female subjects and on the problems that worry women most, such as breast cancer, osteoporosis, menopause, and hormone replacement therapy. Harvard's 122,000-subject Nurses' Health Study and the 167,000-subject Women's Health Initiative are but two examples of the many important research projects that already have provided major dividends for women. All in all, the United States General Accounting Office reports that women currently account for 63 percent of the subjects enrolled in clinical research projects funded by the National Institutes of Health. Reflecting the current emphasis on women's health, the U.S. Department of Health and Human Services has an Office of Women's Health, but there is no similar program for men's health.

When it comes to concentrating on women's health, the federal government is hardly alone. Most medical centers have women's health units, most general medical textbooks have a special section on women's health, and many excellent medical texts are devoted solely to women's health. This trend in scholarly writing has found a counterpart in popular health publications, which boast many excellent books, newsletters, and magazine articles on women's health. In all these areas, though, men hardly are represented.

Where does all this leave men? Doing as well as ever in the basic sciences and clinical practice—but doing as poorly as ever in personal health. Women have made enormous professional progress in medicine without hindering men, but their progress in health has not helped men.

It is time for a change, not a step back to the days of medical inequality, but a step forward to equal progress in health for both sexes. Since doctors already are doing their best for men, the impetus for change will have to come from men themselves.

To begin the process, we founded the *Harvard Men's Health Watch* in 1996, three years after the acclaimed *Harvard Women's Health Watch* was established. At the time, there were no health letters for men and skeptics doubted that men would be interested enough to subscribe. In short order, more than 100,000 men proved them wrong and showed that the time had come for a men's health book as well.

The Harvard Medical School Guide to Men's Health joins the *Harvard Medical School Family Health Guide; Healthy Women, Healthy Lives;* Dr. Walter Willett's *Eat, Drink, and Be Healthy;* and the other Harvard health books. All have common goals: to inform people about health, to empower them to improve, and to motivate them to change.

Men need all three. At the start of the new millennium, the Commonwealth Fund produced a major study on the health practices of American men. The study's title tells its tale: "Out of Touch: American Men and the Health Care System." The survey found that three times as many men as women had not seen a doctor in the previous year; one-third of all men do not have a regular doctor, but only 19 percent of women lack a physician. More results:

- More than half of all men had not had a physical exam or cholesterol test in the previous year.
- Sixty percent of men older than fifty had not been screened for colon cancer within the previous year.

- Forty-one percent of men older than fifty had not been screened for prostate cancer within the previous year.
- Twenty-five percent of men said they would handle worries about health by waiting as long as possible before seeking help; only 18 percent said they would seek care as soon as possible.

The Commonwealth Fund Survey found that men shy away from health care. It also suggested that when men do see doctors, their physicians shy away from discussing sensitive issues. Only 43 percent of men had received advice about exercise from their doctors, and for other issues, the percentage of men who received counseling were even lower: diet, 37 percent; family history of prostate cancer, 31 percent; urinary symptoms, 25 percent; sexually transmitted diseases, 14 percent; and impotence, 10 percent.

The Commonwealth Fund Survey concluded that men had to pay more attention to exercise, diet, smoking, and drinking as well as urinary problems, erectile dysfunction, prostate cancer, sexually transmitted diseases, and depression. We agree.

The Harvard Medical School Guide to Men's Health shares the philosophy of the *Harvard Men's Health Watch:* Knowledge is power. To help provide that knowledge, Part I reviews the unique health needs of men and introduces a unique resource for information, three long-term Harvard studies that have been tracking more than 96,000 men for many years. Part II asks what keeps men healthy—and answers the questions by assembling data from the Harvard studies and other relevant sources. In Part III, the *Guide* turns to what can go wrong, focusing on the diseases that are particularly important to men. Although the book stresses individual responsibility and personal action, it concludes, in the Epilogue, with a brief guide to the health-care system that can help men work with their doctors to achieve better health.

It's a formidable task, but the reward, a longer, healthier, happier life, justifies the effort. Let's get started.

PART I

In Health and Sickness

The Unique Attributes of Men

CHAPTER ONE

What Makes a Man?

IT ALL STARTS WITH THE GENES, or, at least, with the chromosomes. The many similarities between men and women depend on the forty-five chromosomes they share, but the many differences between the genders depend on just one chromosome, the Y, which is unique to men.

Chromosomes are, of course, the repositories of the body's genetic master code, *deoxyribonucleic acid* (DNA). Chromosomes come in pairs, which collectively carry a total of perhaps 30,000 genes. Twenty-two of these pairs are present in both males and females, but the twenty-third pair separates men from women. This final pair contains the sex chromosomes. In women, both members of the pair are X chromosomes, but in men, one is an X, the other a Y (see Figure 1.1).

The Y chromosome is one of the smallest human chromosomes, only about one-third the size of the X. It is also one of the simplest chromosomes, carrying no more than forty genes, or about 2 percent of the number on the X chromosome. And in evolutionary terms, the Y chromosome probably derived from the X some 240 to 320 million years ago, after mammals diverged from the reptiles that lacked sex chromosomes. Adam's rib notwithstanding, males evolved from females.

Small, simple, and derivative—the Y chromosome sounds like a radical feminist's dream come true. Consider, though, the impact of a tiny chunk of DNA that resides on the apparently puny male chromosome. In fact, masculinity does not even depend on the whole Y chromosome. Instead, a single gene, the *sex-determined region Y* (SRY), makes the man. Without SRY's input, all babies would be born looking like girls, even if they had an XY pair of sex chromosomes. SRY directs the production of two hormones during fetal life. One bears the formidable name of *mullarian-inhibiting substance* (MIS); it suppresses the primordial duct system that would otherwise develop into the uterus and fallopian tubes. The other hormone needs little introduction: It is *testosterone*, the chemical that directs the development of a masculine genital tract in the embryo.

"What a piece of work is a man," Hamlet tells us. As usual, Shakespeare

FIGURE 1.1. MALE KAROTYPE

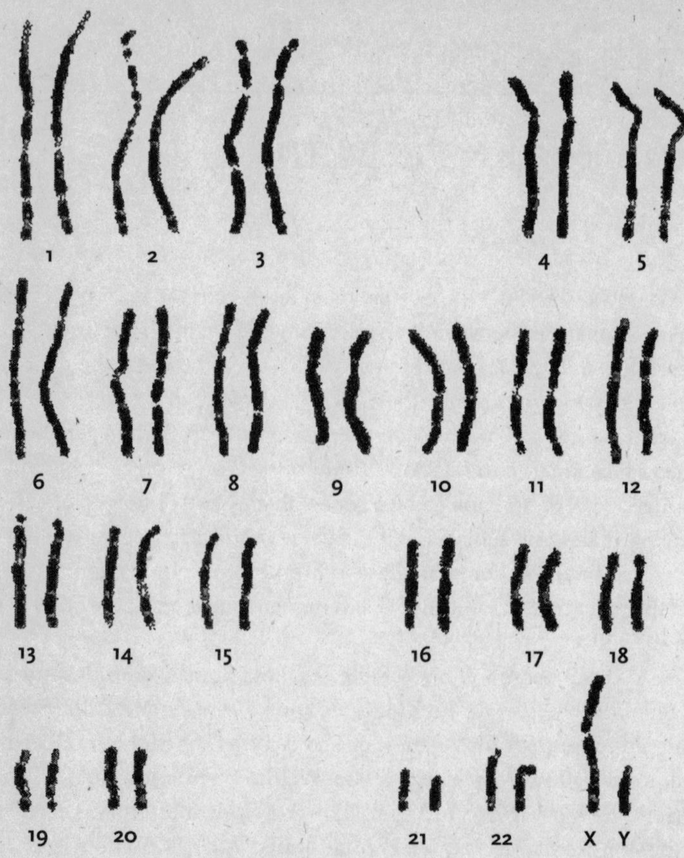

got it right—and four hundred years later, scientists finally have learned that a single bit of DNA is the ultimate craftsman of that work. Even so, there is much more to man than the SRY gene, and the differences between men and women depend on more than Xs and Ys. Since the special health needs of men are related to their unique attributes, we should try to understand what makes the man, and what makes him different from women.

Hormones

In simplest terms, male hormones are *androgens,* and female hormones are *estrogens.* Beyond that simple distinction, though, lies a world of complexity. In fact, all humans have both androgens and estrogens, but men have much more of the former, women much more of the latter. Although the sex hormones produce profoundly different biological effects, they have fundamental structural similarities. Cholesterol is the basic building block of all sex hormones, and in the process of producing androgens and estrogens, the body converts one sex hormone into another.

If the SRY gene gets its way, testosterone production begins early in fetal development and continues throughout life. Although testosterone is the most potent male hormone, it is only one of many androgens. The ancient Greeks provided the name, and they chose well. "Androgen" comes from the words for man-maker, and indeed androgens make the man, or at least his characteristic male traits.

Androgen production requires a complex chain of events (see Figure 1.2). It all begins in the brain, where the *hypothalamus* produces *gonadotropin-releasing hormone* (GnRH, also known as *luteinizing-hormone releasing hormone* or LHRH). Hormones are chemicals that are produced in one part of the body before traveling to another part, where they do their work. GnRH is a true hormone, but it does not have a long commute to work. Instead, it acts on a nearby part of the brain, the *pituitary gland*. In turn, the pituitary secretes two additional hormones, *follicle stimulating hormone* (FSH) and *luteinizing hormone* (LH). FSH and LH were named for their effects on the ovaries, but they are every bit as important for men as for women. In men, they act on the testicles, where LH triggers testosterone production and FSH, acting with testosterone, stimulates sperm production.

Testosterone is produced by the *Leydig cells* of the testicles. The starting point is cholesterol, notorious for its effects on the heart but critical for its role as the building block of all sex hormones, both male and female. After several intermediate steps, cholesterol is converted into *androstenedione*, the hormone that is readily available to Mark McGwire and other athletes as the unregulated "dietary supplement" Andro. Whether androstenedione comes from the body or from a bottle, it is rapidly converted into testosterone.

Testosterone has many direct effects on the male anatomy and metabolism (see Chapter Ten). It is responsible for the deep voice, increased muscle mass, and strong bones that characterize the gender. Testosterone stimulates the production of red blood cells by the bone marrow. The hormone also has crucial, if incompletely understood, effects on male behavior; it contributes to aggressiveness and it is essential for the libido or sex drive, as well as for normal erections and sexual performance. Testosterone stimulates the growth of the genitals at puberty, and it is responsible for sperm production throughout adult life. Finally, and for most men unhappily, testosterone also acts on the liver,

FIGURE 1.2. THE ANDROGEN CASCADE

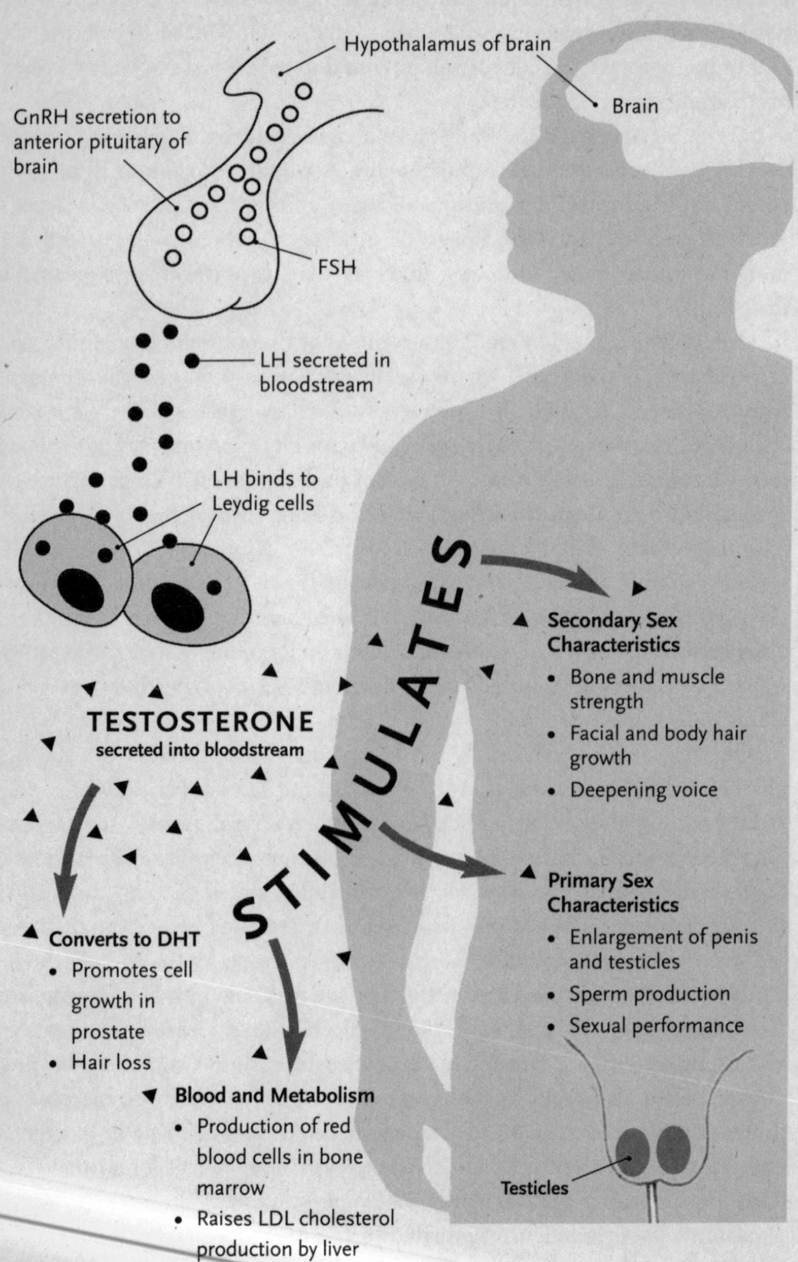

raising the production of LDL ("bad") cholesterol and lowering the amount of HDL ("good") cholesterol.

Although testosterone acts directly on many tissues, some of its least desirable effects do not occur until it is converted into another androgen, *dihydrotestosterone* (DHT). DHT acts on the skin, sometimes producing acne, and on the hair follicles, putting hair on the chest but often taking it off the scalp. Male-pattern baldness is one thing, prostate disease quite another—and DHT also stimulates the growth of prostate cells, producing normal growth in adolescents but contributing to *benign prostatic hyperplasia* (BPH) (see Chapter Eleven) and prostate cancer (see Chapter Twelve) in many older men.

About 95 percent of a man's testosterone is produced in the testicles under the control of LH. The remaining 5 percent is produced in his adrenal glands. Women also make testosterone in their adrenal glands; in both sexes, adrenal hormone production is independent of LH and FSH, and in both, an important precursor of testosterone is *dehydroepiandrosterone* (DHEA), another notorious hormone that is widely popular as a nonprescription "dietary supplement."

Testosterone metabolism has a last complexity; in its final stages, the quintessential male hormone is converted to *estradiol,* a major female hormone. Most of this final conversion takes place in fat cells, which is why obese men (and women) have higher estrogen levels than lean men (and women).

Testosterone and the Life Cycle

In males, testosterone production begins very early indeed, usually at the start of the seventh week of embryonic development, when boys become boys (see Chapter Nine). Testosterone levels remain high throughout fetal life, but they fall just before birth, so they are only slightly higher in newborn boys than girls. Baby boys experience a blip in testosterone production between three and six months of age, but by a year their levels are back down. Between six and eight years of age, adrenal androgen production rises, triggering a transient growth spurt and a bit of body hair, but no sexual development.

At puberty, a surge in GnRH and LH fires up testosterone production—and testosterone stimulates growth of bones and muscles, production of red blood cells, enlargement of the voice box, growth of facial and body hair, enlargement of the genitals, and awakening of sexual function and reproductive capacity. In most young men, testosterone production reaches its maximum at about age sixteen, and levels remain high for the next two to three decades. On average, healthy young men produce about 7 milligrams of testosterone a day.

In some men, testosterone levels remain high throughout life, but in many, they begin to decline at about age forty. Unlike the precipitous drop in hormones that women experience at menopause, however, the decline in men is gradual, averaging just over one percent a year. A 1 percent yearly drop in testosterone production is imperceptible at first, but by age seventy, the average men's testosterone production is 30 percent below its peak. Still, even with an average rate of decline testosterone levels remain within the normal range in at least 75 percent of older men—which is why many men can father children in their eighties and even beyond.

The SRY gene is responsible for testosterone production; in turn, the hormone is responsible for the development of masculine sex organs in the male fetus. But the interaction between genes and hormones does not end at birth. One example of the life-long interaction is baldness. Since men are afflicted but women are not, scientists first assumed it was a sex-linked trait. In fact, it is not. The gene for baldness is transmitted by *autosomal dominant inheritance,* which means that men and women are equally likely to inherit the gene. But since testosterone is required for the baldness gene to do its devious work, the trait is expressed only in men (see Chapter Fourteen).

Not all men are bald, but all men are men. The actions of genes and hormones are responsible for the male reproductive anatomy at birth and for the dramatic changes that occur at puberty.

Reproductive Anatomy

You don't have to know DNA from a doorknob to know that men are different from women, and the difference depends on hormones. Testosterone directs the formation of the male genitalia during embryonic life, the growth of the reproductive organs at puberty, and the function of the reproductive system throughout life.

The male genital tract is complex (see Figure 1.3). The testicles contain the Leydig cells that produce testosterone, the *germ cells* that produce sperm, and the *Sertoli* cells that nurture immature sperm. After about seventy-four days in the testicles, sperm cells enter the *epididymis,* a thin 20-foot-long tube coiled behind each testicle. After another twelve days in transit, the maturing sperm arrive in the *vas deferens,* a muscular tube that travels into the lower pelvis, where it widens into the *ampulla*. The *seminal vesicles* join the ampulla to form

FIGURE 1.3. THE MALE REPRODUCTIVE SYSTEM

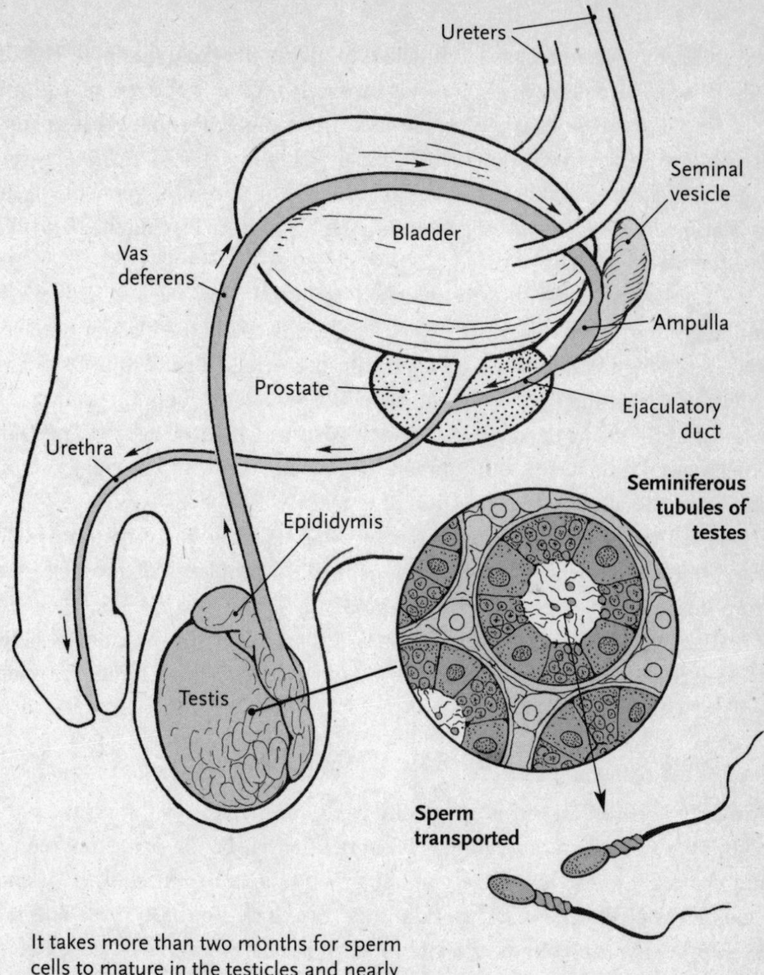

It takes more than two months for sperm cells to mature in the testicles and nearly two weeks for them to travel up through the system. But ejaculation is rapid, and semen contains fluid from the vas, seminal vesicles, and prostate.

a common *ejaculatory duct* that travels through the prostate gland into the *urethra*. Semen contains fluids from three sources; sperm-rich fluid from the vas constitutes about 10 percent of the total volume, fluid from the prostate 20 percent, and fluid from the seminal vesicles 70 percent.

The evolutionary imperative is reproduction, and the entire male sexual apparatus is dedicated to that end (see Chapter Ten). Testosterone is essential for libido, but it is not by itself sufficient to maintain sexual function. The first step is sexual arousal, which depends on erotic thoughts and sensual stimuli. The impulses of arousal are transmitted from the brain through the spinal cord to the nerves in the pelvis and genitals. These nerves, in turn, relay messages to the arteries in the penis; the arteries widen, admitting more blood, and they also compress the veins, preventing the blood from leaving the penis. The result is an erection.

Ejaculation occurs in three stages. First, fluid from the seminal vesicles and vas enter the ejaculatory ducts. Next, the muscles at the bladder neck contract, so semen cannot flow back up into the urine. Finally, muscles in the pelvis, prostate, and penis contract, expelling semen through the urethra. The arteries in the penis narrow, returning the organ to its flaccid state. The entire process is coordinated by the autonomic nervous system and is usually accompanied by the pleasurable sensation of orgasm.

Freud may have overstated the case when he wrote that "anatomy is destiny," but many of the most important medical problems of men originate from disease or dysfunction of the reproductive tract. You can learn how doctors diagnose and treat these difficulties in Part III of this book; even better, you can learn how to prevent many of them from developing in the first place.

The Male Metabolism

Sexuality is complex, but is simplicity itself compared to running the entire body. Digesting food, liberating the energy that all bodily processes require, and channeling it to growth, tissue repair, and locomotion, requires an enormous array of enzymes that work around the clock. To make these enzymes work properly, the body needs vitamins, minerals, hormones, and other cofactors.

Men and women have nearly identical metabolic machines and nutritional requirements. But there are differences; for example, men need more thiamine, riboflavin, niacin, pyridoxine, magnesium, and selenium, while women need more iron and calcium. Even so, these differences are small. Except for the extra iron needed by menstruating women and the additional calcium required by postmenopausal women, the differences depend more on body size and composition than biological distinctions between the sexes.

Men and women metabolize certain chemicals differently. Perhaps the best example is alcohol. Men metabolize alcohol more efficiently. As a result, women have higher blood alcohol levels after drinking, and they are more vulnerable to alcohol-induced liver, heart, and muscle damage. It is an interesting difference, but it does not mean that the Y chromosome confers an invitation to imbibe. On the contrary, men are more likely to abuse alcohol than women—not because of metabolic differences, but because of cultural influences (see Chapter Seven).

One of the most telling metabolic differences between men and women is the way their bodies handle cholesterol—and in this case, at least, women are clear winners. Young women usually have lower LDL ("bad") and higher HDL ("good") cholesterol levels. Hormones account for the disparity: Estrogens improve both cholesterol counts, while testosterone has the opposite effect. After menopause, though, the gap narrows; as a woman's estrogen levels plummet, her cholesterol profile takes on a manly look, and her risk of heart disease rises to rival a man's.

The final metabolic difference between men and women has no winner, but it has two losers. In America, as in most of the industrialized world, both genders have too much body fat; 33 percent of the men and 36 percent of the women in the United States are obese (see Chapter Four).

Excess body fat is bad for both men and women, increasing their risks of heart disease, hypertension, diabetes, gallstones, and certain malignancies, including cancers of the colon, and of the male and female reproductive organs (see Chapter Three). Excess fat is never good, but some body fat is worse than others. In particular, upper body fat that is concentrated around the waist and chest increases the risk of heart attack and stroke. Fat cells in the abdomen and the chest have several unique properties. They have high levels of an enzyme called *lipoprotein lipase;* in everyday terms, this means they are geared up to store energy when the body has an excess of calories—when men gain weight, fat tends to accumulate first around the waist (the "beer belly").

Fat cells also respond differently to hormones. Lower-body-fat cells are more responsive to estrogens. In contrast, abdominal fat is more responsive to the stress hormone *adrenaline.* As a result, abdomen fat cells tend to release large amounts of *free fatty acids,* which are carried directly to the liver, where they impede the normal breakdown of *insulin.* Over time, high insulin levels make the body unresponsive to the hormone, boosting the risk of diabetes. Because insulin acts as a growth factor, high insulin levels may also contribute to the link between abdominal obesity and certain cancers. In addition, free fatty acids stimulate the liver to overproduce *triglycerides,* blood fats that can increase the risk of heart disease. If that were not bad enough, upper-body-fat cells have an enzyme that activates *cortisone,* a hormone that is another potential contributor to hypertension and diabetes.

Men and women handle excess fat differently; men are prone to develop upper body obesity (the "apple shape"), while women are more likely to tote their excess pounds on their thighs and buttocks (the "pear shape"). Women can, of course, develop abdominal obesity, but it is much more common in men. That is why scientists refer to the apple shape as the *android* fat distribution and the pear shape as *gynecoid.*

Body shape is more than a question of aesthetics; it is also an important predictor of health and disease. In these terms, the shape of man is the shape of risk—but it does not have to be that way. In Chapters Four and Five, men can learn how they can shape up for better health.

Manly Muscles and Bones

Men are bigger than women, averaging about 10 percent more in height and 15 to 20 percent more in weight. Even without considering reproductive anatomy, men and women are also shaped differently. Whereas females have a slightly higher risk of being overweight than males, men are more vulnerable to the medical consequences of obesity because of their greater tendency to accumulate abdominal fat. Even when men and women maintain ideal body weight, they exhibit important differences in body composition. Women have more body fat. On average, healthy young women have 20–27 percent body fat as compared to 13–17 percent for average young men. By the same token, men have more muscle.

You do not need an advanced degree in biology to know that men are more muscular than women. But the difference is confined to one of the three types of muscle in the human body. Men have the lead in the *skeletal* or *striated muscles* that power exercise, but the genders are on equal footing in terms of the *cardiac muscle cells* in the heart and the *smooth muscle cells* that line the arteries, intestinal tract, and other internal organs.

Skeletal muscle is the most abundant tissue in the human body. Composed mostly of protein, each muscle is made up of millions of individual muscle cells or fibers. Muscle cells have several unique properties. They are huge, at least in comparison to most other cells in the body, and each muscle cell has many nuclei, the DNA-containing control centers that are usually distributed one to a cell. Perhaps because they have multiple nuclei, skeletal muscle cells cannot divide and multiply in adult life; muscles do not enlarge by growing more cells, but by increasing the size of existing fibers.

Men do not have more skeletal muscle fibers than women, but they do have fibers that are larger and stronger. Although women can increase their muscular strength with regular resistance exercise, men are much more likely to "bulk up" as they exercise. The difference is testosterone; androgens increase the size and strength of skeletal muscle fibers, especially when these fibers are put to work with resistance exercise.

Women's muscle cells will also bulk up if they are exposed to androgens. That's why so many competitive athletes and body builders of both genders succumb to temptation and use androgens to boost performance. It is illegal and it is dangerous. Athletes who abuse androgens are at risk for athletic disqualification and for medical problems ranging from acne and hair loss to infertility, liver disease, heart disease, aberrant behavior, and more.

Men have stronger bones as well as stronger muscles. In part, their bones are stronger because their muscles are stronger. To move the body, muscles contract, thus exerting force on the scaffold of bone that supports the tissues. Bone responds to that force by adding calcium and growing stronger.

Hormones also explain why men have more bone calcium. Sex hormones increase bone mineral content in both genders. Because estrogens drop so precipitously after menopause, older women have a high risk of developing *osteoporosis,* with "thin" bones that are fracture-prone. Because testosterone levels decline much more gradually, falling by only 1 percent a year beyond age forty, older men have a lower risk of osteoporosis. Even when older men become testosterone deficient, they can still convert some testosterone into estradiol, a female hormone that helps keep bones strong in men as well as women.

Despite these advantages, older men cannot rest on their laurels. The average American man will lose twelve to twenty pounds of muscle, 15 percent of bone density, and almost two inches of height as he ages. Although testosterone replacement therapy can blunt these declines, potential side effects make hormone therapy inappropriate for healthy men. But exercise and diet make up the differences. Chapters Four, Five, and Six will explain how you can keep your muscles and bones manly, and healthy, throughout life.

The Minds of Men

Men can be proud of their muscles, but we cannot always be so proud of the things we do with those muscles.

Following in Freud's giant footsteps ("anatomy is destiny"), the biologic model of masculinity attributes male behavior to the genes, hormones, and organs unique to men. Without disputing the importance of biology, the social model of gender attributes behavior patterns to historical, cultural, and familial influences. It is an interesting debate, but it often generates more heat than light. Neither side has a monopoly on truth. In fact, men and women behave differently, and both biological and social factors contribute to those differences.

In twenty-first century America, cultural changes are narrowing the behavioral gap between the sexes. Still, most differences persist; Table 1.1 lists some of the stereotypical differences between men and women:

Table 1.1: GENDER-SPECIFIC PERSONALITY STEREOTYPES

MALE	FEMALE
Stoical	Emotional
Aggressive	Expressive
Ambitious	Compassionate
Analytical	Intuitive
Assertive	Gentle
Successful	Loyal
Competitive	Sensitive
Forceful	Tender
Independent	Interdependent
Domineering	Yielding
Skeptical	Gullible
Cold	Warm
Crass	Refined

Sexual stereotypes, of course, both exaggerate the differences between men and women and tend to perpetuate these differences. But even in a culture that is steadily but slowly becoming more egalitarian, there is more than a grain of truth in these stereotypes. On the whole, men tend to be less social and more independent, less communicative and more active. Men take more risks and are more aggressive. Men may thank these traits for their political dominance and economic success, but they also contribute to the occupational injuries, accidents, substance abuse, and violence that cost so many men their lives (see Chapter Eight). The problem is particularly acute in young men. Among fifteen-to-twenty-four-year-old Americans, for example, the death rate of males is three times higher than females. Motor vehicle accidents and homicides account for much of the differences, but suicides are also more common in teenage boys than in girls, by a ratio of sixteen to eleven.

Cultural expectations and peer pressures certainly account for many behavioral differences between boys and girls and men and women. But hormones also play a role; in particular, testosterone contributes to aggressive behavior, especially in high doses. In addition, neuroscientists are beginning to assemble data that suggest there are structural and functional differences in the brains of men and women. For example, scientists in Germany reported in 2000 that men and women use different parts of their brains to navigate their way out of a maze—and that men are about 28 percent faster at navigation. It's an interesting observation, but the researchers did not offer any explanation for the legendary male reluctance to ask for directions when their navigational skills fail. For whatever reasons, men tend to perform better on certain spatial tasks, but women excel at certain precision manual tasks. Men outperform women on tests of mathematical reasoning, but women do better on arithmetical calculation tests. Males tend to have superior musical and mathematical skills, women enhanced verbal abilities.

These distinctions are far from absolute, and it is far from clear if they depend on biology or culture, nature or nurture. Still, behavior contributes to two of the most important health differences between men and women: the disparities in life expectancies and in the risks of various diseases.

The Longevity Gap

"Why can't a woman be more like a man?" It's a humorous question asked in song by Henry Higgins in *My Fair Lady*. But Higgins would sing quite a different tune if the subject was longevity. When it comes to lifespan, why can't a man be more like a woman?

Women do indeed live longer than men, but why? Can men do anything to catch up?

THE GAP

Much has changed in the United States over the past fifty years. Medicine has changed as much as any field, with dramatic advances in diagnosis and treatment. Changing, too, is the American lifestyle, with its new emphasis on healthier diets and regular exercise and its declining dependence on tobacco. As a result of these developments, life expectancy is also changing, rising slowly but steadily year after year. One thing, though, has not changed: the gender gap. People of both sexes are living longer, but in every year, women have outpaced men. In fact, the gap is getting wider; it has expanded by 60 percent over the past seventy years (see Figure 1.4).

The latest data (2000) from the National Center for Health Statistics tell the story:

Table 1.2: LIFE-EXPECTANCY IN AMERICA

Women	79.5 years
Men	74.1 years
Gap	5.4 years

It's an impressive difference, and it is responsible for the striking demographic characteristics of older Americans. More than half of all women older than sixty-five are widows, and widows outnumber widowers three to one. At age sixty-five, for every one hundred American women, there are only seventy-seven men. At age eighty-five, the disparity is even greater, with women outnumbering men by 2.6 to 1. And the longevity gap persists even into very old age, long after hormones have passed their peak. Even beyond age eighty-five, the average woman will outlive the average man by 1.2 years, which is why female centagenarians outnumber their male counterparts by nine to one.

The gender gap is not unique to America. In fact, every country with reliable health statistics reports that women live longer than men. The observation is at least as old as health statistics themselves, since women outlived men by nearly three years when such data were first recorded in Europe more than two hundred years ago. The longevity gap is present both in industrialized societies (seventy-nine versus seventy-three years in Western Europe and Australia) and in developing countries (fifty-four versus fifty-one years in sub-Saharan Africa);

FIGURE 1.4. LONGEVITY OF MEN AND WOMEN

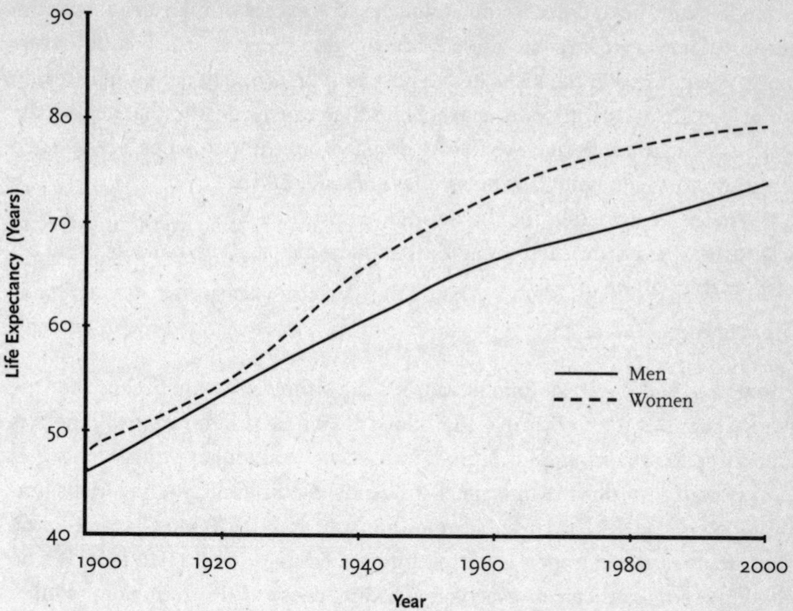

it is a universal observation that suggests a basic biologic difference between the aging process in males and females.

A Lifelong Disparity

Males are different from females from the very moment of conception, and new research suggests that events during fetal life can affect health in adulthood. For example, a low weight at birth increases a man's risk of heart attack and stroke in adulthood. It is possible then, that the levels of sex hormones and other factors at the very beginning of life are partially responsible for events at the very end of life.

Although prenatal factors can increase the risk of disease and death in adulthood, the longevity gap makes its first appearance in embryonic life itself. Sperm cells that contain a Y chromosome can out-swim sperm bearing an X. As a result, 115 males are conceived for every 100 females. But male embryos are more likely to miscarry than females, probably because women who are pregnant with boys are more likely to have defective placentas than women pregnant with girls. As a result, boys outnumber girls by only 104 to 100 at the time of birth. Newborn boys are also more fragile than girls, with a higher risk of prematurity, birth defects, and stillbirths. The excess of male deaths continues in infancy and early childhood, but the difference is small until adolescence, when testosterone kicks in and boys start behaving like men. The result: motor vehicle accidents, homicides, and other violent deaths that send male death rates soaring. By age twenty-five, females outnumber males, and the gap continues to widen with each subsequent decade of life.

What is responsible for the age-old, worldwide, life-long longevity gap? Scientists are not sure, but they agree that many factors, both biological and behavioral, play a role.

Hormones

Estrogen is good, testosterone is bad. It's the simplest way to account for the gender gap, but it's too simple to explain the whole difference. Still, there is something to it. During their reproductive years, women have much less heart disease than men of the same age. Estrogen is the difference—the female hormone lowers LDL ("bad") cholesterol and raises HDL ("good") cholesterol. After menopause, estrogen levels plummet, LDL rises, and HDL falls. It's no wonder, then, that heart disease is the leading cause of death in older women as well as in older men. Even without postmenopausal hormone replacement, women have high estrogen levels for about forty years; that's forty years more than men, and it helps explain the gap.

Estrogen protects women, enhancing their longevity by reducing the risk of heart attack and stroke. Men have much less estrogen. But they have much more testosterone. When it comes to longevity, is that hormone friend or foe? While the very large doses of androgens that are used illicitly by some athletes certainly are hazardous, contributing to acne, aberrant behavior, liver tumors, infertility, and heart disease, that tells us a lot more about the risks of drug abuse than the risks of testosterone. But new evidence suggests that even the normal levels of testosterone produced by a man's body may perhaps contribute to life-shortening diseases.

The prostate is an obvious example. In the prostate, testosterone is converted to dihydrotestosterone (DHT), the hormone that causes up to 80 percent of men to develop benign prostatic hyperplasia (BPH) as they advance in years. BPH is well named; it is a benign enlargement that does not usually shorten life, though it often lengthens urination. But DHT is also the enzyme that drives prostate cancer, the disease that kills about 3 percent of American men.

A man's own testosterone may also contribute to his risk of heart disease and stroke, the first and third leading killers in America. Five mechanisms have been postulated: (1) adverse effects on cholesterol metabolism, including a rise in LDL ("bad") cholesterol and a fall in HDL ("good") cholesterol (2) accumulation of abdominal fat (3) activation of the blood-clotting system and increased red-blood-cell mass (4) spasm of blood vessels (5) direct effects on heart muscle cells, producing enlargement and possible injury. Some of these effects can be produced with testosterone administration in experimental animals and some have been observed in men who abuse androgens. But more study will be needed to find out if a man's normal testosterone can contribute to similar abnormalities in his cardiovascular system.

TRAUMA AND VIOLENCE

Blame it on genes and hormones, or attribute it to societal expectations. For many reasons, men are more aggressive than women. Even in hunter-gatherer societies, males assume the risk of pursuing game while women take on the safer task of collecting vegetable foods. In industrial societies, too, men pursue more dangerous occupations and hobbies. Most dangerous of all are encounters with other men. Even discounting wars, violence and trauma kill far more men than women. Women do face the unique challenge of childbirth, but maternal mortality is low in the modern world and does not begin to offset the male penchant for risk, violence, and trauma.

SMOKING AND DRINKING

In the old days men smoked but women did not. They were good old days for women, but not for men. Times are changing. Many more women use tobacco than they did a generation ago, but the smoking rate of American men is down from 50 percent to 25 percent.

If smoking contributes to the gender gap, why is the gap getting larger even as smoking rates have equalized? Because smoking kills slowly. People who start smoking today will pay a steep price for their habit, but the payment will not come due for many years. Unfortunately, women are now suffering from a generation of tobacco abuse. As recently as 1960, lung cancer was rare in American women. Today, more women are killed by lung cancer (67,000 a year) than by any other cancer, including breast cancer.

At the start of the twenty-first century, smoking is one longevity factor that will not cause men to envy women. In fact, it is an area with plenty of room for improvement by both sexes (see Chapter Eight).

Like smoking, alcoholism traditionally is a male problem that is increasingly shared by women. Small to modest amounts of alcohol protect a man's health, reducing his risk of heart disease (see Chapter Seven). But larger amounts shorten life, increasing the incidence of hypertension, stroke, liver disease, accidents, and various cancers. Heavy drinking contributes to the shortened lifespan of American men.

Diet, Exercise, and Obesity

Meat is bad, veggies good. It's another oversimplification, but it may help explain why women live longer: in most cases, they eat better. In America, real men do not eat broccoli. They should. The masculine ideal of meat and potatoes should give way to vegetables, fruits, grains, and fish. Diet really makes a difference (see Chapter Four).

American men do not get enough exercise. Neither do American women. But in their traditional role, homemakers were always on the move, climbing stairs, carrying laundry, hauling vacuum cleaners, and scrubbing floors. It's another area of rapid change. Modern appliances have replaced muscles at home, and women are joining men in the work force, often in sedentary desk jobs. Still, some of today's older women retain the active patterns of their youth, and they are reaping the rewards of years of exercise. (See Chapter Five.)

Stress and Social Isolation

The hard-driving American male, succeeding at business but raising his blood pressure and clogging his coronary arteries in the process. The calm American woman, busy but happy at home. Both are stereotypes that contain a grain of truth. Type A behavior, anxiety, stress, and hostility have all been implicated as heart disease risk factors, and these traits tend to be more prevalent in men than women. Men who are feeling stress over their shorter life expectancy might be able to narrow the gap a bit by learning to relax (see Chapter Eight).

"No man is an island," wrote John Donne some 400 years ago—but in twenty-first century America, many men seem to be trying hard to be as insular as possible. The American male ideal is the independent, go-it-alone type. But that may not be good for a man's health. People are good medicine. Strong social-support networks reduce the risk of many problems, ranging from the common cold to heart attacks. In some studies, at least, support groups even improve the outcome of cancer patients. In contrast, social isolation has been identified as a heart disease risk factor. Women are in touch with their feelings and with other women. Women may not really be from Venus, any more than men are from Mars, but good interpersonal relationships may help explain why women live longer on Earth.

Iron

In 1992, Finnish scientists shocked the cardiological world when they published a report linking high levels of iron with a greatly increased risk of coronary artery disease. Since women lose iron with each menstrual period, the research fueled speculation that lower blood-iron levels help explain the protection against heart attacks that is enjoyed by premenopausal women. A 1997 Finnish study seemed to corroborate the original findings when it reported that men who donate blood have a lower risk of heart disease than men who do not donate.

Does iron explain the male vulnerability to heart disease? Probably not. Five American studies have examined the question, and each failed to corroborate an association between iron and heart disease. More study will be needed to resolve the conflicting data; at present, although there are many good reasons for a man to donate blood, longevity does not appear to be one of them.

Health Care

Women think about health more than men, and they also do more about it. Women are more diligent about checkups and preventive care. They are better at listening to their bodies and reporting discordant signals to their doctors. Seventy-six percent of the women who responded to a 1998 CNN survey had been tested for health problems within the two prior years, compared with only 64 percent for men. According to the National Center for Health Statistics, American women make 471 million visits to doctors' offices each year, men just 316 million. On average, that means 3.5 annual visits for women, but just 2.4 for men. It is another plus for women, but it's another thing that men can change (see the Epilogue).

Even when men do visit their doctors, they tend to minimize symptoms, gloss over concerns, and even disregard medical advice. It is hard to know why men make poor patients. Busy work schedules and competing responsibilities and interests may play a role, but the macho mentality appears to be the chief culprit. Who can blame men for wanting to be John Wayne? What can convince men to take the simple steps that can protect them from the heart disease and lung cancer that felled the quintessential American he-man?

Why do women live longer than men? The explanation is complex, depending on both biological and behavioral differences between the sexes. In today's changing world, women seem to be acting more like men. When it comes to health, it's a step in the wrong direction. With apologies to Professor

Higgins, it is men who should be more like women, at least when it comes to health habits and health care.

What Makes Men Ill?

Men and women each have medical problems that are unique to their gender. Only men get prostate cancer or testicular cancer and only women face the risk of childbirth and diseases of the female reproductive organs. Although breast cancer is usually considered a female disease, men are not immune. In fact, about 1,500 American men are diagnosed with the disease each year. It is a small number compared with the 204,000 cases in American women, but it is far from trivial.

Certain diseases, while not unique to either sex, have a marked predilection for men or women. For example, migraine headaches, lupus, and other autoimmune diseases that cause vascular inflammation are much more common in women than in men. But men have problems of their own. Table 1.3 lists diseases that strike males disproportionately.

Table 1.3: DISEASES MORE COMMON IN MEN

Disease	Male/Female Ratio
Inguinal hernia	9.5
Aortic aneurysm	5.0
AIDS (in America)	4.0
Gout	4.0
Kidney stones	3.5
Alcoholism	3.3
Bladder cancer	3.0
Rectal abscess	2.5
Emphysema	2.2
Duodenal ulcer	2.2
Nasal polyps	2.2
Heart attack	1.9

Men tend to get different diseases than women, and they often die from different causes. All in all, the death rate is 1.6 times higher in men than in women. A look at the ten leading causes of death in America tells the tale:

Table 1.4: THE LEADING CAUSES OF DEATH IN AMERICA

CAUSE OF DEATH	MALE/FEMALE RATIO
Heart disease	1.8
Cancer	1.4
Stroke	1.2
Chronic lung disease	1.5
Accidents	2.4
Pneumonia and influenza	1.5
Diabetes	1.2
Suicide	4.2
Kidney disease	1.5
Liver disease	1.5

In every category, the "weaker sex" is way ahead. But men can catch up, not by trading in their genes but by learning how to stay healthy.

What Keeps Men Healthy?

Men can't change their chromosomes, and very few would change their hormones, even in quest of health and longevity. Fortunately, they do not have to. A program of diet, exercise, supplements, stress control, and medical care close the gender gap and keep men healthy.

That's what this book is about. Starting with a single gene and moving to its consequences in terms of hormones, reproductive anatomy, metabolism, and behavior we have seen what makes the man. In Part II, we will consider crucial general health issues, focusing on the three large ongoing Harvard studies that have revealed so much about men's health. In Part III, we will explore selected male health problems, including genitourinary diseases unique to men and various disorders that are much more common in men than women. Finally, in the Epilogue, we will review routine medical care, both conventional and alternative.

It's a long journey, but it has great rewards.

CHAPTER TWO

Questions and Answers: The Harvard Men's Health Studies

THERE WAS A TIME when men relied on their doctors for medical facts and advice. To be sure, some information—accurate or not—trickled into our heads at school, through public-health campaigns, and from well-meaning family and friends. But now that trickle of health information has turned into a river. You can hardly open a newspaper or turn on the radio without learning of some new health risk or scientific breakthrough. And if you log onto the web, the river of advice becomes a flood.

Most men want clear answers to simple questions: Should I take aspirin? Is wine really good for me? Should I have a PSA blood test? But simple questions, however important, often have complex answers. How can a man sort through the barrage of health information to get the information he needs?

The short answer is no surprise: Read this book and keep up with new developments by reading our monthly newsletter, the *Harvard Men's Health Watch*. I hope you'll do both, but I hope you'll do more. If you know how researchers arrive at their results and how to determine if their conclusions really apply to you, you will be in the best position to evaluate medical advice. It's a bit complex, but it's worth some thought since you have the ultimate responsibility for the decisions that affect your body. And that's the way it should be. Your health is too important to be left to your doctor or even to your family.

During the past twenty-five years, scientists at Harvard Medical School and the Harvard School of Public Health have been conducting three large studies of men's health. Each of these investigations has produced a great deal of valuable information, and all three are still in progress, looking for answers to the questions that matter most to American men. In the following pages, I will introduce you to these studies and show you how to use them in conjunction with other data to improve your health. But first, we should consider how doctors learn.

Seeking Answers

Human biology is complex, human behavior no less so. To learn about both health and disease, scientists use a variety of methods:

Laboratory Studies—are the test-tube experiments that probe basic mechanisms of health and disease. Fundamental research is absolutely essential, providing the scientific basis for all of clinical medicine. It is also fascinating in its own right but, typically, it is years away from practical application in medical tests and treatments. It's great to keep up with the latest news from the lab, but, in general, you should not rush to change your lifestyle because of test-tube triumphs, however spectacular.

Animal Studies—often bridge the gap between basic research and clinical observations. Scientists have come a long way in planning experiments that are humane as well as productive. They have used animal research to generate enormous benefits for human health. But here, too, perspective is crucial. If you acted on every animal study, your health decisions might begin to resemble the moves of a mouse in a maze.

Human studies bring science into your daily life. As observations of real men, the three Harvard studies are of obvious relevance to your health. Even so, they do not span the entire range of investigative techniques. Here is how researchers can study health in human beings:

> *Case Reports*—are the simplest and most limited type of study. Here, doctors record medical details about individual patients or small groups of patients. Most often they are patients with rare or unusual problems. Case reports can help individual practitioners recognize diseases they have never seen before and they often stimulate basic research of great merit. Still, they are essentially anecdotes: more interesting than useful.
>
> *Observational Studies*—provide systemic, objective information about large groups of patients. Although they differ in the details, major portions of the three Harvard studies of men all belong to this category. In addition, much of the other research that lies behind this book depends on this approach. There are two basic types of observational studies:

- Cohort analysis begins when researchers recruit a group of apparently healthy individuals. Next, the scientists establish health profiles for each member of the group. Their third step is to observe the cohort over time, relying on various combinations of questionnaires, medical tests, and health records to track the group. Finally, the investigators compare members of the cohort who have remained healthy with those who have fallen ill, trying to identify the factors associated with illness.

  Cohort analysis is a powerful technique but it is slow, difficult, and expensive, typically involving thousands of subjects over many years. All three Harvard studies of men's health rely in part on the technique of cohort analysis. I hope you'll agree they are worth all the time, effort, and money that has gone into them. Still, in the era of fiscal restraint and diagnostic urgency, researchers are turning to other methods to supplement cohort analysis.

- Case control studies have the same goals as cohort analyses, but they proceed from the opposite direction. Instead of observing a group of initially healthy people, researchers began case control studies by identifying a group of patients who are already ill. Next, they compare the patients with an equal number of demographically similar healthy people to identify factors that may account for the difference between illness and health. Case-control studies use many fewer subjects, so they are much less difficult and expensive than cohort studies. Because they look back instead of forward, they are also much faster. In general, though, cohort analysis is a more potent investigative tool.

Clinical Trials—Observational studies are essentially passive; researchers keep an eye on people without intervening in their lives. In contrast, clinical trials are active; researchers ask some of their subjects to take medications or undergo procedures while assigning other subjects to different interventions. By comparing outcomes scientists can find out which intervention is best—or, for that matter, if an intervention is better than no treatment at all.

To understand how clinical trials work, we can think back to the very first one. The investigator was Dr. James Lind, the year 1747, thirty-seven years before the founding of Harvard Medical School. A British navy surgeon, Lind believed that citrus fruit could treat scurvy, a common affliction of sailors during long voyages at sea. To find out if his thinking was right, Lind divided his sailors into six groups of two. In addition to the normal ship's diet, each pair received a different supplement: a quart of cider; two spoonfuls of vinegar before each meal; half a pint of sea water; elixir of vitriol; a paste of garlic, mustard seed, and other herbal remedies; or one lemon and two oranges. The treatments lasted for two weeks.

After just six days, though, the sailors who ate citrus fruits had recovered. The others remained ill with the abnormal bleeding and diseased gums, skin, and hair characteristic of scurvy. Despite the success of his experiment, Dr. Lind experienced the same frustration as many of today's scientists: It took the bureaucrats of the British Admiralty fifty years to add citrus fruits to sailors' rations.

Dr. Lind's experiment at sea was a medical landmark, but it would not pass muster today. To meet current standards, Dr. Lind would have to be sure his subjects were participating voluntarily and that they had been fully informed of the study's risks, benefits, and goals. To eliminate bias, he would have to randomly assign the volunteers to the various treatment groups. Dr. Lind would also have to conduct his experiment without knowing which group got which therapy. To meet today's standards, Dr. Lind would have to give his control group (the sailors receiving a normal diet without supplements) a placebo or inert "dummy" treatment that looked just like the test treatment. In a properly designed trial, all the treatments look and taste alike, so neither the subjects nor the researchers can be influenced by prior expectations. That is why scientists call these studies "double-blind."

At the start of the twenty-first century, the *randomized double-blind placebo-controlled* trial is the gold standard for clinical research. It is a high standard, but it is really the only way to prove if an intervention is beneficial. As we will see, it is the way the Harvard study of 21,000 American male physicians found that low-dose aspirin therapy is helpful to healthy men above fifty, while beta-carotene is not.

Meta-analysis—Observational studies and clinical trials are demanding and difficult. As a result, individual studies may not be large enough to produce meaningful results. Meta-analysis is a research technique that attempts to circumvent these problems by pooling individual studies. It is not as easy as it sounds, since researchers have to select studies that are similar, screen them to be sure they are all technically competent, and use sophisticated statistical techniques to analyze the pooled data. It's a new technique that is growing explosively; only sixteen meta-analyses of clinical trials were published in the 1970s, but more than 500 appeared in 1999. Despite their real advantages however, meta-analyses have limitations and flaws of their own.

Consensus conferences—It is not a study method, but it tries to achieve some of the goals of meta-analysis, and more. A consensus conference is a gathering of medical experts who review all the research in an area, debate the results, and issue a summary with guidelines. Sometimes those guidelines are directed to doctors; the American College of Physicians position statements on the PSA blood test is an example. Often, though, the guidelines are aimed directly at you; The American Heart Association's dietary guidelines and the U.S. Surgeon General's exercise recommendations are examples.

Clinical guidelines are written on paper, not chiseled in stone. They are subject to debate and disagreement, and they are revised periodically as new discoveries change the scientific landscape. Still, even if they are not commandments, clinical guidelines are usually solid, balanced recommendations that deserve your attention, and mine.

Interpreting Results: Significance

Medical research generates numbers—but raw data, however massive and impressive, must be analyzed before they are of any use. To accomplish this, scientists apply the standard of statistical significance; it is very strict, but very narrow. Researchers can use various mathematical tests to analyze their data, but they all have the goal of determining whether the findings could result from chance alone. It is a question of probability; if the statistical tests show a 95 percent likelihood that the results did not occur by chance, the results are deemed statistically significant.

The media often abbreviate "statistically significant" as "significant"—but practicing physicians need to take closer look. Results may meet the mathematical tests of significance without being clinically meaningful. The mystery novelist Rex Stout said, "There are two kinds of statistics, the kind you look up and the kind you make up." For doctors, though, the two types are the statistically significant numbers that researchers publish and the clinically significant studies that change medical practice.

For men faced with decisions about their health, the third and most relevant type of significance is personal significance. Here, individual standards predominate. You are likely to find a result personally important if the study was conducted on people like you, if you are at risk for the disease being investigated, and if you are willing to make the changes suggested by the findings. As you learn about the Harvard men's health studies—or any other research—ask if they meet the criteria of personal significance for you.

Interpreting Results: Risks, Benefit, and Causality

If you are like most men, the first question that you'll ask when you read about a disease is "Will it happen to me?" Despite its urgency and simplicity, it is a question that does not have a simple answer. Instead, it usually gets a statistical reply: Compared to an average person, an individual with your numbers is x times more likely to become ill. In this case, x marks *relative risk*. If your relative risk of a heart attack is greater than 1, you are more likely than average to be stricken; a relative risk of 2, for example, means you are 2 times more likely to have an attack. Although even a small risk can be important when your health is involved, you should interpret relative risks below 1.5 with caution, since they may just represent statistical flukes.

Benefit is the converse of risk. If you have a factor that doubles your risk of getting a disease, you may be able to cut your risk by 50 percent by eliminating the predisposing problem. A 50 percent reduction in risk sounds great, and it is—if you have a high risk to begin with. If not, your personal benefit may be marginal.

To learn if a relative risk reduction is likely to help you, consider your *absolute risk*. If your absolute risk of a heart attack is high—say, 20 percent—a treatment that cuts your risk in half will reduce your absolute risk by 10 percent, a big gain. But if your absolute risk is low to begin with—say, 2 percent—the same excellent treatment will produce a net gain of only 1 percent. That's why people at high risk benefit much more from tests and treatments than those who are likely to stay healthy on their own.

Even after epidemiologists identify a potential risk factor by cohort analysis or the case control method, they face additional challenges. First, they must evaluate the relative importance of various factors that are present simultaneously. For example, if a smoker with high blood pressure and high cholesterol has a heart attack, which factor is to blame? To get the answer, researchers turn on their computers and use a statistical technique called *multivariate analysis* to sort it out. In this case, they can report that smoking, hypertension, and high cholesterol all increase risk.

The final and most difficult problem is to establish causality. Although the human mind is quick to assign blame, the mere coexistence of two events does not necessarily mean that one is the cause of another. For example, storks vanished from Europe at about the time the birth rate fell. Did the disappearance of the stork cause the decline in births? No. The two events were associated but did not represent a cause and its effect.

Epidemiologists can use statistics to establish associations, but they cannot determine causality. That subtler task requires several steps. To be judged causally important, an association should be biologically plausible and should be backed up by laboratory or animal experiments. Finally, because even the smartest and best-intentioned scientist is human, it should also show up in several independent studies.

Still want to be an epidemiologist? It is a vitally important science, but it's a risky business.

Reporting Results: Medicine and the Media

The public has a voracious appetite for health information, and the media are eager to feed that hunger. Too often, though, you will get little more than a sound bite. Too often, complex findings are reduced to a headline proclaiming "New Hope" or "No Hope."

To be an informed health consumer, you will have to read behind the headlines. Thoughtful medical journalists can help you do that, but they are a rare breed. About 100 years ago, the soon-to-be British Prime Minister Lloyd George explained that "you cannot feed the hungry on statistics." Today's media should not feed your hunger for health with catchy summaries that transform research findings of statistical significance into simplistic formulas for health.

Unfortunately, some medical researchers also fall prey to temptation and hype their results in press conferences and interviews. Neither is a good forum for communicating new findings, however dramatic. You should focus on results that have been published in peer-reviewed medical journals. Even with this assurance of quality and objectivity, you should note any potential conflicts of interest, particularly when research is funded by pharmaceutical companies and other commercial interests. Feel free to apply these standards to the Harvard studies and the other research cited in these pages.

Changing Results: Frustration and Fortitude

Medicine is a science, and decisions about health should be based on sound scientific evidence. But as a biologic science, medicine lacks the cold precision of physics and chemistry, and as a clinical science it must grapple with the subtleties of psychology and behavior, to say nothing of the economic reality of our times.

"Who shall decide?" asked Alexander Pope in 1732, "when Doctors disagree?" It is a difficult problem today as well. Conflicting opinions can be confusing, even frightening. When new research changes the "rules" that health-conscious people have tried to follow, the result is often frustration and even anger.

Researchers should understand your frustration, but you should understand their methods. New information should always be welcome, even if it casts a doubt on established beliefs. Medical knowledge is like a jigsaw puzzle; we know the outlines quite well, but new insights may reposition or replace some of the smaller pieces. Do not be too upset with the Harvard scientists who told you that the trans fatty acids in margarine are bad for you after all. Instead, be glad that new research can help you fine tune your diet. And if you have been following the broad outlines of a low-fat diet, even the emerging worries about margarine did not mandate major changes in your style of eating.

In preparing this book, I have tried to present the latest information in the context of what scientists have learned over the years. When conflicting data exist, I present both sides of the issue and let you know where I think the weight of the evidence lies. As you'll see, even the Harvard studies contain some conflicting results, not in the forest but in the trees. The studies agree, for example, that exercise is good for you, but disagree about its ability to prevent colon cancer. That's why there are three Harvard studies, not one, and why I will also consider the enormous body of research beyond the Harvard men's health studies.

As you read these pages, see how new information fits into your personal health puzzle before you decide to change your ways. Keep the big picture in mind, and remember to factor in your personal preferences and priorities. If you have lingering questions, discuss them with your doctor. Remember, too, that you should review your lifestyle plans with your family before you attempt to institute important changes. Good health loves company, and resolutions are most likely to succeed when backed by collective willpower.

Introducing the Harvard Studies

The three Harvard studies share certain features: All are observational studies that have been following large cohorts of men for many years but one, the U.S. Physicians' Health Study, is something of a hybrid, since it incorporates randomized clinical trials into the observational format. Because all three cohorts are composed exclusively of men, the studies provide a unique resource for the study of men's health issues. Because all three cohorts are composed of highly educated men, the questionnaires that provide much of the data are likely to have been answered with care and accuracy. But if the homogenous nature of the cohorts is an advantage, it also represents a potential drawback. The results are most relevant to highly educated, middle-class white men in mid to late life, but they are not necessarily as directly applicable to broader groups of American men. Finally, at the risk of being chauvinistic toward my Harvard colleagues, I think it is fair to say that all three studies have been conducted with meticulous care and objectivity. I am willing to take the risk of appearing biased, since I have not participated in any of the studies as an investigator. However, in the interest of full disclosure, I should point out that I have participated in one of the studies as a subject.

Despite their common features, the studies have unique characteristics that merit individual attention.

THE HARVARD ALUMNI HEALTH STUDY

The Alumni Study began at the same time as another, similar project at the University of Pennsylvania. Together, the two are known as the College Alumni Health Study. The Harvard Alumni Study began by identifying approximately 36,500 men who entered Harvard College between 1916 and 1950. Alumni who were still alive in 1962 and 1966 received questionnaires concerning their physical activity and health. In addition, the investigators obtained college archives and alumni office records and official death certificates that could be used to supplement and corroborate the questionnaires. To validate the accuracy of the questionnaires, the researchers interviewed a subset of the men by phone and performed physical examinations on another group.

From the original pool of graduates, the scientists assembled a cohort of 21,582 men who provided enough information on questionnaires in 1962 and 1966 to enable a detailed analysis of their health and their habits. The subjects were reevaluated in 1977, 1988, and 1993, when 11,894 subjects remained available for continued analysis. The Alumni Study, which is still in progress, has focused principally on exercise and its effects on coronary artery disease, strokes, hypertension, diabetes, cancer, obesity, and mortality. The faculty members responsible for the Alumni Study are identified and acknowledged in the bibliography available at www.health.harvard.edu/HMS_mens_health.

The U.S. Physicians' Health Study

Between 1981 and 1984, researchers at Harvard contacted all 261,248 American male physicians who were then forty to eighty-four years of age, inviting them to participate in the study. Approximately half the physicians responded, of whom 59,285 were willing to volunteer. The researchers excluded all the men with histories of heart attacks, strokes, or transient ischemic attacks (mini-strokes), cancer (except mild skin cancers), kidney disease, liver disease, or gout. That left a cohort of 22,071 apparently healthy men who enrolled in the study; a subset of 14,916 participants also provided blood samples that were frozen and stored for analysis at intervals over the ensuing years.

At the start of the study, each participant was randomly assigned to one of four groups: the first took 325 milligrams of aspirin on alternate days, the second took 50 milligrams of beta-carotene on alternate days, the third took both aspirin and beta-carotene, and the fourth took placebos. The aspirin limb of the study was terminated in 1988, the beta-carotene study in 1995. Each participant also provided detailed information about his height, weight, exercise, diet and dietary supplements, smoking, alcohol consumption, and health status, including his cholesterol, blood pressure, and blood sugar. The surveys have been repeated annually, allowing the researchers to track heart disease, stroke, cancer, and overall survival in the subjects. The Physicians' Health Study has fulfilled its original goal of ascertaining the possible benefits of aspirin and beta-carotene, but it continues to provide important information on cardiac risk factors, exercise, diet, alcohol, vitamins, and other issues. The many scientists who have contributed to the study are identified and acknowledged in the bibliography available at www.health.harvard.edu/HMS_mens_health.

The Health Professionals Follow-Up Study

The newest and largest of the three Harvard Studies of men began in 1986; like the other studies, it continues today. The initial cohort was composed of 51,529 dentists, optometrists, osteopaths, podiatrists, pharmacists, and veterinarians who were between the ages of forty and seventy-five when they enrolled in the study. The participants provided detailed information about their age, marital status, height and weight, ancestry, smoking, physical activity, medications, symptoms, and illness. The dietary questionnaire was particularly comprehensive; it covered 131 foods and beverages and elicited specific information on portion size, frequency of eating, and individual brands. The surveys have been repeated every two years; the researchers have contacted family members and reviewed death certificates to obtain information about the small number of men who did not respond to the questionnaires. In addition, 33,137 participants provided samples of their toenail clippings for subsequent chemical analysis.

The Health Professionals Study has focused on nutrition and health with particular attention to cardiovascular disease, prostate cancer and BPH, colon cancer, and other intestinal diseases. The many scientists responsible for the study are identified and acknowledged in the bibliography available at www.health.harvard.edu/HMS_mens_health.

Beyond Harvard

The three ongoing Harvard studies provide unique insights into men's health. Together, they have evaluated more than 95,000 men, a database of unparalleled dimensions. Because they have concentrated on heart disease, stroke, diabetes, cancer, prostate disease, and longevity, they deal with the health issues that matter most to men. Since they focus on diet, exercise, alcohol, and supplements, they can show men how to help themselves achieve better health and longer lives.

The Harvard studies are a marvelous resource for health-conscious men, but they occupy just one orbit in the universe of health information. In the chapters that follow, I hope to show you how those studies can help you stay well, but I will also call on the wider world of research to bolster the effort. In discussing the specific findings of the studies, I will refer to them in shorthand as the Alumni Study, the Physicians' Health Study, and the Health Professionals Study. By the end of this book, you should be able to recognize both the considerable strengths and the acknowledged limitations of the Harvard studies. Perhaps then you will be able to decide if you agree with James Barnes, who said, "You can always tell a Harvard man, but you can't tell him much."

CHAPTER THREE

Perils and Problems: Three Leading Killers of American Men

EVEN IF THEY DO NOT LIVE AS LONG AS WOMEN, American men can be proud of the progress that has added more than twenty-five years to their average life expectancy over the course of the twentieth century. But pride should not breed complacency. To make further gains, men will have to improve on many fronts. Good health habits, lifestyle changes, and simple supplements can have a dramatic effect on each of the three leading causes of death: coronary artery disease, stroke, and cancer. This chapter will explain these formidable foes, and the next four will present solutions to the threats they pose. Looking beyond these three diseases, subsequent chapters will discuss preventive strategies that can protect against the other major killers of American men—and improve the quality of life in the process.

Coronary Artery Disease

Heart disease is an example of what is best about American medicine and what sadly is lacking in American health. The good news is that the heart disease death rate fell by a remarkable 60 percent between 1950 and 2000; the bad news is that heart disease remains the leading killer of American men—and American women, too.

About 1 million Americans will have heart attacks this year, and one-third will die as a result. It does not have to be that way. Coronary artery disease is so common that most men assume it is an inevitable part of the aging process—but it is not. In fact, heart disease is largely preventable. The key is to understand the factors that put you at risk, then take steps to reduce your risk. You will have to do the work, but the Harvard men's health studies can help guide your efforts.

What is Coronary Artery Disease?

Although the blockages that lead to heart attacks are small and localized, coronary artery disease is actually just one manifestation of *atherosclerosis,* a disease that involves the whole body. Atherosclerosis usually is translated as "hardening of the arteries," but the disease is much more complex. Modern science has learned that the ancient Greek words that go into the name are surprisingly accurate: *athere* means porridge or gruel, and in atherosclerosis the middle layer of an artery becomes filled with soft, mushy material; only later does the artery develop *sclerosis* or stiffness and hardening.

The process starts when low-density lipoprotein cholesterol (LDL, the "bad" cholesterol) penetrates the wall of an artery (see Figure 3.1). If all goes well, high-density lipoprotein cholesterol (HDL, "good" cholesterol) will reverse the process, carrying cholesterol away from the artery for eventual disposal by the liver. But if LDL accumulates in the artery wall, it becomes a target for oxygen free radicals, the high-energy molecules generated by the body's metabolism. When free radicals bombard cholesterol, they turn it into *oxidized LDL,* much as they turn fat rancid.

Oxidized cholesterol gets atherosclerosis started. Until recently, doctors assumed that the fatty plaques of atherosclerosis were simply passive deposits of cholesterol, and that the largest plaques were the most dangerous. Neither assumption is correct. In fact, oxidized cholesterol triggers active inflammation in the artery wall. *T-lymphocytes* and *macrophages,* special white blood cells that are key components of the body's immune system, leave the blood, migrate into the artery wall, and gobble up the oxidized LDL. When macrophages ingest bacteria and viruses, they kill the microbes, but in the case of cholesterol, the reverse is true: the lipid-laden macrophages enlarge to become *foam cells,* then rupture, releasing oxidized cholesterol into the artery wall where it can perpetuate the cycle of damage. In response to all the inflammation, smooth muscle cells in the artery wall enlarge and attempt to form a hard cap over the inflammatory plaque.

Large plaques with firm caps are serious: they narrow coronary arteries, reducing the flow of blood. Such plaques cause *angina,* the chest pain that develops when the heart muscle cannot get the oxygen-rich blood it needs. But these large, firm plaques don't usually cause heart attacks. Instead, smaller, softer plaques are the culprits. They rupture, triggering the formation of a blood clot or *thrombus* on the disrupted plaque's surface. It is the clot that finally blocks the artery, killing the heart muscle cells that depend on the artery to supply oxy-

FIGURE 3.1. ANATOMY OF A HEART ATTACK

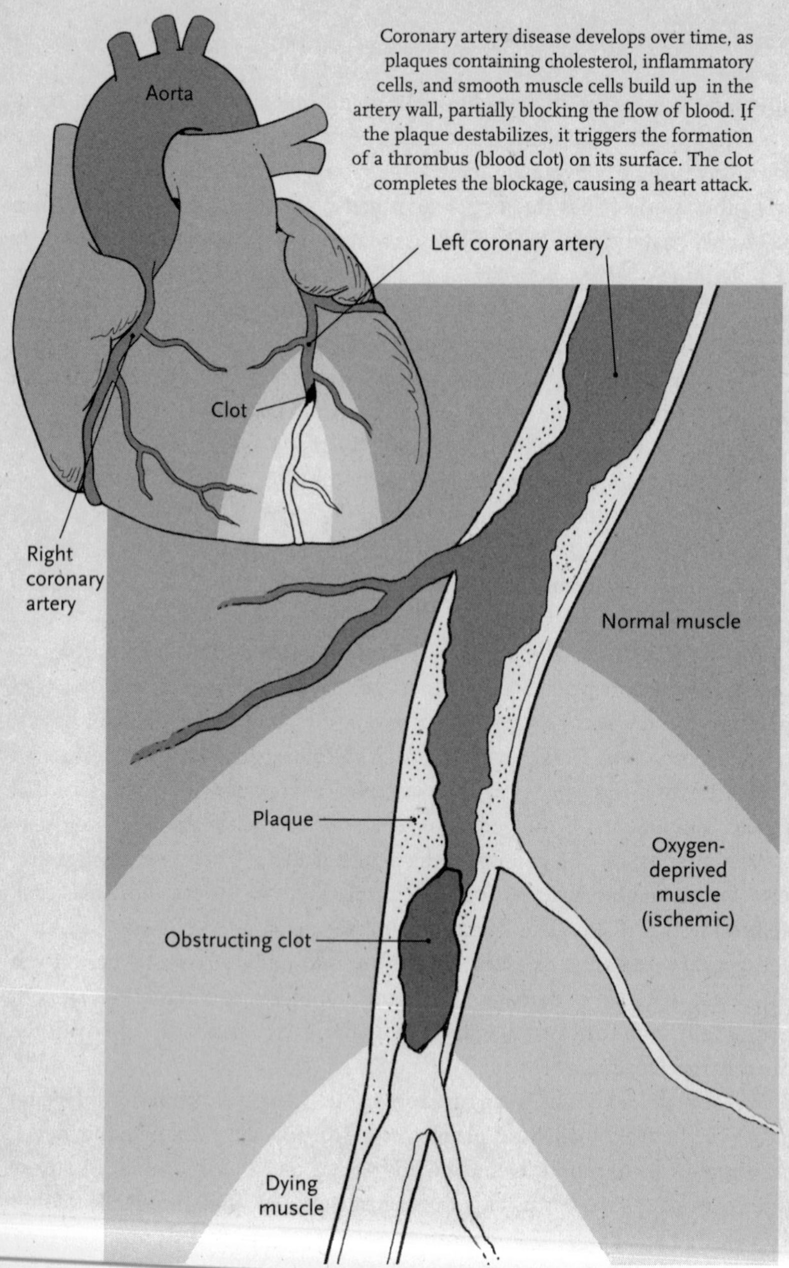

gen (see figure 3.1). And if enough muscle cells are damaged, the heart may never recover, suffering a lethal rhythm disturbance or a permanent inability to pump properly.

RISK FACTORS

Heart attacks are sudden and swift, but atherosclerosis is predictable and slow. America's heart disease epidemic began in the 1920s and 1930s. From the earliest days of the epidemic, doctors suspected that the male gender, advancing age, a family history of heart disease, and diabetes were important contributors to coronary artery disease—but they did not begin to suspect smoking, the most dangerous risk factor of all, until the 1950s. Similarly, cholesterol was not implicated until the 1960s, and it took another twenty years before research began to document the crucial next step, that lowering cholesterol will reduce risk.

During the sixty years of the coronary disease epidemic, scientists have identified ten major factors that contribute to the problem:

Table 3.1: STANDARD CARDIAC RISK FACTORS

FACTORS THAT CANNOT BE MODIFIED
Male Gender
Family History
Advancing Age
FACTORS THAT CAN BE MODIFIED
Tobacco Exposure
Abnormal Cholesterol
High LDL Cholesterol
Low HDL Cholesterol
High Blood Pressure
Lack of Exercise
Diabetes
Obesity
Psychological Factors
Stress and Anger
Depression and Isolation

It's an important list, particularly since the most dangerous risk factors can be improved by simple lifestyle changes, backed up, if necessary, by medications to improve cholesterol, lower blood pressure, and regulate diabetes. But as important as it is, the list is not complete. It's by no means rare for a person with an excellent risk-factor profile to have a heart attack. It is natural and appropriate for such an individual to ask, "Why me?" Scientists finally are starting to answer the question by identifying new cardiac risk factors—and the Harvard men's health studies are making important contributions to the effort. It's a work in progress, but Table 3.2 shows some of the newly appreciated cardiac risk factors.

Table 3.2: NEW CARDIAC RISK FACTORS

Homocysteine

Inflammation and Infection

Clotting Factors

Blood Fats

- Lipoprotein (a)
- Triglycerides

To see how your health stacks up, have a look at each of the risk factors:

Male Gender—It's simple enough, unfortunately: To be a man is to be at risk. Because the Harvard men's health studies do not include women, they cannot evaluate the relative risks of males and females. But the Framingham Heart Study has been following a mixed gender cohort since 1949. Fifty years later, in 1999, the study estimated the lifetime risk of developing coronary heart disease in Americans. Men who are healthy at age forty have a 48.8 percent chance of developing the disease during the remainder of their lives; for forty-year-old women, the lifetime risk is 34.9 percent. Even people who stay healthy until age seventy are not immune; for them, the risk is still 34.9 percent for men and 24.2 percent for women.

As you may recall from Chapter One, the gender gap depends on biology (estrogens and cholesterol levels) and behavior (smoking, exercise, diet, and stress and social isolation). Unfortunately for them, women are catching up to men in the dubious race toward heart disease. Women tend to get their heart attacks about ten years later than men, but heart disease is now the leading cause of death in American women as well as in men. Men tend to survive heart attacks better than women, but among patients with congestive heart failure, women have a better outcome.

All in all, a healthy middle-aged man reading this book has a one in two chance of developing coronary artery disease; for a seventy-year-old the risk is one in three. With odds like that, you probably will want to pay close attention to the other risk factors.

Age—If you are under forty-five, you may take some comfort in the fact that heart attacks are rare in your age group. If you are like the rest of us, you will be more impressed by the fact that four out of every five heart attacks occur after age sixty-five.

Advancing age is a risk factor that you would not dream of modifying. But before you accept the inevitability of a heart attack in your golden years, remember the advice of the great seventeenth century physician, Thomas Sydenham: "A man is only as old as his arteries." You can keep your arteries young—and your risk low—throughout life.

Family History—Heart disease runs in families, but the relationship is complex. Families share genes but they also share health habits, such as smoking and patterns of diet, exercise, and drinking. Families also tend to share medical problems that increase cardiac risk; obesity, diabetes, and abnormal cholesterol levels are examples. The Health Professionals Study accounted for the clustering of risk factors and still found that family history increases risk; a man with a parent who had a heart attack before age seventy is 2.2 times more likely to suffer a heart attack than a man whose parents had healthy hearts.

Smoking—It is the most important cardiac risk factor (and the most dangerous cancer risk factor), but you don't need Harvard scientists to explain what to do. Do not smoke cigarettes or, for that matter, cigars or pipes. Do not succumb to the newest threat to young men, chewing tobacco, either. And do your best to avoid second-hand smoke, which accounts for more than 50,000 premature deaths in the U.S. each year.

Cholesterol and Blood Fats—It is a well-known risk factor, but it is also an area of important new insights. Even as the tragedy of atherosclerosis was beginning to take center stage in medical research, LDL cholesterol was identified as the villain of the piece. The higher your LDL cholesterol, the higher your risk of atherosclerosis. It is a central tenet of cardiology that was confirmed by observation of the Physicians' Health Study in 1991 and 1996.

Where villains lurk, heroes can be found. In the drama of atherosclerosis, HDL cholesterol is the hero; the higher your HDL, the lower your risk. It's a new wrinkle that has changed the way doctors think about cholesterol. Although HDL is still complicated, it is perhaps the only area of atherosclerosis that has actually gotten a bit simpler—and we can thank the Physicians' Health Study for that. Until the 1991 report from Harvard, doctors thought there were two types of HDL, one protective but the other not. Blood tests on 14,916 men in the Physicians' Health Study changed that by showing that both forms of HDL are protective.

How does your cholesterol measure up? There are two ways to make that judgment. The first and more widely used relies on the latest guidelines of the American Heart Association. It places particular emphasis on the LDL cholesterol and on the presence or absence of other cardiac risk factors. The second method depends largely on data from the Framingham Heart Study; it gives equal weight to the total cholesterol and HDL and generates a simple easy-to-understand cardiac risk ratio. To see where you stand, you have to know your total cholesterol, LDL, and HDL.

For the first method, you also have to know if you have any other risk factors. These include: age above forty-five for men (fifty-five for women), cigarette smoking, a family history of coronary artery disease before age fifty-five in a father or brother or age sixty-five in a mother or sister, and high blood pressure, even if it is controlled by medication (see Table 3.5, page 49). An HDL below 40 also counts as a risk factor, but an HDL above 60 entitles you to subtract one risk factor. Table 3.3 shows how these risk factors can help you interpret your cholesterol.

Although the goals are most stringent for men who need help the most, every man should try to get his LDL as low as possible and his HDL as high as he can. If you need medication to reach your goals, you should continue the healthy lifestyle that is so important to your heart and overall health: Do not smoke (see Chapter Eight), eat properly and control your weight (Chapter Four), get regular exercise (Chapter Five), and consider low-dose aspirin, limiting alcohol use, and using supplements (Chapters Six and Seven).

Table 3.3: INTERPRETING YOUR CHOLESTEROL

YOUR CURRENT RISK FACTORS	YOUR SUGGESTED LDL GOAL	YOUR CURRENT LDL LEVEL	SUGGESTED THERAPY
Fewer than 2	130	Below 190	Lifestyle Modification
		190 or higher	Medication
Two or More	130	Below 160	Lifestyle Modification
		160 or higher	Medication
Coronary artery disease, other types of atherosclerosis, or diabetes	100	Above 100	Medication

The Framingham method requires a little math, but since it depends only on your total and HDL cholesterol levels it is easier to understand:

$$\text{Risk Ratio} = \frac{\text{Total Cholesterol}}{\text{HDL Cholesterol}}$$

After you do the simple math, use Table 3.4 to estimate your risk.

Table 3.4: YOUR CARDIAC RISK RATIO

RATIO	RISK
6.5	High
5.0	Above average
4.5	Average
4.0	Below Average
3.0	Low

Two ways to evaluate your blood fats may seem like one too many, but new research is adding additional subtleties. In 1996, for example, the Physicians' Health Study found that *triglycerides* also contribute to risk in men. Each 25-

point rise in triglycerides boosts risk by 10 percent. Men with the highest triglyceride levels are 2.5 times more likely to suffer heart attacks than men with the lowest levels. Normal triglyceride levels are 150 mg/dl, but unlike cholesterol, triglycerides have to be measured after a twelve to fourteen hour overnight fast to be accurate.

Another area of risk research is focusing on a blood fat called *lipoprotein(a)*. Although some research suggests that elevated lipoprotein(a) levels are independent predictors of risk, the Physicians' Health Study did not find the test useful. Few doctors are currently checking lipoprotein(a) levels. It is just as well, since these levels are hard to change. Genetics are the major determinants of lipoprotein(a) levels; unlike LDL, HDL, and triglycerides, diet and exercise appear to have little influence. Even the statin drugs, such as lovastatin (Mevacor) and atorvastatin (Lipitor), do not lower lipoprotein(a) levels—though they certainly protect against heart disease, chiefly by reducing LDL levels.

Hypertension—High blood pressure ranks just below smoking and cholesterol on the cardiac risk parade—and since one-quarter of all American men have high blood pressure, it is a major risk indeed.

Blood pressure seems mysterious to many people, but it is really very simple. Your blood pressure is the force that propels blood through your arteries, and it depends on two factors, the strength of your heart's pumping action and the resistance in your body's arteries.

Blood pressure readings seem no less obscure—but they are actually just as straightforward. Your doctor will measure two pressures with each blood pressure check. The higher number is your *systolic blood pressure;* it is the pressure in your arteries during the time your heart is actually pumping blood. But after each beat, your heart muscle relaxes and fills with blood to prime the pump for the next beat. Your *diastolic blood pressure* is the pressure in your arteries in the interval between heartbeats; it is the lower of the two readings. By convention, the systolic pressure is given first. For example, if your systolic blood pressure is 120 and your diastolic is 80, your doctor will tell you your reading is "120 over 80" and he will record it in your chart as 120/80.

Doctors have been monitoring blood pressures for more than a century. It didn't take long for them to realize that hypertension is a major cause of heart attacks, strokes, and kidney failure. Even so, two very important factors about blood pressure did not emerge until very recently. First, there is no "normal" blood pressure; instead, the risk of the disease is continuously related to blood pressure across its entire range. Put simply, the higher your blood pressure, the higher your risk. Second, both your systolic and diastolic blood pressures are important. For many years, doctors overlooked systolic readings, concentrating therapy on the diastolic pressure alone. It did not make much sense, and it didn't identify the people who need treatment most. In fact, both numbers count.

All three Harvard men's health studies have important messages about blood pressure for you.

The Physicians' Health Study has helped to quantify the risk of hypertension and to set goals for your blood pressure. The study found that high blood pressure is a major contributor to cardiovascular disease in men, increasing the risk of heart attack 1.78 times and the risk of cardiovascular death 2.1 times. Even "borderline" systolic blood pressures between 140 and 160 are dangerous, increasing the risk of cardiovascular death by a factor of 1.56.

The moral of the Physicians' Health Study is that you would do well to keep your blood pressure below 140/90. Your doctor can prescribe a vast array of medications to get you there, but you would be better off in terms of side effects, expense, and overall health if you could do it on your own. And even the many men with high blood pressure who need medication should be sure to implement the simple lifestyle changes that will help reduce blood pressure.

Table 3.5: INTERPRETING YOUR BLOOD PRESSURE

CATEGORY	SYSTOLIC BLOOD PRESSURE (MMHG)	DIASTOLIC BLOOD PRESSURE (MMHG)
Optimal	120 or lower	80 or lower
Normal	121–129	81–85
High normal	130–139	86–89
Hypertension		
Stage 1	140–159	90–99
Stage 2	160–179	100–109
Stage 3	180 or higher	110 or higher

What if your systolic blood pressure is in one category but your diastolic is in another? Use the higher category to determine your status. For example, if your blood pressure is 162/85, you have Stage 2 hypertension.

The Alumni Study highlights the benefit of regular exercise. Like the Physicians' Health Study, it found that hypertension nearly doubles a man's risk of developing coronary artery disease. But it also found that men who exercise regularly are 35 percent less likely to develop hypertension than sedentary men. And the Alumni Study found that obesity is another important contributor to hypertension, increasing risk by 78 percent among men who are 20 percent overweight.

The Health Professionals Study focuses on another health practice that has a major impact on blood pressure: diet. It found a high intake of potassium, magnesium, and fiber is associated with a lower blood pressure; calcium also seems to help, though to a lesser degree. The study did not implicate a high intake of sodium as a cause of hypertension, but other studies identify salt as an important culprit.

The Harvard studies tell you that blood pressure control is crucial to good health and that lifestyle changes can help attain that control. In the next few chapters you will learn to put diet and weight control (Chapter Four), exercise (Chapter Five), prudence in your use of alcohol (Chapter Seven), and smoking cessation and stress control (Chapter Eight) to work for you.

Lack of Exercise—Most doctors now know that sedentary living increases the risk of heart attack, but when the Alumni Study first presented its evidence back in 1978, it was big news: regular exercise reduced the risk of suffering a heart attack by 36 percent. Another important finding in that initial investigation was that genetic endowment does not explain the protective effect of exercise. Men who were varsity athletes as undergraduates did not enjoy protection unless they continued to exercise over the years. And in a 1993 publication, the Alumni Study provided encouraging news for men who were sedentary in youth; exercise can reduce a man's death rate by 23 percent even if he does not begin to exercise until middle age.

The Alumni Study set the bar high. It found maximum benefit from vigorous sports performed for three to four hours a week. The study also triggered an explosion of research into exercise and health. During the past two decades, many studies have corroborated the cardiac benefits of exercise, but they have added the reassuring news that even more modest activity is beneficial. New research—including the three Harvard studies—also demonstrates that exercise protects against diabetes, stroke, obesity, osteoporosis, and certain cancers, as well as heart disease. Chapter Five will fill in the details.

Diabetes—In 2001, the Physicians' Health Study reported that the presence of diabetes increases the risk of a heart attack every bit as much as a history of previous coronary artery disease. Diabetics are two to three times more likely to die from heart attacks than nondiabetics. In all, diabetes accounts for about 30,000 cardiac deaths in the United States each year. If that were not bad enough, diabetes is an important chronic disease in its own right, all too often leading to strokes, peripheral artery disease that threatens the legs, kidney failure, and visual loss. It is a major problem, particularly since 7.5 million American men have diabetes, and their numbers are increasing every year.

Diabetes is a disorder of the metabolism of *glucose,* the sugar in blood that fuels the body's metabolism. After a meal, the carbohydrates, fats, and proteins in food are digested in the intestinal tract, then absorbed into the bloodstream. Blood sugar levels rise after meals, but the sugar will not do any good unless it gets into the body's cells. Insulin, produced by the pancreas, is the hormone that opens the door, allowing glucose to enter cells. In diabetes, the door does not open properly, leaving too much sugar in the blood and not enough in the body's cells.

There are two kinds of diabetes. In Type 1 diabetes, the pancreas does not produce enough insulin; Type 1 usually starts abruptly, usually before age forty and often before age twenty. Patients with Type 1 diabetes require insulin injections to prevent dehydration, coma, and death. In contrast, Type 2 diabetes begins gradually later in life. Most patients with Type 2 diabetes produce plenty of insulin, but their tissues resist the action of the hormone, so blood sugar levels rise. But some develop this disease as their bodies' insulin-making machinery gradually grinds to a halt. Many oral medications are effective for Type 2 diabetes, though some patients with the disorder need insulin. Type 2 diabetes is about fourteen times more common than Type 1, and it is on the rise as Americans eat more, exercise less, and gain weight.

Although diabetes tends to run in families, it is not a strictly hereditary disease. In fact, a man's risk of diabetes depends more on his habits than his relatives. The Physicians' Health Study emphasized the importance of exercise: Men who exercise at least once a week are 36 percent less likely to develop Type 2 diabetes than sedentary men, and men who exercise five or more times a week enjoy a 42 percent risk reduction. The benefits of exercise do not depend simply on weight loss, since physical activity protects both men who are obese and those who are lean.

Obesity and diet are the other important lifestyle contributors to Type 2 diabetes. The Health Professionals Study confirmed the importance of obesity, finding that a simple measurement of waist size could predict a man's risk of diabetes. The study also found that a diet that contains little fiber but lots of carbohydrates that boost blood sugar levels rapidly increases the risk of diabetes. A third observation of note is that a modest intake of alcohol may actually reduce a man's risk of diabetes.

Many men with Type 2 diabetes do not know they have the disease. To find out if diabetes may increase your risk of heart disease, simply have your blood sugar checked after you have fasted for at least eight hours; a result of 126 mg/dl or higher indicates diabetes. Another test that can be obtained without fasting is the *glycosylated hemoglobin* (Hb_{A_1C}); a result above 7.0 suggests diabetes.

Exciting new research from the late 1990s demonstrates that good blood sugar control reduces the complications of diabetes. Chapters Four and Five will show you how to attain those goals.

Obesity—A quick visit to a Coronary Care Unit will persuade you that obesity is a cardiac risk factor, but it has taken years for epidemiologists to persuade themselves that the link is valid. That's because obesity increases cholesterol, blood pressure, and blood sugar, all of which are major cardiac risk factors on their own. But using the advanced technique of multivariate analysis, researchers became convinced that obesity is an independent risk factor. All in all, a 10 percent gain in body fat increases the risk of heart attack by about 25 percent. Abdominal obesity—the shape that overweight tends to take in men—is particularly hazardous.

The Alumni Study found that men who maintain ideal body weight have a 35 percent lower risk of heart disease than men who are obese. The Health Professionals Study found that obesity is directly linked to the risk of heart disease in men younger than sixty-five; as compared to lean men, men who were mildly, moderately, or severely overweight were 1.7, 2.6, and 3.4 times more likely to develop heart disease, respectively. Among older men, abdominal obesity was the strongest predictor of risk. The study also identified sedentary living as a major cause of obesity. In particular, long hours spent in front of a TV screen were linked to excess poundage.

Affecting about one of every three men, obesity is a weighty problem in America—and it is a growing concern as we enter the twenty-first century. Chapter Four will help you calculate your body fat. Even more important, Chapters Four and Five will explain how you can shed excess pounds.

Psychological Factors—Mental factors occupy last place among the ten traditional cardiac risk factors, not because they are unimportant, but because they are hard to quantify. Still, researchers have long suspected that men with the so-called Type A personality ("hurry sickness") have an increased risk of heart disease; other indicators of stress that increase risk include hostility and suppressed anger. More recently, social isolation and depression have been identified as cardiac risk factors. Although depression is more common in women, it is more likely to be heartbreaking for men. The Health Professionals Study found that phobic anxiety is a strong predictor of fatal coronary artery disease, but that strong social networks may help men survive heart attacks. The Alumni Study reports that exercise helps fight depression; other investigators agree, and many suspect that exercise helps dissipate stress as well. Chapter Eight will help you identify and control heartfelt emotions.

It has taken years for researchers to identify the ten standard cardiac risk factors, but they have not stopped there. In fact, more than 200 additional factors have been studied and more are likely to crop up. At present, three new factors appear particularly crucial, and the Harvard studies have had an important role in elucidating each of them. They are:

Homocysteine. It's a natural substance that is present in many foods and is also synthesized by the body itself. In normal amounts, it is essential for health, but in high amounts it increases dramatically the risk of heart attack and stroke. In some people, high levels result from inherited abnormalities, but in others, a poor diet is the culprit. It's *homocysteine*—but the description also applies to cholesterol. Indeed, in some studies high levels of homocysteine increase cardiac risk every bit as much as high levels of cholesterol.

Despite these similarities, cholesterol and homocysteine are chemically distinct. Homocysteine is not a fat, but an *amino acid*, one of the twenty nitrogen-rich compounds that are the building blocks of all the body's proteins. Homocysteine is produced from *methionine*, another sulfur-containing amino acid. Under normal circumstances homocysteine is rapidly converted into other amino acids, keeping blood levels low. Among other things, the metabolism of homocysteine depends on three B vitamins: B_6 (pyridoxine), B_{12} (cobalamin), and folic acid.

How risky is a high homocysteine level? Estimates vary, but two studies of men show that they can be very important. In 1992, the Physicians' Health Study was one of the first to raise the alarm. Among 14,916 apparently healthy men who were observed for five years, elevated homocysteine levels were associated with a threefold increase in the risk of heart attack, even after cholesterol, smoking, high blood pressure, and other risk factors were taken into account. In 1998, a British study of 21,520 men reported nearly identical results. After accounting for other risk factors, men with the highest homocysteine levels were 2.9 times more likely to develop coronary artery disease than men with the lowest levels. For perspective, a 5-point rise in homocysteine appears as dangerous as a 20-point rise in total cholesterol, each increasing risk by about 20 to 40 percent.

Why is homocysteine such a powerful risk factor? New research suggests that high levels accelerate atherosclerosis in at least four ways: by producing toxic damage to the *endothelial cells* that line the inner surface of arteries, by increasing the activity of oxygen free radicals, by stimulating the enlargement of smooth muscle cells in the middle layer of arterial walls, and by accelerating the clotting process.

The fourfold nature of homocysteine's threat explains why it has deleterious effects beyond the heart. The Physicians' Health Study, for example, found that high homocysteine levels increases the risk for stroke (see below) and *thrombophlebitis* (blood clots in veins).

As with cholesterol, healthy people have a wide range of homocysteine levels. The "normal" range is 5 to 15 micromoles per liter (mmol/L), but levels below 10 are safest. Although most doctors routinely measure cholesterol levels, few measure homocysteine. That is likely to change as homocysteine blood tests become easier, cheaper, more reliable, and more widely available. But since most people can lower their homocysteine levels with measures that are simple, safe, and inexpensive, many authorities recommend instituting treatment in everyone without bothering to diagnose the abnormality in some. The Physicians' Health Study and the Health Professionals Study agree that the key is an adequate intake of folic acid; vitamins B_6 and B_{12} also seem to help. Chapter Four will explain how to get these B vitamins from your diet, and Chapter Six will discuss the potential benefits of vitamin supplements.

Homocysteine research today is about where cholesterol research was thirty years ago: Scientists know that high levels predict risk, but they do not yet know if lowering levels reduces that risk. Time will tell. In the meanwhile, a diet rich in vegetables, fruits, and fortified grains supplemented by a daily multivitamin makes sense for most men.

Inflammation and Infection. Inflammation is the "itis" in prostatitis, appendicitis, and bronchitis. It can show up in any part of the body because it is one of the most basic biologic responses to injury. Infection is the most common cause of that injury, but allergies, immunologic reaction, and trauma can also trigger inflammation.

In coronary arteries, oxidized LDL cholesterol produces injury and inflammation. The tiny proteins that perpetuate inflammation in the artery wall spill out into the bloodstream, traveling to the parts of the body. The liver responds by producing proteins of its own, including *C-reactive protein* and *fibrinogen,* a clotting factor that is discussed below.

The Physicians' Health Study identified C-reactive protein as a cardiac risk factor in 1997, when it reported that apparently healthy men with high levels were 2.9 times more likely to develop heart attacks than men with low levels, even after other risk factors were taken into account. The finding has been confirmed in subsequent studies from around the world. It has already helped doctors establish a progression for cardiac patients and it may soon help guide therapy. In 1999, the study reported that elevated levels of C-reactive protein were linked to a series of correctible cardiac risk factors, including smoking, cholesterol, hypertension, obesity, and homocysteine. In another report, the Physicians' Health Study demonstrated that the treatment with low-dose aspirin reduces the risk of heart attack by 55 percent in men with high C-reactive protein levels. Underscoring the importance of inflammation in coronary artery disease, the study has recently implicated two other inflammatory markers, *IL-6* and *ICAM-1,* as cardiac risk factors.

Scientists are also exploring the possibilities that infection may contribute to the inflammation of atherosclerosis. The leading candidate is *Chlamydia pneumoniae,* a tiny bacterium that usually causes pneumonia or bronchitis. Although many studies in humans and animals have linked the bacterium with atherosclerosis, others—including the Physicians' Health Study—disagree. Adding to the uncertainty, three trials have suggested that antibiotics that target Chlamydia pneumonia may help treat men with coronary artery disease, but two others disagree. Much larger trials that should settle the question are in progress, but the results will not be available for several years. The chlamydia story is a work in progress. Meanwhile, the Physicians' Health Study has provided evidence against the role of two viruses, *herpes* and *CMV,* that had previously been touted as possible causes of atherosclerosis.

Clotting Factors. The final act in the tragic drama that leads to a heart attack is the formation of a blood clot that completes the blockage of a partially narrowed artery. Since clotting, or thrombosis, is the final coup, abnormalities of the blood clotting system might be able to predict risk—and they do.

Doctors can measure blood factors that promote clotting as well as factors that help dissolve clots. The Physicians' Health Study reported recently that men with high levels of the clotting protein fibrinogen had a twofold increase in the risk of heart attack. Fibrinogen is also boosted by inflammation and it may help explain how inflammation in a distant part of the body may increase the risk of heart attacks. Several studies have suggested that chronic peridontal disease is just that sort of inflammation, but in a 2001 report, the Physicians' Health Study found no link between gum infection and heart attacks.

Scientists can also measure factors that help dissolve clots; low levels of *thrombomodulin* and a reduced *fibrinolytic capacity* have been implicated as risk factors. The Physicians' Health Study found that the clot-busting system appears to gear up long before a heart attack, suggesting that the body is attempting to fight back. Interestingly, exercise (see Chapter Five) and low-dose alcohol (see Chapter Seven), two of the things that reduce heart attack risk, exert part of their protective action by boosting the body's clot-busting system.

Fourteen risk factors—and the list keeps growing. It is a long list because atherosclerosis is so complex. And it's a daunting list, refleeting the fact that heart disease remains the number one killer of American men. But it is also an encouraging list, since the scientists who are finally zeroing in on the causes of heart disease tell us that you can modify eleven of the fourteen risk factors to reduce your risk of heart disease. Although some men need medication to achieve optimal risk reduction, all will benefit from a healthy diet and good exercise (see Chapters Four and Five), many will benefit from low-dose aspirin and nutritional supplements (see Chapter Six), and some will benefit from low-dose alcohol (see Chapter Seven). Even better, the program that will help prevent heart disease will also provide protection against two other major illnesses that threaten your health, stroke and cancer.

Stroke

Although the symptoms of strokes and heart attacks are entirely different, the two illnesses share many common risk factors. That's because both are caused by damage to the arteries that supply oxygen-rich blood to vital organs. And the two problems have even more in common: Both are leading causes of death and disability, and both can often be prevented by simple lifestyle changes backed up, when necessary, by medications.

About 730,000 Americans have strokes every year; 72 percent are above age sixty-five and 59 percent are men. About 62,000 die, making stroke the nation's third leading cause of death, and many of the survivors suffer prolonged, even permanent disabilities. Nearly one-third require assistance in caring for themselves.

An American's risk of dying from a stroke has declined even more dramatically than the risk of a fatal heart attack, falling some 70 percent since 1950. But that does not mean the problem is solved; we have done well so far, but we can do better.

DIFFERENT STROKES

There are two major types of strokes, *ischemic* and *hemorrhagic* (see Figure 3.2). Hemorrhagic strokes are less common but more cataclysmic. They occur when a blood vessel in the brain bursts, spilling blood into the brain or the fluid that surrounds it.

Ischemic strokes, which account for about 80 percent of the total, result when an artery that supplies blood to the brain becomes blocked by a clot. This can happen in either of the two ways. In a *thrombotic stroke,* the clot forms in a diseased artery within the brain itself. In an *embolic stroke* the clot forms outside the brain, then breaks away and is carried by the blood to the brain, where it lodges in a previously normal artery. Most emboli originate on atherosclerotic plaques in the carotid artery or aorta or in the heart itself.

The term stroke is derived from a Middle English word meaning blow or sudden attack. Indeed, most strokes wreak their havoc abruptly. Even so, many are preceded by warning symptoms called *transient ischemic attacks* or TIAs. The symptoms of TIAs resemble those of strokes, but they resolve completely within twenty-four hours because blood flow is restored before brain cells die. But since many patients with TIAs go on to have strokes, it is essential for men who experience warning symptoms to get medical attention. TIAs can produce abrupt, painless visual loss in one eye, slurred speech, or an inability to understand or use words. They may also produce clumsiness, weakness, or numbness of the face, arm, or leg on one side of the body. Less often, TIAs can cause abrupt but transient dizziness, usually accompanied by loss of balance, double vision, or slurred speech. A typical TIA lasts just two to fifteen minutes, and half of all patients are back to normal in less than an hour.

FIGURE 3.2. ANATOMY OF STROKES

HEMORRHAGIC STROKE

- **20% of strokes**
- **Caused by ruptured blood vessels followed by blood leaking into tissue**
- **Usually more serious than ischemic stroke**

ISCHEMIC STROKE

- **80% of strokes**
- **Caused by blockages in brain blood vessels**
- **Brain tissue dies when blood flow is blocked**

Subarachnoid hemorrhage

- A bleed into the space between the brain and the skull
- Develops most often from an aneurysm, a weakened, ballooned area in the wall of an artery
- Severe headache is often the first symptom

Embolic stroke

- Caused by emboli, blood clots that travel from elsewhere in the body to the brain blood vessels
- 60% of strokes among Americans are embolic strokes
- 25% of embolic strokes are related to atrial fibrillation, an irregular heart rhythm

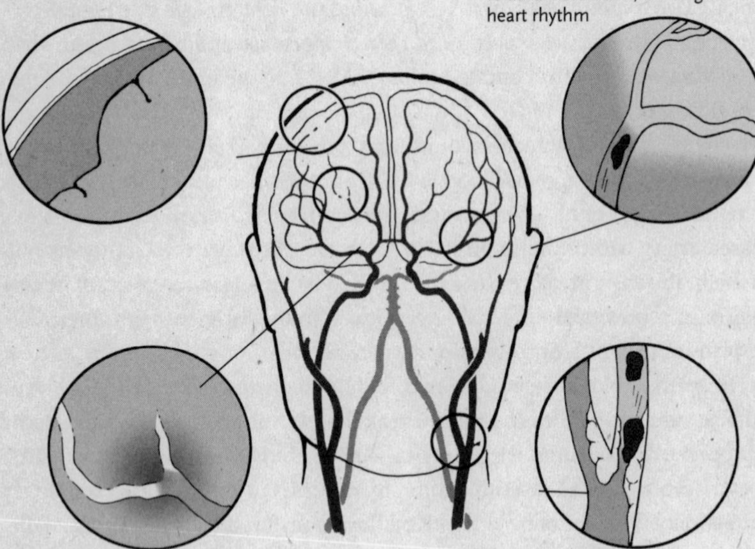

Intracerebral hemorrhage

- A bleed from a blood vessel inside the brain
- Often caused by high blood pressure and the damage it does to arteries

Thrombotic stroke

- Caused by thrombi, blood clots that form where an artery has been narrowed by atherosclerosis
- Most often develops when part of a thrombus breaks away and causes a blockage in a "downstream" artery

A TIA is a call for prompt diagnosis and aggressive preventive measures. But men do not have to wait for TIAs to take steps to reduce their risk of stroke. In fact, the best time for you to start is now.

CAUSES AND PREVENTION

Hypertension. The most powerful stroke risk factor is high blood pressure. In the Physicians' Health Study, for example, high blood pressure increased the risk of stroke by 220 percent, and even Stage 1 systolic hypertension (systolic blood pressures of 140–159) increased risk by 140 percent. All in all, if you reduce your blood pressure by just 6 points, you will cut your risk of stroke by about 40 percent and your risk of heart disease by 15 percent. Chapters Four and Five will present a program that puts even better blood pressure reduction within easy reach.

Tobacco. Tobacco is the second major cause of strokes. The Physicians' Health Study found that men who smoke more than a pack a day are two and half times more likely to have a stroke than nonsmokers; smoking less than a pack a day is only slightly less hazardous, doubling the risk of stroke.

Cholesterol. Elevated cholesterol levels increase the risk of ischemic, but not hemorrhagic, strokes. A 1996 study found that patients with ischemic strokes are likely to have the same cholesterol profiles as patients with coronary artery disease: high total cholesterol, LDL cholesterol, and triglycerides, and low HDL cholesterol. The Physicians' Health Study reported that measurements of homocysteine and lipoprotein(a) do not add to this risk profile. Four independent meta-analyses, including one performed by researchers associated with the Harvard studies, found that lowering blood cholesterol levels with a statin drug can reduce the risk of stroke by 24 to 31 percent. Chapters Four and Five will explain how you can use lifestyle changes to improve your cholesterol results.

Diabetes and Obesity increase the risk of stroke, much as they increase the risk of heart attack. Both risk factors show up in many studies, and they have been confirmed by the Physicians' Health and the Health Professionals studies. To date, however, no research has proved that controlling blood sugar or shedding excess pounds will reduce the risk of stroke. Even without such proof, it is a logical assumption, and both improvements will surely help your heart and your health.

Lack of Exercise. Another atherosclerosis risk factor that increases the chances of suffering strokes as well as heart attacks is lack of exercise. A 1998 report from the Alumni Study shows that regular exercise can really help. Men who burn 1,000 to 2,000 calories a week have a 24 percent lower risk of stroke than sedentary men. Exercising to the tune of 2,000 to 3,000 calories a week will reduce risk by a whopping 46 percent. And you do not have to go to a gym to get the exercise you need; stair climbing, gardening, dancing, and cycling are among the many activities that help, but light exercise such as bowling is much less beneficial. If walking is your choice, hit the road for thirty minutes five times a week for good protection, or double your commitment for maximal benefit.

Cardiovascular Diseases. People with various cardiovascular diseases have an increased risk of stroke. Examples include atherosclerosis of the aorta or carotid arteries, an irregular heart rhythm called *atrial fibrillation,* and previous heart attacks. If you have any of these problems, check with your doctor about preventive action. Most often, medication that inhibits clotting, such as aspirin (Chapter Six) or *warfarin* (Coumadin), will do the trick, but some men with severe narrowing of the carotid artery may benefit from surgical repair of the artery.

New Risk Factors. Some of the new cardiac risk factors also appear to have a role in stroke. The Physicians' Health Study has reported that elevated levels of C-reactive protein are linked to an increased risk of stroke, as is activation of the body's clot-busting protein *t-PA.*

Diet. It is not yet clear if men can use new risk factor information to reduce their risk of stroke, but the Health Professionals Study suggests that old-fashioned dietary changes can go a long way toward achieving that goal. Among 43,738 men who were observed for eight years, a high intake of potassium (averaging 4,300 milligrams a day) reduced the risk of stroke by 38 percent as compared with men who averaged only 2,800 milligrams a day. Men at the highest risk of stroke because of hypertension enjoyed the greatest benefit. Fruits and vegetables offered the best protection; nine servings a day provide the optimal amount of potassium, and the risk of ischemic stroke declined by 6 percent for each portion of fruits and vegetables consumed on an average day. Citrus fruits and juices, leafy green vegetables, and cruciferous vegetables such as broccoli, cabbage, and cauliflower were the most beneficial, but potatoes and legumes were not protective. In the Health Professionals Study, eating cereal also decreased the risk of stroke.

Fruits and vegetables provide antioxidant vitamins as well as potassium. But the Health Professionals Study cautions men against relying on vitamin supplements alone. In a 1999 report, the study found no benefit from supplements of vitamin E, vitamin C, or carotenes.

Alcohol. Until recently, doctors believed that drinking was linked to an increased risk of stroke. Indeed, heavy drinking raises blood pressure and boosts the risk of hemorrhagic strokes. But two 1999 studies show that light drinking is another matter. The Physicians' Health Study found that men who consume one to seven drinks weekly are about 20 percent less likely to suffer ischemic strokes than men who average less than one drink a week. Similarly, in a case-control study of 1,816 men and women, researchers from Columbia University found that mild drinking—up to two drinks a day—was associated with a 49 percent reduction in the risk of ischemic strokes, even after other risk factors such as heart disease, high blood pressure, diabetes, smoking, and obesity were taken into account. As in the case of heart attacks, though, larger amounts of alcohol were associated with increased risk. Despite the good news about low-dose alcohol, the recent studies do not necessarily mean that drinking is right for you. Chapter Seven will help you decide this for yourself.

Cancer

About one in every three Americans will develop a malignant disease during the course of a lifetime. During this year alone, more than 1,285,000 Americans will learn that they have invasive cancer and at least 555,000 will die of the disease. It is a frightening statistic, but it does represent some progress, since the overall cancer mortality rate in the United States has declined by more than 3 percent since 1990. To make further progress, scientists will have to learn more about the molecular biology of cancer and doctors have to develop better methods of diagnosis and treatment. Research in these areas is complex and expensive, and advances are likely to be frustratingly slow. But a third avenue for progress is already wide open, since people have simple yet effective ways to reduce their risks of succumbing to the nation's second leading killer.

What is Cancer?

Cancer is not one disease, but many. More than 100 types of human cancers have been identified, but only about a dozen are common and four (lung, prostate, breast, and colorectal) account for more than half of all cancer deaths.

The different types of cancer have varied causes and unique characteristics. Still, all cancers share two basic properties. The first is unregulated cell growth; the second is the ability to invade normal tissues and spread to other parts of the body.

Each cancer begins with a single malignant cell. That cell divides without restraint through at least thirty generations before it grows to the 1 billion cancerous cells that typically constitute the smallest detectable tumor mass. Another ten generations brings the tumor to the 1 trillion cell population that is usually lethal to the body's 30 trillion healthy cells. In the course of growing to a maximum weight of one to two pounds, the typical malignant tumor spreads to adjacent tissues and invades blood vessels and lymph channels, which carry the cells to distant organs where they grow as *metastases*. Cancer kills by interfering with vital functions of normal cells and by producing general wasting or *cachexia*.

Normal Cell Growth

Cell division is a necessity. It is required for growth and to replace dying cells and repair damaged tissues. In health, the body has an intricate set of mechanisms to control and regulate the process, so cells divide and grow only when they should.

The signals that trigger a cell's growth do not originate in the cell itself, but in its neighbors: it's the way the body preserves the normal architecture of its tissues. When new cells are needed in the neighborhood, cells secrete small protein *growth factors*. The growth factors latch onto the surface of the target cell, where they trigger messenger molecules that travel deep into the cell, telling the DNA in the nucleus that it is time to reproduce.

One set of genes stimulates cell growth (*proto-oncogenes*), while another (*suppressor genes*) inhibits growth. Another type of checks and balances is the process of *apoptosis* or genetically programmed cell death, which tells healthy cells that it is time for them to self-destruct, making way for the arrival of new cells.

It's a complex process. To keep it running properly, each cell has an internal clock that regulates the individual components of cell growth, turning them on and off at appropriate times.

GROWING PROBLEMS

Cancer develops when the mechanisms that control cell growth fail. Imbalances that result in unchecked cell growth can occur at many stages of the regulatory process. In some cases, the problem is an excess of stimulatory growth factors; for example, the Physicians' Health Study found that men with the highest levels of *insulin-like growth factor-1* (*IGF-1*), are 4.3 times more likely to develop prostate cancer than men with the lowest levels; men with intermediate levels had intermediate risk. In other cases, the normal genes undergo mutations that transform them into *oncogenes,* genes that cause unrestrained cell division. Also very common are DNA changes that block the action of suppressor genes, preventing them from checking cell growth; about half of all cancers, for example, involve a failure of the *p53* gene that is supposed to halt cell division. Another newly identified cause of excessive growth is a failure of apoptosis, so that cells do not commit suicide when they should. Newly recognized, too, are failures in the cell clock that allow the growth cycle to escape control. A normal cell only divides fifty to one hundred times before it dies. That is because it loses a bit of DNA, called a *telomere,* from the tip of its chromosomes with each cell division; after a while, so much DNA has been lost that the cell can no longer divide. But in cancer cells, an enzyme called *telomerase* repairs the chromosomal damage, rewinding the cell's clock so it can continue to divide indefinitely. Scientists have recently identified the gene responsible for telomerase, raising the hope that therapy to correct the defect may be developed soon.

SPREADING PROBLEMS

Abnormal cell growth is only one part of the cancer equation; the other is tissue invasion and spread to other organs. In healthy tissues, cells are held together by *adhesion molecules;* in cancerous tissues, adhesion molecules are absent or ineffective. But cell detachment is not the only abnormality that allows cancer to spread. Normal cells that detach remain adrift until they kill themselves off by apoptosis, but cancerous cells are able to survive in solitude, then invade blood vessels and travel to other organs. Once they have arrived at their unhappy destination, cancer cells have some final tricks up their sleeves. They have surface molecules that allow them to adhere to healthy cells, and they trigger *angiogenesis,* or the growth of new blood vessels that nourish the tumor. This is the crucial step that is blocked by the experimental cancer drugs *endostatin* and *angiostatin,* which are being studied by Harvard professor Judah Folkman and his colleagues at Children's Hospital Medical Center with promising early results.

FIGHTING BACK

It's axiomatic: The more things can go wrong, the more they will go wrong. The processes that control cell growth are enormously complex, with many opportunities for error. Indeed, errors are common, but most people do not get cancer. That's because the body has so many checks and balances as well as natural defenses against cancer.

DNA is at the heart of the matter, since abnormal genes are ultimately responsible for cancer. In fact, DNA abnormalities crop up all the time, but each cell has a set of enzymes to repair abnormal DNA. Even when a gene is beyond repair, it does not cause cancer all by itself; six or more errors are needed to produce most malignancies. Moreover, only about one of every ten thousand cancer cells has what it takes to detach, invade, spread, adhere, and grow as a metastasis. Finally, the body's immune system is able to detect and kill many cancer cells. That's because they have unique surface proteins that function as *antigens;* the immune apparatus recognizes tumor antigens as foreign and abnormal. It mobilizes special lymphocytes called *natural killer* (NK) cells that attack and kill tumor cells. It produces *cytokines* that damage, and then kill, cancer cells. The immune system also produces *antibodies* that latch onto tumor cells, preparing them for destruction by *antibody dependent cellular cytotoxicity* (ADCC). It is a good defense network, but it is far from perfect. Still, new experimental cancer treatments are seeking ways to bolster the system with *immunotherapy.*

TIPPING THE SCALES

In health, cell growth and cell death are precisely matched. When imbalances occur, they are detected and corrected. Even when errors sneak through, the body can seek and destroy malignant cells.

In cancer, however, the body's checks and balances fail. Many things can tip the scales in the wrong direction:

Heredity. Some people inherit an oncogene from a parent; examples include the recently identified prostate cancer genes, *HPC 1* and *HPC 2*. Colon cancer can also run in families; the Health Professionals Study found that men with two or more siblings or parents with the disease are nearly three times more likely to develop colon cancer than men whose close relatives are free of the disease. All in all, more than twenty hereditary forms of cancer have been identified, but they account for only about 1 percent of all malignancies.

Oxidative Damage. Oxygen free radicals bombard DNA, causing gene mutations. A person's DNA sustains an estimated 10,000 oxidative hits per day. Most are repaired, but cancer may result if antioxidants fail. That is why the antioxidants in fruits and vegetables are attracting so much attention. The Health Professionals Study, for example, found that high intakes of *lycopene,* the most potent antioxidant in the carotene family, and *selenium,* a mineral with antioxidant properties, are linked to a substantial reduction—up to 38 percent—in the risk of prostate cancer.

External Toxins. Environmental poisons can damage DNA, thwart repair mechanisms, or both. The most important toxin is the most obvious, tobacco smoke. At least sixty other *chemical carcinogens* have been identified. Some occur in the workplace, while others can contaminate soil, water, and air, where they can account for the relatively uncommon community clusters of cancer.

Radiation. Ionizing radiation is most dangerous; nuclear energy, medical X-rays, and the natural gamma radiation in cosmic rays are examples, as is *radon,* a naturally occurring radioactive gas that causes lung cancer in high doses. *Ultraviolet radiation* packs much less punch, but prolonged exposure can cause DNA damage and cancer; that's why excessive sunlight leads to *malignant melanomas* and other skin cancers. Despite popular concerns, however, *electromagnetic radiation* around high-voltage power lines and *radiofrequency radiation* from cellular phones and microwave ovens do not convey enough energy to cause cancer.

Viruses. Once considered a major cause of cancer, viruses appear responsible for only a minority of human cancers. Examples include the *hepatitis B* and *C* viruses that can cause liver cancer and the *human papillomavirus* that is sexually transmitted and can cause genital tract cancers. The *human immunodeficiency virus* (HIV) opens the door to many cancers by destroying the body's immune defense mechanisms.

Chronic Inflammation and Infections. Helicobacter pylori, the bacterium that causes ulcers, has been linked to stomach cancer, but it is the only known bacterial cause of cancer. In addition, some people with chronic inflammation are susceptible to cancer; an example is the intestinal inflammation that increases the risk of colon cancer in patients with severe ulcerative colitis.

Hormones. Sex hormones trigger the growth of cells in the reproductive organs; excessive hormone levels—or unusual tissue sensitivity—can stimulate uncontrolled growth. It is the way that the male hormone *testosterone* promotes prostate cancer.

Medical Therapies. Anticancer drugs and radiation treatments do their good work by damaging cancer cells. Unfortunately, they can injure normal cells as well, sometimes transforming them into new malignancies. The powerful drugs that allow transplants to survive can also lead to cancer by suppressing the immune system.

Nutritional Factors. In rare instances, spoiled food is the culprit. *Aflatoxins* produced by a fungus that can contaminate peanuts and corn is an example. Also uncommon are cancers promoted by food additives or preservatives, such as *nitrates* that can be converted in the body to carcinogenic *nitrosamines.* Neither spoilage nor preservatives are important factors in the United States, and, although pesticide residues are a concern, they also do not appear to be major offenders. However, the high temperatures characteristic of charcoal broiling may produce carcinogenic chemicals such as *polycyclic aromatic hydrocarbons* (PAHs) that may promote intestinal cancers.

Paradoxically, common foods are a much greater worry. A simple excess of calories produces obesity, which increases the risk of many cancers. For example, the Alumni and Health Professionals studies have both linked obesity, particularly abdominal obesity, to an increased risk of colon cancer. Dietary fat, itself calorie-dense, has also been implicated. The Health Professionals Study found that men who eat large amounts of fat are nearly two times more likely to develop prostate cancer than men who eat only small amounts; the saturated fat found in animal products is responsible for the increased risk. Alcohol is another dietary cause of cancer; men who drink too much have an increased risk of certain cancers.

Dietary Deficiencies. Diets low in fruits, vegetables, and fiber have been linked to many malignancies.

THE BIG PICTURE

Oncogenes, cell clocks, neovascularization, these terms are enough to make a person's head swim. At the cutting edge of cancer research, molecular biology offers real hope that one day soon doctors will have the tools they need to detect and cure cancer. But you do not have to wait for breakthroughs in basic science to bring help. Instead, you can protect yourself now by correcting the big things that damage DNA.

Researchers at the Harvard School of Public Health, where the Harvard men's health studies are headquartered, have recently issued a report on the factors that cause cancer deaths (see Table 3.6). Look over the list and you will see why experts believe that up to 75 percent of cancer deaths in the United States could be prevented.

Table 3.6: THE CAUSES OF CANCER

RISK FACTOR	% OF CANCER DEATHS
Smoking and tobacco use	30
Obesity and diet (red meat vs. fruits and vegetables)	30
Lack of exercise	5
Carcinogens in workplace	5
Viruses (hepatitis, papilloma)	5
Family history of cancer	5
Body size (taller, bigger people get more cancer)	5
Women's reproductive factors (late or no childbearing, late menopause, early periods)	3
Excessive alcohol consumption	3
Poverty (aside from bad diet)	3
Environmental pollution	2
Excessive exposure to sun	2
Medical procedures, drugs	1
Salt, food additives	1

Source: *Harvard Report on Cancer Prevention,* International Association of Cancer Registries.

Can cancer really be prevented? It sounds like a utopian dream, but it is not. In fact, simple preventive measures can substantially reduce a man's risk of developing many kinds of cancer. And many of the lifestyle changes that protect against heart attack and stroke will also help prevent cancer. The next four chapters will discuss the health practices that can do so much to combat the three great perils of heart disease, stroke, and cancer. It really works: healthful living is what keeps men healthy.

PART II

What Keeps Men Healthy?

CHAPTER FOUR

The Answers: Diet

THE TWENTIETH CENTURY WITNESSED revolutionary changes in the American way of life. Although computer-driven technologies have been responsible for the most visible developments, dietary changes have been far more important for health. And while most technological advances have improved man's life, quite the reverse is true of America's new way of eating. At the start of the twentieth century, the average American diet was based on fresh, minimally processed vegetable foods, but at the start of the twenty-first century, the American diet centers around highly processed foods of animal origin.

Over forty years ago, Harvard Professor John Kenneth Galbraith observed that "more die in the United States of too much food than of too little." Although he is an economist, the good professor was right. As a nation, we are consuming far more calories, fat, cholesterol, refined sugar, animal protein, sodium, and alcohol than is healthful—and we are also getting far less fiber and far fewer vitamins and complex carbohydrates than we should.

You do not need a computer to figure out how the modern diet has affected health. To a considerable degree, it is responsible for many of the chronic diseases that afflict American men, including obesity, high blood pressure, heart disease, stroke, and diabetes. Diet also has a major impact on prostate cancer, colon cancer, and other malignancies. Even if a man escapes these major battles, he may well eat himself into gallstones, hemorrhoids, hernias, and diverticulosis.

Nearly two hundred years ago, the French jurist Jean Anthelme Brillat-Savarin said, "Tell me what you eat, and I shall tell you what you are." Today's doctors and nutritionists can do even better; tell them what you eat, and they will tell you what you'll get. During the past twenty-five years, thousands of men have been telling Harvard researchers what they eat and how they are. Now these scientists can help tell you what to eat to stay healthy.

Calories

Although it's a seven-letter word, it has nearly assumed the role of a four-letter epithet. But, despite all the nutritional pejoratives heaped upon it, the calorie is just a unit of energy. Every food has a specific energy value, and every human activity has a certain energy cost; both can be measured as calories. And calories do count; men who consume more calories than they burn up will gain weight, but men with a negative energy balance will reduce.

How many calories do you need to stay in balance? It is surprisingly hard to say; genetic, metabolic, and behavioral variables make it difficult to calculate a man's exact energy requirements. As a rough guide, though, a sedentary man needs about thirteen calories per pound of body weight each day; moderate physical activity boosts the daily requirement to sixteen calories per pound, and men who exercise vigorously burn up about eighteen calories a pound each day. On average, then, a 150-pound man who consumes between 2,000 and 2,700 calories a day will keep his weight stable.

The caloric value of nutrients varies considerably: carbohydrates and proteins have four calories per gram, alcohol has seven, and fats pack nine calories per gram. Because it is so calorie-dense, dietary fat is the most potent nutritional determinant of body weight.

A pound of adipose tissue (body fat) contains about 3,500 calories. To lose a pound of fat in a week, a man must achieve an energy deficit of 500 calories a day, either by eating less or by exercising more. Sustainable weight loss, though, is not actually an either/or proposition; instead, success depends on a combination of a disciplined diet and diligent exercise. It is not quick or easy, but it is very important; obesity has a major impact on health, and none of it is good.

Obesity

Line up with four other American men. Look to your left, then to your right. If you are five average men, one of you is obese and two more are overweight. Now look in a mirror; if you are one of the many, many Americans who needs to lose weight, read on. And even if you are trim at present, you may want to learn how to stay that way.

WHAT IS OBESITY?

Whether your concern is health or aesthetics, the important issue is not how much you weigh, but how much of your body's weight is fat. In medical terms, obesity is defined as an excess of body fat.

It is easy to measure body weight, but difficult to measure body fat. Underwater weighing is the traditional method, but *magnetic resonance imaging* and *bioelectrical impedance testing* have replaced it for most obesity research. Unfortunately, none of those methods is suitable for clinical use, but *skin fold thickness* measurements can be used to estimate body fat. Many health clubs have skin fold calipers, but most men can get an even better idea of where they stand simply by using a scale and a yardstick to measure weight and height, then doing a simple calculation to determine their *body mass index* (BMI).

The BMI may sound like a new wrinkle but it has actually been in use since 1869. Although it is less accurate in highly muscular men and in men over sixty-five, the BMI has emerged as the best overall indicator of obesity and medical risk. To calculate your BMI, just follow four steps: (1) Measure your height in inches (without shoes) and your weight in pounds (without clothing); (2) Multiply your weight by 700; (3) Divide that number by your height; (4) Divide again by your height. Or, if you are mathematically challenged, you can simply look up your BMI in Table 4.1.

IDEAL BODY WEIGHT

What should you weigh? Your tailor may have one answer, your insurance agent another, and your family a third. Each opinion may have some merit, but the Harvard men's health studies can do even better by helping you determine the BMI that is best for your health.

The Health Professionals Study has identified the health risks associated with a high BMI. Diabetes tops the list; even a modestly elevated BMI of 28 will quintuple a man's risk of diabetes, and a BMI of 35 boosts his risk by an astonishing 4,200 percent. If the risk of heart disease is less dramatic, it is no less important. In the Health Professionals Study, obese men with BMIs above 33 were 3.4 times more likely to develop heart disease than men with lean BMIs below 23. Even within the "healthy" BMI range of 22–25, the study found that men with less body fat have a lower risk of diabetes. The study also established a link between increasing amounts of body fat and stroke, hypertension, and gallstones. Some of these associations are displayed in Figure 4.1. As for cancer, the Health Professionals Study found that obesity increases a man's risk of

Table 4.1: YOUR BODY MASS INDEX

HEIGHT	BODY WEIGHT IN POUNDS													
							Overweight				**Obese**		**Very Obese**	
4'10"	91	96	100	105	110	115	**119**	**124**	**129**	**134**	**138**	**143**	**167**	**191**
4'11"	94	99	104	109	114	119	**124**	**128**	**133**	**138**	**143**	**148**	**173**	**198**
5'	97	102	107	112	118	123	**128**	**133**	**138**	**143**	**148**	**153**	**179**	**204**
5'1"	100	106	111	116	122	127	**132**	**137**	**143**	**148**	**153**	**158**	**185**	**211**
5'2"	104	109	115	120	126	131	**138**	**142**	**147**	**153**	**158**	**164**	**191**	**218**
5'3"	107	113	118	124	130	135	**141**	**146**	**152**	**158**	**163**	**169**	**197**	**225**
5'4"	110	116	122	128	134	140	**145**	**151**	**157**	**163**	**169**	**174**	**203**	**232**
5'5"	114	120	126	132	138	144	**150**	**156**	**162**	**168**	**174**	**180**	**210**	**240**
5'6"	118	124	130	136	142	148	**155**	**161**	**167**	**173**	**179**	**186**	**216**	**247**
5'7"	121	127	134	140	146	153	**159**	**166**	**172**	**178**	**185**	**191**	**223**	**255**
5'8"	125	131	138	144	151	158	**164**	**171**	**177**	**184**	**190**	**197**	**230**	**262**
5'9"	128	135	142	149	155	162	**169**	**176**	**182**	**189**	**196**	**203**	**236**	**270**
5'10"	132	139	146	153	160	167	**174**	**181**	**188**	**195**	**202**	**207**	**243**	**278**
5'11"	136	143	150	157	165	172	**179**	**186**	**193**	**200**	**208**	**215**	**250**	**286**
6'	140	147	154	162	169	177	**184**	**191**	**199**	**206**	**213**	**221**	**258**	**294**
6'1"	144	151	159	166	174	182	**189**	**197**	**204**	**212**	**219**	**227**	**265**	**302**
6'2"	148	155	163	171	179	186	**194**	**202**	**210**	**218**	**225**	**233**	**272**	**311**
6'3"	152	160	168	176	184	192	**200**	**208**	**216**	**224**	**232**	**240**	**279**	**319**
6'4"	156	164	172	180	189	197	**205**	**213**	**221**	**230**	**238**	**246**	**287**	**328**
BMI	19	20	21	22	23	24	**25**	**26**	**27**	**28**	**29**	**30**	**35**	**40**

colon cancer. Although obesity in adulthood was not associated with prostate cancer, obesity in childhood appeared to predict an increased risk of developing the disease later in life. And if the threat of diabetes, heart attack, stroke, and colon cancer is not enough to convince you that thin is better, consider a new finding of the Health Professionals Study: Obesity increases the risk of impotence. All in all, a man with a 42-inch waist is twice as likely to develop erectile dysfunction as a man with a 32-inch waist.

FIGURE 4.1. BMI AND THE RISK OF DISEASE

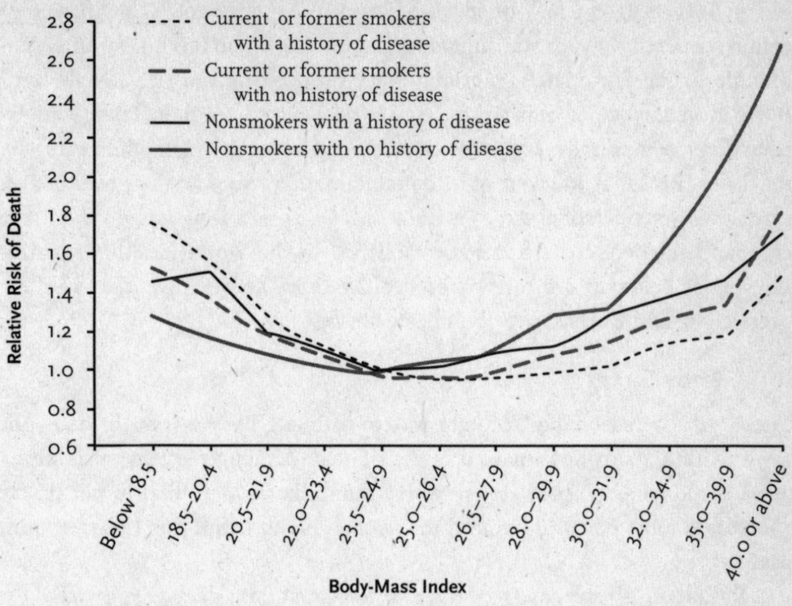

Obesity is linked to mortality as well as morbidity, to death as well as disease. The Health Professionals Study found a direct link between a man's BMI and his mortality rate. Even a rise from a BMI below 23 to a BMI between 23 and 24.9 was linked to a 21 percent increase, and the death rate continued to rise with increasing BMIs, so men above 30 had a 97 percent higher rate than men below 23. In its analysis of nonsmoking men, the Alumni Study reported similar results. The study also found that men who gain weight as they age have a higher mortality rate than men who maintain a steady BMI. The Health Professionals Study determined the factors that predict weight gain. No surprise here: the culprits are less time exercising, more time watching TV, and eating between meals.

You do not have to be a Harvard man to suffer the consequences of obesity. A 1997 study of 7,735 British men pegged the ideal BMI at 22; above that very lean level, each increase of 1 BMI point was associated with a 10 percent increase in the risk of heart disease and in the overall mortality rate. Other studies of men agree: in Japan the ideal BMI was 22.5 and in Framingham, Massachusetts, it was 22.6. In a 1999 study of over 1 million American adults, the American Cancer Society found that men with BMI of 23.5–24.9 had the lowest mortality rates (see Figure 4.1).

A BMI of 22–24 may be ideal, but is it realistic for you? The answer, of course, depends on your starting point, but for most men it is an extremely demanding goal. Fortunately, mortality rates do not begin to rise steeply until BMIs exceed 25–26, so it is fair to set your goal at 25. Even then, tailor your expectations to your body. Try to recall your weight over the years, then estimate the lowest BMI that you were able to maintain for a year above age twenty-five; set that as your personal target, with a BMI of 25 as a long-range vision. For comparison, check the standards established by the World Health Organization: BMIs below 25 are considered healthy, those between 25 and 30 reflect overweight, and BMIs above 30 indicate obesity.

Ideal Body Shape

The BMI is a reasonably accurate way to estimate body fat, but it does not say anything about how that fat is distributed. Although excess fat is never good, some types of body fat are worse than others. Men tend to put on fat where it is most harmful, around the abdomen and trunk (see Chapter One, page 15).

To find out if you have too much of the worst fat, calculate your waist-to-hip ratio. First, with your abdomen relaxed measure your waist at its narrowest, which is usually at the navel. Next, measure your hips at their widest, usually at the bony prominence. Finally, divide your waist size by your hip size to learn your ratio.

$$\frac{\text{Waist size (inches)}}{\text{Hip size (inches)}} = \text{ratio}$$

How does your ratio translate into health risk? The risk of heart attack and stroke increases progressively in men with ratios above 1.0 (for women, the danger begins at 0.8), and the risk is substantial. For example, men with ratios above 1.0 have twice the death rate of those with ratios below 0.85. According to the Health Professionals Study, men with ratios above 0.98 are 2.3 times more likely to suffer strokes than men with ratios below 0.89. That is a big effect from just a few inches.

The waist-to-hip ratio is a powerful predictor of a man's risk of heart disease and stroke. But an even simpler index is the waist circumference itself—a waist size above 40 inches increases a man's risk for complications, and a 46-inch waist increases risk substantially.

CONTOUR CONTROL

"Imprisoned in every fat man," wrote Cyril Connolly, "a thin one is wildly signaling to be let out." Signals notwithstanding, it is not so simple.

Americans spend millions of dollars on gadgets and plans guaranteed to take inches off one part of the body or another. Every one of those dollars is wasted. There is just no way to "spot reduce." It is true that abdominal fat can be removed surgically by liposuction or apronectomy ("tummy tuck"), but there is little reason to think that a surgically-produced cosmetic improvement in your waistline will translate into metabolic improvements that will protect your heart and blood vessels. In fact, although surgery can remove fat from beneath the skin, it cannot remove the deeper fat around the abdominal organs. And in most cases, patients rapidly regain the fat that was removed surgically.

There just is no quick fix. But, there is a slow fix; the same lifestyle that is so good for your health will help you shed pounds and inches, not quickly perhaps, but steadily and substantially. The key to waist control is a combination of diet and exercise.

To lose body fat, put less fat into your body. Try to keep your intake to 20 to 30 percent of your total caloric consumption. Substitute high-fiber foods that are filling but less caloric; aim for at least 30 grams of dietary fiber per day. Eat complex carbohydrates instead of simple sugars, but do not overdose on "good" calories, either. To lose weight, it is important to limit portion size and reduce your caloric intake.

Even if you cut down on fat and calories, it will be nearly impossible to maintain weight loss without exercise. Aim for at least thirty minutes of vigorous exercise or forty-five minutes of moderate exercise nearly every day. If you are serious about weight loss, you may find yourself doing even more. Chapter Five will explain the details.

SLIM DOWN; SHAPE UP

Weight control is like playing a violin. You can have a Stradivarius of a diet, but without the bow of exercise, you will not hear the music of weight loss. It takes time, however, to learn to play. Change gradually, but progressively. Improve your diet slowly, but steadily. In time, your tastes will change and you will come to enjoy low-fat, high-fiber, vegetable-based foods. Build up your exercise little by little so you will avoid injuries and have fun. Weight loss is never easy, but men with abdominal obesity actually have an edge, since upper-body fat is a bit easier to shed than lower-body fat. A healthful lifestyle should be seen as an opportunity, not a punishment. Take the opportunity to change your ways; you'll improve your health, enjoy life more, and change the shape of man.

Fat and Cholesterol

First came the bad news: As the average American's consumption of fat and cholesterol increased during the first half of the twentieth century, his risk of heart attack and stroke also rose to record levels. Next came the good news. Eating less fat and cholesterol can reduce that risk. It is true and it works—but it is not the whole story. In fact, scientists are now learning of important differences among the dietary fats; many are living up to their reputation as villains, but a few may prove to have a positive, if not heroic, effect on health.

New research constantly modifies old beliefs. New and complicated information requires some understanding of chemistry, but it is important information with practical implications for diet and health.

The Fats in Foods

Nearly all the fats in the human diet are in the form of *triglycerides*—three individual *fatty acids* bound together in a single large molecule. Because dietary triglycerides are so large, they cannot be absorbed directly into the blood. Instead, the pancreas and intestines produce *lipases,* enzymes that break down the dietary fat into individual fatty acids that are absorbed into the bloodstream.

The human diet contains many fatty acids. Although each has unique properties, they fall into several major families that produce characteristic effects on blood cholesterol levels and health. For cooks, the distinction is simple: foods contain either fats, which are solid at room temperature, or oils, which are liquid. In general, fats come from animal sources such as meat and dairy products, while oils come from vegetable products. But for chemists, the situation is more complex: animal fats are high in *saturated fatty acids,* as are four vegetable oils (see Table 4.2), while most other vegetable oils contain *unsaturated fatty acids.* In broad terms, saturated fatty acids raise blood cholesterol levels and increase the risk of heart disease, while unsaturated fats do not. But new research indicates that it is not quite so simple. In fact, the unsaturated fatty acids are themselves quite diverse, with some having effects that are deleterious, while others appear beneficial.

WHAT ARE FATTY ACIDS?

Structurally, fats are simple molecules built around a series of carbon atoms (C) linked to each other in a chain. Dietary fats are composed of long chains containing twelve to twenty-two carbons.

Each carbon atom must form four bonds to other atoms. The carbon at one end of the chain is surrounded by three hydrogens and another carbon. The carbon at the other end of the chain has two bonds to oxygen (O), one to an oxygen-hydrogen pair (OH) and the fourth to another carbon; this is the acid group that puts the acid in fatty acids.

In *saturated fatty acids,* each of the interior carbon atoms is bonded to two hydrogen atoms as well as two other carbons. All of the bonds available for hydrogens are filled, or saturated, with hydrogen.

In *unsaturated fatty acids,* some of the hydrogens are missing. Because each carbon must have four bonds, a double bond between neighboring carbon atoms replaces the missing hydrogens. *Monounsaturated fatty acids* have one double bond between carbons. *Polyunsaturated fatty acids* have two or more double bonds.

The health effects of fatty acids depends on how many double bonds are present and on the location of the double bonds. Unsaturated fatty acids are classified according to the number of carbons between the three-hydrogen end of the molecule and the first double bond. In *omega-3 fatty acids,* the first double bond is three carbons from the end; in *omega-6 fatty acids,* the first double bond is six carbons from the end.

In nearly all the unsaturated fatty acids in natural foods, the carbon chain assumes a curved shape called the "cis" configuration. But, when food manufacturers add hydrogen atoms back to polyunsaturates, the shape of the chain becomes straightened to the "trans" configuration. *Trans fatty acids* are found in the partially hydrogenated vegetable oils present in processed foods, such as stick margarine, potato chips and other fried foods, puddings, and commercial baked goods, such as crackers and cookies.

WHAT ABOUT CHOLESTEROL?

Cholesterol is not a fatty acid but a *sterol,* a waxy substance with a complex ring-like structure. Cholesterol is present only in animal tissues; all foods derived from plants are cholesterol-free.

Plants do not have any cholesterol. But they do have sterols, closely related substances that have a key role in plant cell membranes. More than forty sterols have been identified in vegetables oils and whole grains, but the amounts are small.

For more than fifty years, scientists have known that plant sterols can lower blood cholesterol levels, but they could not figure out how to incorporate sufficient amounts into the human diet. Enter Finnish food chemists. In the 1990s, they learned how to make plant sterols palatable. Ironically, perhaps, the process involves adding hydrogen—but instead of producing harmful trans fats, it produces *stanols*. Stanols have nearly twice as much cholesterol-lowering power as sterols, and esterified stanols dissolve in fat, allowing manufacturers to incorporate them into margarine, salad dressing, and other foods. It is enough to give food chemistry a good name.

It has also given certain margarines a good name. Benecol was the first to incorporate plant stanols, Take Control the second. On average, people who use two tablespoons a day will reduce their LDL cholesterol by 14 percent.

Essential Fatty Acids

For all their notoriety, fats and cholesterol are crucial for good health. Cholesterol is present in human cell membranes and is the backbone for cortisone, testosterone, and the other steroid hormones manufactured by the body. Fatty acids are also incorporated into cell membranes; each type of fatty acid affects cell function differently. In addition, fatty acids are stored in triglycerides in the body's adipose tissue, which provides insulation, protects and cushions vital organs, and functions as the body's principal energy depot.

The body can make all the cholesterol it needs; that is why strict vegetarians stay healthy even though their diets contain no cholesterol at all. The body can also produce most of the fatty acids it needs simply by converting one fat into another. But there are two exceptions: Because the body cannot produce *linoleic* acid (an omega-6) or *alpha-linolenic acid* (an omega-3), a dietary supply of these two polyunsaturated fatty acids is essential for health, though only small amounts are needed.

The Fats in Foods

People eat foods, not fatty acids. Even if you do not know a double bond from a double bogey, you should know which foods contain the major families of fats.

Table 4.2: THE FATS IN FOODS

SATURATED FATS

Animal	**Vegetable**
Dairy fats	Coconut
Meat and poultry	Cocoa butter
Tallow	Palm oil
Lard	Palm kernel oil

TRANS FATTY ACIDS

Margarine
Fried foods
Commercial baked goods
Snack foods

CHOLESTEROL

Dairy products
Egg yolks
Meat (especially organ meats, fatty and prime cuts)
Poultry (especially the skin)
Shellfish (especially shrimp)

MONOUNSATURATED FATS

Omega-9
Olive oil
Canola oil
Safflower oil (hybrid)
Sunflower oil (hybrid)

POLYUNSATURATED FATS

Omega-6	**Omega-3**	
	Fish	*Vegetables*
Corn oil		
Safflower oil (regular)	Mackerel	Canola oil
Sunflower oil (regular)	Tuna	Walnuts
Soybean oil	Salmon	Flaxseed
Cottonseed oil	Sardines	Rapeseed
	Others	Wheat germ
		Soybean oil

SPECIFIC FATTY ACIDS

Each family of fats contains a number of individual fatty acids. Here are some of the most important:

- *Palmitic acid* (sixteen carbons; saturated) is the major fat in the meat and dairy products.
- *Oleic acid* (OA; eighteen carbons; monounsaturated, omega-9) is the major fatty acid in olive oil (73 percent) and canola oil (53 percent).

- *Elaidic acid* (eighteen carbons; monounsaturated, omega-9); its structure is identical to oleic acid with one very important difference. It is a trans fatty acid, the major trans fat in margarine and fried foods.
- *Linoleic acid* (LA; eighteen carbons; polyunsaturated, omega-6), is one of the essential fatty acids; it is the major constituent of corn oil (58 percent) and soybean oil (51 percent).
- *Alpha-linolenic acid* (ALA; eighteen carbons; polyunsaturated, omega-3) is the other essential fatty acid. It is found most abundantly in flaxseed oil (50 percent) and canola oil (11 percent); olive oil, walnuts, and wheat germ provide lesser amounts.
- *Eicosapentaenoic acid* (EPA; twenty carbons; polyunsaturated, omega-3) and *docosahexaenoic acid* (DHA; twenty-two carbons, polyunsaturated, omega-3) are the two major fatty acids in fish. The greatest amounts are in oily, dark-fleshed fish that live in deep, cold waters, such as mackerel, herring, striped bass, and Atlantic salmon.

Health Effects

When you go for a physical, your doctor will not measure your fatty acids, but will check your cholesterol. The fats in your diet have an important effect on your blood cholesterol levels. They also influence other less-well-known biologic functions that may turn out to be as important as cholesterol in determining your risk of cardiovascular disease. Here is an overview of how various fats affect your body.

Body Fats and Blood Lipids.

- *LDL cholesterol.* LDL is the "bad" cholesterol; the higher your level, the greater your risk of coronary artery disease. Three dietary factors will elevate your LDL cholesterol: saturated fat, trans fat, and cholesterol itself. Surprisingly, perhaps, saturated and trans fatty acids will raise your LDL even more than dietary cholesterol. Mono- and polyunsaturates do not have a major effect on LDL cholesterol levels. Plant sterols and stanols, found in new margarines such as Benecol and Take Control, can lower LDL cholesterol levels.
- *Oxidized LDL cholesterol.* Although LDL is the villain of the piece, it does not damage arteries in its natural form. Instead, LDL is bombarded by *oxygen free radicals;* the *oxidized LDL* that results is what ac-

tually causes atherosclerosis (see Chapter Three). Monounsaturated fatty acids, particularly oleic acid, help protect LDL from oxidation. That is why olive oil, canola oil, and the new hybrid sunflower and safflower oils are getting a good name. In contrast, linoleic acid, the major polyunsaturate in most other vegetable oils, appears to make LDL more susceptible to oxidative damage.

- *HDL cholesterol.* HDL is the good cholesterol. The higher your level, the lower your risk of coronary artery disease. Trans fatty acids lower HDL cholesterol, but saturated fat does not; it is what makes stick margarine even worse than butter. Mono- and polyunsaturates do not affect HDL directly, but a very low intake of these fats can reduce HDL levels. HDL levels tend to fall when dietary fat levels provide less than 15–20 percent of calories, particularly when certain carbohydrates replace fat in the diet (see Carbohydrates, page 88). All in all, the current evidence seems to favor dietary fat in the low (20–30 percent) but not ultralow (10–15 percent) range.
- *Blood triglycerides.* Fish oils tend to reduce blood triglyceride levels.

Dietary Fats and Human Biology. Dietary fatty acids have biologic effects that can influence several stages in atherosclerosis as well as several other important diseases.

- *Inflammation and immunity.* The omega-3 polyunsaturates have anti-inflammatory properties that may have a protective role in atherosclerosis.
- *Blood clotting.* The omega-3 polyunsaturates in fish oils reduce clot formation by inhibiting *platelets,* the fragmentary blood cells that initiate the clotting process. In addition to platelets, clot formation depends on a series of blood proteins. In high amounts, all dietary fats can increase some of these clotting factors; that's why even the "good" fatty acid should be consumed in moderation.
- *Endothelial function.* The endothelium is composed of a thin layer of cells that line the inner wall of blood vessels (see Chapter Three, Figure 3.1). Endothelial cells help keep tissues healthy by widening arteries when more blood flow is needed. In high amounts, all the fatty acids can impair endothelial function.

- *Arrhythmias.* Arrhythmias are abnormalities of the heart's pumping rhythm. The omega-3 polyunsaturates in fish oil appear to reduce arrhythmias.
- *Body weight.* When it comes to calories, all fats are created equal—equally undesirable, that is. A high-fat diet increases the risk of obesity and its complications. It is a good reason to be judicious with all fats, even the more desirable ones such as olive and canola oils.

Researchers are accumulating more and more information about how various dietary fats affect human biology. But do these factors actually influence health?

Dietary Fat and Heart Disease. For decades, doctors have known that people who eat large amounts of fat have an increased risk of heart disease; saturated fat and cholesterol have been the chief offenders. That is why the American Heart Association suggests reducing dietary fat to less than 30 percent of calories, saturated fat to less than 10 percent, and cholesterol to less than 300 milligrams a day. These old guidelines still apply, but Harvard studies and other new research efforts are providing important qualifications.

In 1996, the Health Professionals Study confirmed that eating saturated fat and cholesterol is bad for the heart. In comparison to the men who ate the least amount of saturated fat, the men who ate the most were 20 percent more likely to suffer heart attacks and 2.2 times more likely to die from heart disease. Similar results were observed for the other well-known dietary culprits: the men who consumed the most cholesterol and total fat had the highest risk of developing heart disease. Men with poor diets may have other negative habits, but lack of exercise, smoking, obesity, and other nondietary risk factors did not explain the results.

It is hardly news that eating fat is bad for the heart. But the Health Professionals Study did break new ground in finding that eating fat and cholesterol is not as bad as it seems if dietary fiber is also considered. Dietary fiber reduces the risk of heart disease (see Carbohydrates and Fiber, page 88). In fact, a low-cholesterol diet did little to reduce the risk of heart attack unless it was also accompanied by an increase in dietary fiber—in which case it worked very well indeed.

Along with other research from Harvard and elsewhere, the Health Professionals Study found that eating large amounts of trans fatty acids is linked to an increased risk of having a heart attack. The effect was substantial, amounting to a 60 percent increase in risk, but as for total fat and cholesterol, it was partially neutralized by the effects of a high fiber diet.

Although the Health Professionals Study's 1996 report confirmed that a high intake of cholesterol was linked to an increased risk of heart disease, a 1999 report from the study gives men who like eggs a bit of breathing room. Except in diabetics, eating up to one egg a day did not appear to increase a healthy man's risk of suffering a heart attack or stroke. Each egg yolk contains about 200 milligrams of cholesterol, but it also contains healthful nutrients such as B vitamins and essential amino acids. It is good news—but don't let it scramble your dietary plans. One egg a day is okay, but larger amounts may not be.

Saturated fat, cholesterol, and trans fatty acids really do belong on your "caution" list—but can any other fat actually help protect your heart? The Health Professionals Study identified one that may; alpha-linolenic acid, an omega-3 polyunsaturated fat found in canola oil and certain nuts and seeds. The Harvard-sponsored Nurses' Health Study agrees. In its 1999 study of 76,283 women, it reported that a high intake of alpha-linolenic acid was linked to a 45 percent reduction in the risk of dying from coronary artery disease.

Studies from other parts of the world are also raising the possibility that certain fats can be healthful, at least in moderation. For years, doctors have been intrigued by the "French paradox." Despite a high intake of fat, people living in Southern France have a lower than predicted risk of heart disease. The same paradox has been observed throughout the Mediterranean basin, even in a country as poor as Albania. Researchers speculate that the protective effect may depend on a high intake of oleic acid, the monounsaturate present in olive oil. Even the enthusiasts, however, acknowledge that other aspects of the Mediterranean lifestyle may also contribute to protection, including a low intake of saturated fat, a high intake of fruits, vegetables, grains, and wine, and lots of physical exercise.

Even granting the complexities of the Mediterranean diet, several recent observations suggest that monounsaturated and omega-3 polyunsaturates may be protective, at least in moderate amounts. For example, studies in New Zealand and in the Antarctic have demonstrated that incorporating canola oil into margarine and using it for cooking can improve blood cholesterol levels. More importantly, the Lyon Heart Study tested a diet high in alpha-linolenic acid (the omega-3 polyunsaturate) and low in linoleic acid (the omega-6 polyunsaturate) in 605 patients with coronary artery disease. The high omega-3 diet was associated with a 72 percent reduction in heart attacks and cardiac deaths and a 56 percent reduction in the risk of dying from any cause during the four-year study period.

Although the Health Professionals Study demonstrated a protective effect of omega-3 fatty acids from plants, it did not find a clear benefit from large amounts of the omega-3s in fish. Eating five to six portions of fish per week did not provide any more protection against heart attacks than one to two portions per week.

The Physicians' Health Study calculated fish consumption in two ways. Like the Health Professionals Study, it obtained dietary histories, but it also measured the levels of fish fatty acids in the men's blood. Neither method suggested that fish consumption protects against heart attacks—but the Physicians' Health Study found that eating fish at least once per week was associated with a decreased risk of sudden death, probably because of protection against abnormal heart rhythms. The Physicians' Health Study also found that eating fish was associated with a lower over-all death rate. All in all, many studies suggest that fish should be part of a healthful diet, and new data even suggests that fish oil supplements may help (see Chapter Six).

Dietary Fat and Neurologic Disease. Although the link is not as strong as for heart disease, high blood cholesterol levels do increase the risk of stroke—and lowering cholesterol with a "statin" drug reduces risk by about 25–30 percent (see Chapter Three). But certain fats may actually help protect the brain. For example, a 1995 study of 192 American men found that high blood levels of alpha-linolenic acid were associated with a reduced risk of stroke.

Dietary fats may also influence the incidence of memory loss. A 1999 study found that a high intake of mono-unsaturated fat appeared to reduce the risk of dementia. Similarly, in 1997, researchers from the Netherlands reported that a high intake of saturated fat or of linoleic acid (the omega-6 polyunsaturate in vegetable oil) seemed to increase the risk of cognitive impairment, while a high intake of omega-3s from fish appeared protective.

Although the Harvard men's health studies have not yet reported on how dietary fat affects the brain, the Health Professionals Study investigated a related problem, visual impairment. It found that a high total intake of fat appears to increase a man's risk of *age-related macular degeneration*, but a high consumption of fish appears protective.

Dietary Fat and Cancer. Obesity increases the risk of cancer; because fat is so calorie-dense, high fat diets are associated with both obesity and cancer. In addition to this indirect link, dietary fat has a direct impact on two cancers in men.

The evidence is strongest for prostate cancer, and in 1993 the Health Professionals Study provided one of the clearest demonstrations of that evidence. It reported that the men who ate the most fat were 1.79 times more likely to develop advanced prostate cancer than were men who ate the least fat. But not all fats were equally harmful; animal fat was linked to the disease, but vegetable fat was not. Red meat was the chief culprit. Men who ate the most beef, bacon, pork, and lamb were 2.6 times more likely to develop prostate cancer than men who ate the least. Men who ate chicken with the skin were at increased risk, but men who omitted the skin were not. Butter, mayonnaise, and many salad dressings also appeared to increase risk.

The Health Professionals Study implicated saturated fats as a prostate cancer risk factor, but it also found that a high intake of alpha-linolenic acid was associated with advanced disease. The Physicians' Health Study agrees with both observations. It reported that men who eat red meat at least five times a week are 2.5 times more likely to develop prostate cancer than men who eat it less than once a week. The Physicians' Health Study also found that men with high levels of alpha-linolenic acid in their blood are up to 3.4 times more likely to develop prostate cancer than men with very low levels.

Red meat is easy to blame, but alpha-linolenic acid poses a dilemma, since it is the omega-3 fatty acid in canola oil and nuts that seems to reduce a man's risk of heart attack and stroke. In 1993 and 1994, two Harvard studies raised concern about this essential fatty acid and prostate cancer. Between 1997 and 2001, four smaller studies echoed that concern—but two additional investigations reported no link, and one from the Netherlands found that a high intake of alpha-linolenic acid was associated with a decreased risk of prostate cancer. But if the omega-3 from vegetables poses a dilemma, the omega-3s from fish do not. Three studies from around the world have linked a high consumption of fish with a decreased risk of prostate cancer.

It is clear that more research is needed to sort out the complex link between dietary fat and prostate cancer. At present, the weight of evidence strongly implicates saturated fat from animal sources as a risk factor, but the status of vegetable fat is up in the air.

More research is also needed to clarify how dietary fat affects colon cancer. The Health Professionals Study found that a high intake of saturated fat appeared to increase the risk of *adenomas,* the benign polyps from which colon cancer develops. Curiously, perhaps, saturated fat was not linked to an increased risk of colon cancer itself, but man's old medical nemesis, red meat, was associated with colon cancer. Clearly, there is more to meat than saturated fat.

FACING THE FATS

How much fat should you eat and what types of fats should you favor? It would be nice if there were a simple answer to this important question, but there is not. In this active field of research, doctors do not yet agree on the answers. In the last analysis, the answer will vary from man to man, depending on factors such as blood cholesterol levels, body weight, risk factors for heart disease and cancer, and personal preferences.

It is a work in progress, but some guidelines already have emerged. A low-fat diet that provides 20 to 30 percent of calories from fat appears best. It is particularly important to reduce your intake of saturated fats from meat and dairy products and of trans fatty acids from processed foods made with partially hydrogenated vegetable oils. A low intake of cholesterol is also important, if less critical. In moderation, certain fats may be helpful. The monounsaturates in olive oil and the omega-3s in fish, nuts and possibly canola oil appear desirable. But even if they prove beneficial, you should get these fats from foods rather than supplements (see Chapter Six). Table 4.2 will help you identify the fats and calories in various foods.

Above all, remember while fat is important, it is only part of the equation. To reduce your risk of heart disease, hypertension, and certain cancers, it is important to eat lots of fruits, vegetables, and whole grains that provide vitamins and fiber. Read on to learn the details.

Carbohydrates and Fiber

For most of humanity's 40,000-year history, men did not have much choice about what they ate. Food was scarce, and folks ate whatever they could get their jaws on. About 10,000 years ago, men learned to cultivate crops and domesticate animals. Dietary choice was born, but even way back then, men made choices that were not always wise. The agricultural-era diet reduced dietary diversity and began to substitute high-fat animal foods for lean game and wild vegetables, nuts, seeds, fruits, and berries. Over the millennia, cultural norms, commercial imperatives, and personal tastes determined how men

Table 4.3: THE FAT AND CHOLESTEROL IN SELECTED FOODS

	Portion Size	Total Calories	Total Fat (grams)	Saturated Fat (grams)	% Calories From Fat	Total Cholesterol (milligrams)
High in saturated fat and/or cholesterol, and/or trans fatty acids; undesirable.						
Dairy Products						
whole milk	8 oz	150	8	5	48	33
yogurt, plain	6 oz	105	6	4	47	21
cottage cheese	4 oz	117	5	3	39	17
sour cream	1 oz	61	6	4	87	12
cream cheese	1 oz	99	10	6	90	31
Ricotta cheese (whole milk)	1 oz	197	15	9	67	58
Ricotta cheese (part-skim milk)	1 oz	156	9	6	52	25
Cheddar cheese	1 oz	114	9	6	74	30
Parmesan cheese	1 oz	129	9	5	59	22
Swiss cheese	1 oz	107	8	5	65	26
feta cheese	1 oz	75	6	4	72	25
egg yolk	1	63	6	2	80	272
ice cream (premium)	1 cup	349	24	15	61	88
ice cream (regular)	1 cup	269	14	9	48	59
margarine	1 tbsp	100	11	2	100	0
Meats (cooked)						
hot dogs (beef)	1	158	14	6	82	31
Bologna (beef)	3 slices	312	28	12	82	58
salami (beef)	3 slices	262	20	9	71	65
chuck roast	3 1/2 oz	350	26	11	67	99
ground beef	3 1/2 oz	272	19	7	61	87
corned beef	3 1/2 oz	251	19	6	68	98
rib roast	3 1/2 oz	225	12	5	47	80
T-bone steak	3 1/2 oz	214	10	4	44	80
liver	3 1/2 oz	161	5	2	27	389
lamb chop	3 1/2 oz	215	9	4	39	215
bacon	3 1/2 oz	576	50	18	78	85
ham	3 1/2 oz	178	9	3	46	92
veal cutlet	3 1/2 oz	271	11	5	37	128
Poultry						
duck	3 1/2 oz	201	11	4	50	89
chicken (with skin)	3 1/2 oz	253	16	4	56	91
Seafood						
shrimp	3 1/2 oz	99	1	trace	10	195
Vegetable Products						
coconut meat	1 oz	187	18	16	88	0
Baked Goods						
croissant	1	235	12	4	46	13
donut	1	210	12	3	51	20
chocolate chip cookies	1	143	6	2	1	54
cream pie	1 slice	455	23	15	46	8

Table 4.3: THE FAT AND CHOLESTEROL IN SELECTED FOODS *(cont.)*

	Portion Size	Total Calories	Total Fat (grams)	Saturated Fat (grams)	% Calories From Fat	Total Cholesterol (milligrams)
Baked Goods (cont.)						
apple pie	1 slice	405	18	5	40	0
chocolate cake	1 slice	235	8	4	31	37
pound cake	1 slice	110	5	3	41	64
waffle	1	245	13	5	48	102
Grain Products						
granola	1 cup	595	33	6	50	0
Snacks and Sweets						
pizza	1 slice	290	9	4	28	56
French fries	10 strips	156	8	4	46	9
potato chips	1 oz	147	10	3	62	0
salted crackers	4	50	1	trace	18	4
chocolate	1 oz	145	9	5	56	6
Sauces and Dressings						
mayonnaise	1 tbsp	99	11	2	100	8
Russian dressing	1 tbsp	76	8	1	92	4
Hollandaise sauce	1/2 cup	353	34	21	87	94
Moderate to low in fat, saturated fat, and cholesterol; acceptable in moderation.						
Dairy						
low-fat milk (1%)	8 oz	102	3	2	23	10
frozen yogurt	1 cup	216	2	0	8	0
sherbet	1 cup	270	4	2	13	14
Poultry						
chicken (without skin)	3 1/2 oz	205	10	3	43	91
turkey (without skin)	3 1/2 oz	126	4	1	24	112
Seafood						
lobster	3 1/2 oz	98	1	trace	6	72
cod	3 1/2 oz	105	1	trace	9	55
flounder, sole	3 1/2 oz	99	1	trace	9	58
Grain Products						
egg noodles	1 cup	160	2	1	11	50
Baked Goods						
bran muffin	1	125	6	1	43	24
oatmeal cookie	1	46	3	trace	37	14
Miscellaneous						
peanut butter	1 oz	95	8	1	76	0
popcorn (oil popped)	1 cup	55	3	trace	49	0
pretzels	1 oz	10	trace	trace	0	0
lo-cal French or Italian dressing	1 tbsp	20	1	trace	45	0
margarine, soft	1 tbsp	50	5	1	90	0
nondairy creamer, light	1 tbsp	10	1	0	100	0

High in unsaturated fats; acceptable in moderation.

pecans	1 oz	187	18	2	89	0
peanuts	1 oz	164	14	2	76	0
pistachios	1 oz	164	14	2	76	0
sunflower seeds	1 oz	165	14	1	77	0
sunflower oil	1 tbsp	125	14	1	100	0
safflower oil	1 tbsp	125	14	1	100	0
corn oil	1 tbsp	125	14	2	100	0
avocado	1	305	30	4	88	0

High in monounsaturated fat; desirable in moderation.

olive oil	1 tbsp	125	14	2	100	0
canola oil	1 tbsp	125	14	1	100	0
walnuts	1 oz	182	18	2	87	0

High in omega-3 oils; desirable in moderation.

mackerel	3 1/2 oz	262	18	4	62	75
salmon	3 1/2 oz	216	11	2	46	87
tuna (fresh)	3 1/2 oz	184	6	2	31	49
trout	3 1/2 oz	105	4	1	26	73
halibut	3 1/2 oz	140	3	trace	19	41

Low in fat and cholesterol; desirable.

Dairy Products						
skim milk	8 oz	86	trace	trace	5	4
buttermilk	8 oz	99	2	1	20	9
lowfat yogurt (plain)	6 oz	94	trace	trace	3	3
lowfat cottage cheese	4 oz	82	1	1	13	5
egg white	1	16	trace	0	0	0
egg substitutes	2 oz	15–60	0–3	0	0–45	0
frozen yogurt (nonfat)	1 cup	175	0	0	0	0
Baked Goods						
whole wheat bread	1 slice	70	1	trace	13	0
bagel	1	200	2	trace	9	0
pita	1/2 shell	165	1	trace	5	0
English muffin	1	140	1	trace	6	0
pancake	1	60	2	trace	30	16
fig bar	1	52	1	trace	17	5
Grain Products						
rice	1 cup	225	1	trace	2	0
spaghetti	1 cup	155	1	trace	6	0
oatmeal	1 cup	145	2	trace	15	0
Beans						
garbanzo beans	1 cup	269	4	trace	14	0
lima beans	1 cup	217	1	trace	3	0
kidney beans	1 cup	225	1	trace	3	0
split peas	1 cup	231	1	trace	3	0
Vegetables						
potato (baked)	1	220	trace	trace	0	0
broccoli	1 spear	50	1	trace	25	0
carrot	1 wedge	30	trace	trace	0	0

Table 4.3: THE FAT AND CHOLESTEROL IN SELECTED FOODS (*cont.*)

	Portion Size	Total Calories	Total Fat (grams)	Saturated Fat (grams)	% Calories From Fat	Total Cholesterol (milligrams)
Vegetables (cont.)						
lettuce	1 wedge	20	trace	trace	0	0
mushrooms	1 cup	20	trace	trace	0	0
squash	1 cup	35	1	trace	30	0
tomato	1	25	trace	trace	0	0
Fruits						
apple	1	80	trace	trace	0	0
banana	1	105	1	trace	8	0
berries	1 cup	80	1	trace	11	0
dates	10	230	trace	trace	0	0
melon	1/4	40	trace	trace	0	0
orange	1	60	trace	trace	0	0
Snacks						
popcorn (air popped)	1 cup	30	trace	trace	0	0
graham crackers	2	55	1	trace	9	0
rye crackers	2	56	1	trace	0	0
gum drops	1 oz	100	trace	trace	0	0
hard candy	1 oz	110	trace	trace	0	0
gelatin	1/2 cup	70	0	0	0	0
angel food cake	1 slice	160	1	0	6	0
nonfat mayonnaise salad dressings and cheese substitutes		variable	0	0	0	0–10

Principal Source: *Nutritive Value of Foods*, U.S. Department of Agriculture.

chose their foods. But in the twentieth century, nutritional science came of age and health considerations finally began to influence dietary choices.

In twenty-first century America, though, it can still be hard for a man to know what to eat. The commercial and cultural pressures are stronger than ever, generally pulling men in the wrong direction. When doctors and nutritionists try to tug people toward a healthy diet, they often seem to be pulling in many directions at once. Most of the debate has centered on dietary fat, but a consensus is finally emerging as scientists have learned that not all fats are alike. Some fats are worse than others, and some even seem to be beneficial, at least in moderation.

But now that fats are finally being sorted out, a new controversy is developing. Just as health-conscious Americans were learning to replace dietary fats with carbohydrates, diet books and talk shows are demonizing carbs as the true agents of heart disease and obesity.

What's a person to do? The answer is not a return to fat or a flight to protein. The right choice is still carbohydrates—but to exercise that choice in a healthful way, men must understand that like fats, not all carbohydrates are alike. In fact, some carbohydrates are much better than others.

WHAT ARE CARBOHYDRATES?

In chemical terms, carbohydrates are easy to understand. They are all composed of just three elements, carbon, hydrogen, and oxygen. But carbohydrates differ in how these elements are strung together, and that is what determines how they affect the body.

CARBOHYDRATES IN THE BODY

Carbohydrates are essential for health. They are a vital source of the energy that fuels the body's metabolism, and they are crucial constituents of *nucleic acids* (the genetic master code), *cell membranes,* and *glycoproteins,* including *prostate specific antigen* (PSA) and many important enzymes.

Glucose is the currency of the body's carbohydrate economy. It is the sugar that circulates in the blood and then enters the body's cells to fuel the metabolism and power exercise. In liver and muscle cells, glucose can be converted into a much larger carbohydrate, *glycogen,* which is stored away until the body needs to mobilize its energy reserves.

Insulin is the hormone that allows glucose to enter cells. Blood glucose levels rise after meals. In response, the pancreas secretes insulin; the faster the blood sugar rises, the more insulin levels rise in response. In diabetes, however, the system is out of balance, and blood sugar levels are too high. In Type 1 (juvenile) diabetes, the problem is that the pancreas does not release enough insulin, but in the much more common Type 2 (adult-onset) diabetes, the major problem is that the body's tissues resist insulin's action.

Even in nondiabetics, insulin is the key to how the body responds to dietary carbohydrates. Carbohydrates that boost the blood sugar quickly provoke the release of much more insulin than carbohydrates that raise the blood sugar slowly. Insulin puts the sugar to work in cells, but high insulin levels also appear to have adverse effects, lowering HDL ("good") cholesterol levels and increasing the risk of *atherosclerosis,* which leads to heart attacks and strokes.

The body's metabolism is complex, but its key message is clear: Foods that raise the blood sugar slowly are more healthful than foods that boost blood sugar levels quickly.

Carbohydrates in the Diet

Plants are the major dietary sources of carbohydrates. The only important carbohydrates that originate from animal sources are the *lactose* in milk and the modest amounts of glycogen in meat, poultry, and liver.

Dietary carbohydrates come in three varieties: simple carbohydrates, complex carbohydrates, and fiber. Despite many important differences, simple and complex carbohydrates all have the same energy value, four calories per gram. It is one of the nice things about carbs, which are less calorie-dense than alcohol (seven calories per gram) or fat (nine calories per gram). Because fiber is indigestible it has no caloric value, but it certainly has lots of health value.

There are two types of simple carbohydrates: *monosaccharides,* which contain just one sugar molecule, and *disaccharides,* which contain two sugar molecules joined together. Glucose is a monosaccharide, as are *fructose* (fruit sugar) and *galactose.* Notable disaccharides include *sucrose* (table sugar, composed of glucose and fructose), *lactose* (milk sugar, composed of glucose and galactose), and *maltose* (the fundamental building block of starch and glycogen, composed of two glucose molecules).

Complex carbohydrates are *polysaccharides,* composed of many simple sugars strung together into long strands. Starches are the complex carbohydrates in plants, glycogen the complex carbohydrate in animal tissues.

Dietary fiber is a special type of complex carbohydrate. Found only in plants, fiber is a mix of very long strands of sugars linked into branching chains. The most healthful sources of fiber are the bran of whole grains, the stems and leaves of vegetables, and fruits, seeds, and nuts. Although there are many types of fiber, they all belong to two broad categories, soluble and insoluble. Both are important for health, but soluble fiber has special benefits for the metabolism: it slows the absorption of other carbohydrates so that blood sugar levels rise more gently, and it helps lower LDL ("bad") cholesterol levels. Even without these benefits, insoluble fiber is a health asset because it increases the water content of feces, making the stools bulkier and easier to eliminate.

Carbohydrates in Foods

Since all the carbohydrates in foods are converted into glucose in the body, it seems logical that they would all have the same impact on health. But in this case, at least, logic is misleading; carbohydrates differ in how quickly they are converted into blood glucose, and foods differ in how many nutrients they provide along with their carbohydrates.

Simple Sugars. The least desirable carbohydrates are the simple sugars. They are absorbed quickly and they are empty calories, lacking other nutrients. Unfortunately, the average American gets about 20 percent of his calories—about half his total carbohydrate intake—from simple sugars. That is a lot of sugar, about 150 pounds a year for the typical adult. America seems to have an insatiable sweet tooth; sugar consumption doubled between 1900 and 2000, and the rise shows no signs of slowing.

Sugar is everywhere. We start the day with sugar-coated cereals, grab some candy for a quick pickup, and choose sugary morsels for desserts and snacks. We quench our thirst with soda, forgetting, perhaps, that the average soft drink contains ten teaspoons of added sugar. All these foods are full of simple sugars, high in calories, and low in other nutrients. Sugary foods are not filling, which is why it's so easy to gobble down four or five pieces of candy in the blink of an eye.

You don't have to forswear all sweets to be healthy, but you should limit your consumption of simple sugars to less than 10 percent of your total caloric intake. For the average man, it works out to about 50 grams of sugar a day; or about twelve teaspoons of table sugar, hardly a Spartan ration. Remember, though, that it is not enough to cut down on table sugar or sucrose. Try to limit your consumption of other simple sugars that show up on food labels as glucose, dextrose, maltose, mannitol, sorbitol, honey, corn syrup, maple syrup, and molasses. "Natural" or "brown" sugar is no better than ordinary white table sugar; by any name, sugar is just as sweet.

Complex Carbohydrates. Because complex carbohydrates must be broken down into simple sugars before they are absorbed, they raise the blood sugar slowly. That alone makes them a big step up nutritionally, and when they are present in unrefined foods, they are accompanied by vitamins, minerals, and other valuable nutrients. In addition, unrefined foods are filling, so it is harder to overdose on them.

Unfortunately, complex carbohydrates have gotten a bad rap in today's America. Cultural bias may be part of the reason. Since starchy foods are plentiful and abundant, beans, rice, noodles, whole grain breads, and legumes are staples in the developing world but are often scorned in affluent societies.

From a health viewpoint, we have it backward. Starchy foods are actually less fattening than foods high in sugar or fat, and they are much more nutritious.

If you succeed in reducing your consumption of simple sugars to 10 percent of your day's calories, make up the difference by increasing your complex carbohydrates to 45 to 55 percent.

Fiber. Found in unrefined vegetable foods and unrefined grains, fiber will not give you calories, but will promote your health. Unfortunately, milling and processing remove the fiber from grains, discarding many healthful vitamins, minerals, and oils along with the bran.

Although dozens of complex plant carbohydrates function as dietary fiber, they all belong to two categories, *soluble* and *insoluble;* both are important for health. Insoluble fiber draws water into the intestines, making the feces bulkier and easier to pass; it helps promote intestinal health by reducing the risk of hemorrhoids, diverticulosis, and hernias (see Chapter Nine). Soluble fiber has less effect in the intestines but more influence on the metabolism. It slows the stomach's emptying, producing a feeling of fullness that may help prevent overeating; it slows the absorption of carbohydrates, reducing insulin levels; and it binds bile acids, lowering LDL ("bad") cholesterol levels. Both types of fiber are good for health; fiber-rich foods contain a mix of the two, but a few are particularly valuable for their soluble fiber (see Table 4.4).

The Health Professionals Study found that dietary fiber reduces a man's risk of heart disease. Over a six-year period, men who ate the most fiber had enjoyed a 41 percent reduction in heart attacks compared with men who ate the least fiber. This substantial protection did not require a man to munch on bran from dawn to dusk; in fact, men in the high-fiber group consumed 28.9 grams of fiber a day, the low-fiber men, 12.4 grams. That means the men who were protected from heart disease were consuming the amount of fiber recommended for all Americans, while the men at greatest risk were eating the same amount as their average countrymen. All in all, for each 10 gram increase in a man's daily fiber intake, his risk of heart disease drops by 19 percent—and just one bowl of high-fiber cereal can provide those 10 grams of protection (see Table 4.4).

It is a long way from the stomach to the heart, and since fiber is not absorbed into the bloodstream, it does not even make the trip. How does it reduce the risk of heart disease? Doctors are not sure, but several mechanisms appear to be involved. For one thing, soluble fiber lowers LDL cholesterol. In addition, the Health Professionals Study found that when a high fiber diet is accompa-

Table 4.4: SOURCES OF DIETARY FIBER

Food	Serving Size	Fiber Content (To nearest gram)	Calories
Grains and Flours			
buckwheat	1 cup (cooked)	11	340
whole rye	1 cup (cooked)	11	314
whole wheat	1 cup (cooked)	10	400
barley (s)	1 cup (cooked)	8	700
brown rice	1 cup (cooked)	5	230
oats (s)	1 cup (cooked)	3	132
white rice	1 cup (cooked)	trace	225
refined wheat	1 cup (cooked)	trace	420
Baked Goods			
Ry Krisp	1 square	5	55
Graham cracker	4 squares	2	120
bran muffin	1	2	100
whole wheat bread	1 slice	2	61
pumpernickel bread	1 slice	1	66
bagel	1	1	145
Pasta			
spaghetti	1/2 cup (cooked)	1	155
Legumes			
baked beans (s)	1/2 cup (cooked)	9	155
kidney beans (s)	1/2 cup (cooked)	7	110
navy beans (s)	1/2 cup (cooked)	6	112
dried peas (s)	1/2 cup (cooked)	5	115
lima beans (s)	1/2 cup (cooked)	5	64
lentils (s)	1/2 cup (cooked)	4	97
Greens			
kale	3 1/2 oz	6	50
turnip greens	3 1/2 oz	4	27
spinach	3 1/2 oz	3	22
endive	3 1/2 oz	2	23
romaine lettuce	3 1/2 oz	2	23
iceberg lettuce	3 1/2 oz	1	13
Vegetables, raw			
carrot	1 medium	4	30
tomato	1 medium	2	20
mushrooms	1/2 cup	2	10
bean sprouts	1/2 cup	2	15
celery	1/2 cup	1	10
green pepper	1/2 cup	1	10
cucumber	1/2 cup	trace	8
Vegetables, cooked			
potato (with skin)	1 medium	3	106
sweet potato	1 medium	3	160
parsnips	1/2 cup	3	51
brussels sprouts (s)	1/2 cup	3	28
broccoli (s)	1/2 cup	3	20
zucchini	1/2 cup	2	11
turnip	1/2 cup	2	17
string beans	1/2 cup	2	16
asparagus	1/2 cup	1	15
cauliflower (s)	1/2 cup	1	5

Table 4.4: SOURCES OF DIETARY FIBER *(cont.)*

Food	**Serving Size**	**Fiber Content (To nearest gram)**	**Calories**
Fresh Fruits			
apple (with skin) (s)	1 medium	4	81
pear (with skin)	1 medium	4	90
orange (s)	1 medium	3	62
banana	1 medium	3	115
raspberries	1/2 cup	3	35
strawberries	1/2 cup	2	23
peach (with skin)	1 medium	2	37
cantaloupe	1/4 melon	1	30
cherries	10	1	49
grapes	1/4 cup	1	50
plum	1 medium	1	20
Fruits, Dried			
figs	6	19	255
prunes (s)	6	8	120
dates	6	4	140
apricots (s)	6	4	120
raisins	1/4 cup	3	106
Nuts and Seeds			
peanuts (s)	10 nuts	1	105
almonds	10 nuts	1	79
filberts	10 nuts	1	54
popcorn (air popped)	1 cup	1	54
Breakfast Cereals			
All Bran Extra Fiber	1 oz	14	50
Fiber One	1 oz	13	60
All Bran	1 oz	10	70
Bran Buds	1 oz	10	70
100% Bran	1 oz	9	70
Oat Bran (hot) (s)	1 oz	6	110
Bran Flakes	1 oz	5	90
Corn Bran	1 oz	5	98
Raisin Bran	1 oz	5	110
Oatmeal (s)	1 cup	4	108
Shredded Wheat	1 oz	3	90
Wheaties	1 oz	3	110
Cheerios	1 oz	2	110
Corn Flakes	1 oz	trace	110
Dietary Supplements			
wheat bran	1 oz	12	70
wheat germ	1 oz	3	62
psyllium (Metamucil, Perdiem, Fiberall, and others (s)	1 tsp. or 1 wafer	4	varies
methylcellulose (Citrucel and others)	1 tsp.	2	varies

(s) Indicates good source of soluble fiber.

Principal Source: Diet, Nutrition, and Cancer. *Prevention: The Good News.* U.S. Department of Health and Human Services.

nied by a high intake of potassium and other minerals from fruits and vegetables, it tends to lower blood pressure, reducing the risk of stroke as well as heart attack. Finally, the study has determined that a high intake of fiber helps control diabetes, and a new international study from the United States and Germany found that it can actually lower blood insulin levels.

Dietary fiber is good for the heart and metabolism, and it is also good for the intestinal tract. Nearly every mother's son was taught that "roughage" prevents constipation. Mom was right—again! By reducing constipation and straining, dietary fiber helps prevent hernias and hemorrhoids. The Health Professionals Study found that a high-fiber diet can reduce a man's risk of *diverticulosis* by 42 percent; insoluble fiber was particularly helpful. That is a big benefit, particularly since half of Americans over age sixty have diverticulosis, a condition involving the lower colon that can cause pain, bleeding, or infection and inflammation.

Dietary fiber is healthful but it is not a panacea. Ever since the 1960s epidemiologists theorized that dietary fiber was responsible for the low incidence of colon cancer in Africans who ate traditional diets. The Health Professionals Study casts doubt on the theory, finding no protection against colon cancer from dietary fiber, even though a high-fiber diet was linked to a reduction in adenomas, the benign tumors from which colon cancer arises.

The Health Professionals Study has important things to say about dietary fiber, but it does not stand alone; in fact, studies in men and women from around the globe confirm that dietary fiber is important for cardiovascular, metabolic, and intestinal health.

CHOOSING YOUR CARBOHYDRATES

It is important to reduce your intake of simple sugars and to increase your consumption of complex carbohydrates and fiber. But to make the best choices, you need another piece of information called the *glycemic index*. It is a measure of how quickly a food raises the blood sugar. Remember that rapid rises in blood sugar call forth large amounts of insulin, and that high levels of insulin seem to lower HDL cholesterol and raise the risk of heart disease. Foods with a low glycemic index raise the blood sugar slowly and are the most desirable carbohydrates. In general, they are also rich in complex carbohydrates and dietary fiber.

For many people, the glycemic index is a new tool. Even men who feel comfortable in the complex world of omega-3s and trans fatty acids may find yet another number daunting. But the glycemic index is an important and practical way to classify carbohydrate-rich foods, which is why it is a standard method for planning diabetic diets in Canada, Australia, England, and France. Unfortunately, the glycemic index has not caught on in America, largely because many nutritionists think it is too complex for consumers already struggling to face their fats.

In fact, the glycemic index is very easy to understand. It is simply a measure of how quickly a food raises the blood sugar level. The standard is glucose itself, which is assigned the maximum score of 100. Foods that score below 100 raise the blood sugar more slowly than glucose; the lower, the slower. To date more than 600 foods have been rated; for the test, the portions are adjusted so that each contains the same amount of carbohydrate. Some labs also measure blood insulin along with blood sugar levels.

Table 4.5 lists the glycemic index of some common foods, and it contains some major surprises. It is easy to see why white bread has a higher number than whole grain bread, but harder to understand why potatoes have a higher glycemic index than some candy bars. The reason for the apparent contradictions is that the glycemic index does not depend solely on the distinction between simple and complex carbohydrates. In fact, complex carbohydrates that are fully gelatinized can be rapidly digested and absorbed, which is why potatoes and many processed breads and cereals have high numbers. In contrast, the complex carbohydrates in foods made from unprocessed grains are in a form that is slowly absorbed, as are the carbohydrates in many beans and dairy products. The biggest surprise of all is that some candy products have a modest index despite having lots of sugar, either because they contain fats that slow sugar absorption or because they are made with fructose, a sugar that has little effect on blood glucose. It's why diabetics should be encouraged to eat fruit (but not Mars bars).

Does the glycemic index matter? The Health Professionals Study says it does. In 1997, it reported that the glycemic index of a man's diet helps determine his risk of Type 2 diabetes; men whose diets contained foods with a high glycemic load were 1.37 times more likely to develop diabetes than men who ate foods with a low glycemic load.

Recent research from England suggests that the glycemic index of foods may also play an important role in determining the level of HDL ("good") cholesterol. For several years, doctors have known that a severe reduction in dietary fat (below 16 percent daily calories) has the paradoxical effect of lowering the HDL cholesterol. The new study may resolve the paradox. It suggests that the problem lies not with the very steep reduction in dietary fat, but with the

Table 4.5: THE GLYCEMIC INDEX (GI) OF SELECTED FOODS

	Least Desirable: High GI (70 and above)		Intermediate: Moderate GI (56–69)		Most Desirable: Low GI (55 and below)	
Breads	French	95	rye	65	pumpernickel	41
	white	70	sourdough	57	heavy mixed grain	30–45
Cereals	puffed rice	90	Cream of Wheat	66	oatmeal	53
	corn flakes	84	Bran Chex	58	All Bran	42
	Cheerios	83				
	Rice Krispies	82				
	Shredded Wheat	70				
Potatoes	white	87	new	58	yams	54
	instant mashed	86				
	mashed	72				
Rice	white	72	brown	66		
Sweets	honey	91	Mars Bar	65	fructose	22
	jelly beans	80	refined sugar	64		
	Life Savers	70	oatmeal cookies	57		
Dairy			ice cream	61	yogurt	33
					skim milk	32
Fruit			pineapple	66	orange juice	49
			banana	61	orange	43
					apple	36
					strawberries	32
					peach	28
Pasta, legumes, and grains					baked beans	43
					pasta	38
					chick peas	36
					kidney beans	33
					lentils	28
					barley	22
					soy beans	18

carbohydrates that replace the banished fat. Doctors in London investigated 1,420 British adults, studying the glycemic index of their diets as well as their dietary fiber, fat, and alcohol consumption and their tobacco use. The dietary evaluation was meticulous, requiring all participants to weigh and measure all the food and drink they consumed for a seven-day period. The researchers visited all the volunteers in their home, where they measured their heights, weights, and blood pressures and obtained blood samples to determine LDL and HDL cholesterol levels.

As expected, the participants who ate the least total fat, saturated fat, and cholesterol had the lowest LDL levels. But although a low-fat diet had the expected favorable impact on the LDL, it did not help the HDL. On the contrary, the people who ate the least fat had the lowest HDLs. Smoking, alcohol, and obesity did not account for the lower-than-expected HDLs. Instead, the glycemic index explained the results; a high glycemic index was associated with a low HDL cholesterol level. It's an important confirmation of the 1997 MR. FIT study of American men that did not measure the glycemic index, but found that high intakes of sucrose (table sugar) were associated with low levels of HDL cholesterol. A 2001 study of 13,907 American adults provides still more evidence. As in the smaller British study, people whose diets contained food with the highest glycemic index had the lowest HDL levels, even after body fat, smoking, exercise, alcohol use, and dietary fat were taken into account. And a recent report from the Harvard-sponsored Nurses' Health Study looked beyond cholesterol numbers to the actual risk of heart disease; over a ten-year period, it found that women whose diets provided the highest glycemic load from refined carbohydrates were three times more likely to develop heart disease than those with low-glycemic diets.

To help choose your carbohydrates, have a look at Table 4.5, but interpret it thoughtfully. Man does not live by carbohydrates alone, and the glycemic index is not the only thing that determines a food's healthfulness. Glycemic index notwithstanding, a baked potato is surely more healthful than a Mars bar; vitamins, minerals, and fiber should make the choice easy. Remember, too, that the carbohydrate content of a food and the size of your portion are also important considerations. The glycemic index of honey is about three times higher than that of some whole-grain breads—but if you eat a pound of bread, you'll get a higher total *glycemic load* than from a thin spread of honey on a slice of the bread.

Don't use the glycemic index to plan your entire diet. Instead, use it to compare foods within the same category. Since many of the carbohydrates in the Western diet come from bread and cereal, the index is particularly useful here—and its lesson is simple: favor unrefined, coarsely ground foods over highly processed foods. Table 4.6 provides some examples.

The glycemic index may seem new to Americans, but it really amounts to a numerical endorsement of old dietary habits—very, very old, in fact. Cultivated grains entered the human diet ten thousand years ago but processed,

Table 4.6: CHOOSING YOUR CARBOHYDRATES

INSTEAD OF	CONSIDER
white bread	whole grain bread
Cream of Wheat	oatmeal
corn flakes	All Bran
white potatoes	yams
white rice	beans, pasta
fruit juice	fruit
tropical fruits, such as bananas	Temperate-climate fruits, such as apples

finely ground, and highly refined foods did not appear until the modern era. When it comes to choosing their carbs, at least, forward-looking men should look backward—way back to the natural foods best suited to human nature.

Protein

Proteins are vital constituents of the human body. They provide the structural framework for bones and the contractile power for muscles. Proteins form the enzymes that make the metabolism work and the antibodies that fend off infections. They are also essential for growth and for the repair of tissues damaged by injury or illness. Proteins are the backbone of life.

Men recognized the importance of proteins long before they knew an enzyme from an antibody. For many years, high-protein foods were considered the most beneficial for health in general and for athletic prowess in particular. It's a theory that has been challenged by nutritionists, but it has been revived recently by diet plans that promote high-protein foods for weight loss and health.

Protein is a good thing, a very good thing, in fact—but can men get too much protein? How much protein is enough, and what kinds are best? What are the facts about proteins?

WHAT ARE PROTEINS?

Proteins are large molecules built from small subunits called *amino acids.* All amino acids are composed of carbon, oxygen, and nitrogen molecules; a few also contain sulfur. The nitrogen makes amino acids unique, distinguishing them from carbohydrates and fats.

About 100 amino acids are strung together to make an average-size protein, but a protein is much more than a linear chain of amino acids. In fact, each protein has a unique, complex, folded or twisted three-dimensional structure. Scientists do not know what determines how a protein assumes its final configuration, but they do know the structure is every bit as important as the sequence of amino acids within the protein.

The human body manufactures perhaps 100,000 different proteins, each produced under the direction of one or more genes. All the proteins in the body are at work serving a structural or metabolic function, but all are in flux, being degraded and resynthesized continually. In the average-size man, about ten ounces of protein are broken down every day, but the amino acids are recycled to build new proteins. In addition, about one ounce of protein is lost from the body every day, passing out through the feces, urine, and skin.

Proteins in the Diet

To maintain health, you must eat enough protein to replace and maintain your body's proteins. It is a crucial task, but it takes surprisingly little to do the job. The average 150-pound man's body contains perhaps three pounds of amino acids, and as little as two ounces of protein in his daily diet will provide plenty of material to refurbish his body's supplies.

Like the proteins in your body, the proteins in your diet are composed of chains of amino acids. But the proteins in food are too large to be absorbed from the intestinal tract. Instead, they are digested into units of one, two, or three amino acids that are absorbed into the bloodstream, then carried to the liver, muscle, and other tissues where they are reassembled into proteins. The tens of thousands of proteins in the body are built from just twenty amino acids. How can just twenty subunits build so many different proteins? The differences among proteins depend on the sequences in which their amino acids are linked; it's the way just twenty-six letters can form all the words in the English language.

Not all dietary proteins contain all twenty amino acids. But your body does not actually need to get all twenty from food, since it can manufacture eleven of them from carbon, hydrogen, and nitrogen. Still, nine amino acids must come from your diet. The best way to get all nine *essential amino acids* is to eat a variety of foods that contain a balanced mix of amino acids. Animal protein does have the advantage of having the amino acid combinations needed by our animal bodies. No single vegetable food contains sufficient amounts of all nine essential amino acids. Beans, for example, are low in *methionine.* But by eating a combination of vegetable foods, you can get all the amino acids you need; rice, for example, is high in methionine.

The Perils of Protein Deficiency

Without enough dietary protein, the body's tissues will weaken. If the deficiency is severe or prolonged, the body will break down its own proteins faster than they can be rebuilt. The result is tissue wasting and weakness that is most notable in the body's most protein-rich tissue, muscle.

Fortunately, dietary protein deficiency is very rare in developed countries. The average American man, for example, gets more than twice as much protein as he needs. But people who are ill or elderly can suffer protein malnutrition; protein supplements can help these individuals, particularly when they need extra amino acids to repair a fractured hip or recover from surgery.

Unfortunately, dietary protein will not do much for the people who are burdened by severe wasting illnesses, such as AIDS or advanced cancer. That's because these patients suffer from *cachexia,* a metabolic response to illness characterized by excessive muscle wasting and insufficient protein synthesis. New research, though, suggests that they may benefit from therapy with *androgens* such as *testosterone,* because these male hormones increase muscle growth. Even in health, androgens explain why men have bigger muscles than women, and why they need more dietary protein.

The Pitfalls of Excess Protein

Can too much of a good thing be harmful? The answer for dietary fat and carbohydrates is yes, for protein, maybe.

Protein has four calories per gram, exactly the same as carbohydrates. Although the body does not store excess calories as protein, it can and does convert the carbon, oxygen, and hydrogen from amino acids into fats, which always seem to pile up where they are least welcome. Popular theories notwithstanding, proteins are fattening.

Fat has no nitrogen. What becomes of the nitrogen from excess dietary protein when it is stored away as fat? It is excreted in the urine—but that is not the end of the story. In fact, for the kidneys to excrete extra nitrogen, they have to work extra hard. In animals, long-term protein excess leads to enlarged kidneys and premature aging of these vital organs. Doctors do not know if the same thing occurs in humans, but they do know that patients can slow the progression of certain kidney diseases by reducing the amount of protein they eat.

As nitrogen enters the urine, it carries calcium and sodium along with it. The extra urinary calcium can increase a man's risk of osteoporosis and kidney stones (see Chapter Thirteen). On the other hand, the sodium loss is a good thing, explaining why high protein diets appear to lower blood pressure.

YOUR PROTEIN REQUIREMENTS

Since dietary proteins are not completely digested and absorbed, the average man should eat about two ounces of protein a day, to replace the loss of one ounce of protein a day.

Healthy men should aim to get about 0.8 grams of daily protein for each kilogram of body weight; that's about .36 grams per pound. Here's how it rounds out:

BODY WEIGHT	DAILY PROTEIN REQUIREMENT (GRAMS)
120	43
140	50
160	58
180	65

Men who weigh above 180 pounds will do quite well with 65 grams (about two and a quarter ounces) of protein per day. Athletes may be an exception. Since they have larger muscles that are working harder, they may benefit from a 20 percent increase in daily protein. Higher amounts are perfectly safe in the short run, though they may have adverse effects in the very long run.

Unless you have special problems, such as advanced kidney disease or liver disease, you do not have to count up the proteins in your diet. A balanced diet will give you all the protein you need, and if you keep your dietary protein to about 15 percent of your total daily calories, you will not get too much. To help guide you, Table 4.7 lists the protein content of various foods.

Table 4.7: DIETARY SOURCES OF PROTEIN

Food	Serving Size	Protein Content (to nearest gram)	Calories	% Calories from Protein
Legumes				
soybeans	1 cup	20	235	34
black beans	1 cup	18	225	32
garbanzo beans	1 cup	18	270	27
kidney beans	1 cup	16	230	28
split peas	1 cup	16	230	28
lima beans	1 cup	16	260	25
lentils	1 cup	16	215	30
Vegetables				
potato	1 medium	5	220	9
broccoli	1 spear	4	40	40
corn	1 ear	3	85	14
carrot	1 medium	1	30	13
tomato	1 medium	1	25	16
Fruits				
apple	1 medium	trace	80	–
banana	1 medium	1	105	4
orange	1 medium	1	60	7
pear	1 medium	1	100	4
strawberries	1 cup	1	45	9
Grain Products				
barley	1 cup	16	700	9
pasta	1 cup	7	190	15
rice	1 cup	5	230	7
coffee cake	1 slice	5	230	7
bran muffin	1 medium	3	125	10
bread	1 slice	2	65	12
Meat				
steak	6 oz	51	348	59
pork	6 oz	48	550	35
veal	6 oz	46	370	50
hamburger	6 oz	40	490	33
Poultry				
chicken	6 oz	54	280	39
Fish				
tuna (water-packed)	6 oz	60	270	89
sardines	6 oz	40	350	46
haddock	6 oz	34	350	39
Dairy Products				
skim milk	1 cup	8	85	38
whole milk	1 cup	8	150	21
yogurt (low-fat)	8 oz	12	145	33
Cheddar cheese	1 oz	4	70	23
cottage cheese	1 cup	28	235	48
egg	1 medium	6	80	30

Principal Source: *Nutritive Value of Foods,* U.S. Department of Agriculture.

WHAT PROTEINS ARE BEST?

Although animal foods contain the best mix of amino acids, they are not necessarily the best sources of protein. That is because foods contain more than just protein; the only pure protein food is the albumin in egg whites. In the case of animal protein, the extra nutrients are often saturated fat and cholesterol—high in calories and potentially harmful for the heart. But in the case of vegetable protein, the extras are often complex carbohydrates and dietary fiber.

The typical American man eats more protein than he needs, and it's the wrong kind of protein; two-thirds comes from animal foods and just one-third from vegetable foods, when the ratio should be exactly reversed.

Excessive animal protein means excessive saturated fat, cholesterol, and calories. It also means deficiencies of complex carbohydrates and dietary fiber. This combination of excesses and deficiency is the link between the Western diet and Western diseases such as prostate cancer, colon cancer, obesity, diabetes, high blood pressure, heart disease, and stroke.

Although many vegetable proteins are healthful, one deserves special mention. Soy is a mainstay of the Asian diet, and it may help explain the low risk of prostate cancer and heart disease in that part of the world.

Soy is an excellent source of protein. One cup of the beans provides about 20 grams, and soy contains all 11 essential amino acids. Soy is also rich in fiber and it contains the mono- and polyunsaturated fatty acids that contribute to cardiac health. Soy also has *isoflavones,* the chemicals that may reduce the risk of prostate diseases, both benign and malignant. Add the B vitamins, potassium, and calcium that are plentiful in soy, and you have got a truly excellent food.

Doctors are not sure that soy actually protects the prostate, but they know that eating 25 grams or more a day will lower your cholesterol by about 9 percent.

Soy is making its way into the nutritional mainstream. Look for ways to add it to your diet. Along with other vegetable proteins, it is an example of how you can get the protein you need without going hog wild.

Water

Water is present in all the body's tissues; about half of a man's weight is made up of water. Water is required for all the body's processes. On average, you need about a quart of water for each 1,000 calories you burn. For most men, that means an intake of about two quarts a day, but it doesn't all have to come from beverages. In fact, about 60 percent of the body's needs are met by the water contained in food. In ordinary circumstances, just a pint and a half of water will make up the difference.

Thirst is a reliable guide to your fluid needs, but it has an important drawback: it is slow. By the time you feel thirsty, your body will be dry. During the time it takes to quench your thirst, you may suffer some of the consequences of dehydration, such as impaired concentration, irritability, headache, and fatigue. It's temporary, but unpleasant. Fortunately, you can stay ahead of the game by anticipating special fluid needs. Think ahead and drink ahead.

When will you need extra water? Here are some factors to keep in mind:

Exercise. When you exercise, your muscles generate heat. To get rid of that heat, you will sweat. In warm, humid weather, you will sweat prodigiously, losing up to a quart and a half of fluid per hour. To stay ahead, drink six to eight ounces of water before you start working out, and take similar amounts at frequent intervals. After you finish exercising, spend some time at the water fountain before you shower. If you drink enough you will not feel thirsty—or, for that matter, grumpy or tired. You'll know you have enough when your urine is clear and abundant. Or you can simply check your weight before and after exercise, minus your sweaty clothes, of course. For each pound of weight you lose, you will need to drink a pint of fluid. Despite the popularity of sports drinks that contain sugar and potassium, plain old water is best.

Climate. It is obvious that you will lose water in sweat when it's hot and/or humid. It is not so obvious, though, that you will also need more water when it's cold and dry. That's because you lose water through your lungs every time you exhale. In an average climate, it amounts to a pint a day, but when the air is dry you will lose substantially more water.

Air Travel. Dry air is responsible here, too. You will enjoy your trip more if you drink even before you are thirsty. Don't overdo it, though, especially if you have a window seat.

Illness. Diarrhea calls for extra fluids. Less obvious, perhaps, is the fact that you will need more fluid every time you have a fever. That's because your body's metabolism speeds up by about 7 percent with each degree of fever. You may not feel like drinking when you're feverish, but you really should try to sip enough to prevent dehydration. Water is best for fever, but if you have copious diarrhea you will need to replace minerals and sugar, too. It is actually a good time to use sports drinks, or you can make your own by adding one-half of a teaspoon of honey or sugar and a pinch of salt to a glass of fruit juice, or by dissolving one-quarter of a teaspoon of baking soda in eight ounces of water or a carbonated beverage.

EXTRA BENEFITS OF EXTRA FLUIDS

Bladder cancer is a special problem for men, since three of every four cases occur in males (see Chapter Thirteen). The Health Professionals Study found that extra water may help. Men who averaged more than two and a half quarts of fluid a day had half the risk of bladder cancer as men who drank less than half as much. In all, each eight ounces of daily fluid appears to lower the risk of bladder cancer by 7 percent. All types of fluid were helpful, but water was the best of them all.

A high intake of fluids may protect the bladder by keeping the urine dilute. The Health Professionals Study also found that high fluid intake reduces a man's risk of kidney stones, which is three and a half times higher in men than women. But not all beverages were equally protective against stones. Coffee, tea, wine, and beer were all better than water, while apple juice and grapefruit juice actually increased the risk of kidney stones.

TOO MUCH OF A GOOD THING?

It is possible to drink too much, but it is not easy. Healthy kidneys can match your intake ounce for ounce, all the way to several gallons a day, and even beyond. But under special circumstances, even two quarts a day can be too much. For example, diuretics are medications designed to thwart the kidneys' control mechanisms, causing them to excrete extra sodium. If patients force fluids in a misguided effort to keep up, they may develop *hyponatremia,* an excess of water that can dilute the blood sodium concentration to dangerously low levels. The same thing can happen to patients with various conditions that cause them to retain water. Finally, psychological disorders that impel people to drink huge amounts of fluid can also result in water intoxication.

WATER VS. WATER

Environmentalists at the start of the twenty-first century share the concern of Coleridge's Ancient Mariner of 1798: "Water, water everywhere, nor any drop to drink." America's fresh water supply is at risk. In many parts of the country, water is being consumed by people, animals, and industry faster than it can be replaced by nature. To make matters worse, people, animals, and industry have dumped pollutants into much of the nation's water supply.

Does that mean you should install a water purifier or drink bottled water? Not necessarily. The Clean Water Act has already produced dramatic improvements in water purity, and more are expected. But even now, municipal water is processed and tested to be sure it is safe. If your house has old, leaded plumbing or its own well, you will have to run your own tests. Otherwise, you can rely on your town's water—in most cases, in fact, the standards for community water are higher than for bottled designer water, which tastes better to some but is expensive for all.

Vitamins

Few topics on nutrition are as controversial as vitamins. On the one hand, the supplement industry has fostered extravagant—and scientifically unsubstantiated—claims for the health benefits of vitamins. At the other extreme, academic physicians have argued that there is no evidence that supplementary vitamins add to a well-balanced diet. In medical terms, the doctors are far closer to being right—but evidence is emerging that modest supplementary doses of certain vitamins may be beneficial, particularly for individuals whose diets are not ideal, for patients with chronic illnesses, for those at risk of atherosclerosis, and for older people. In Chapter Six I will discuss vitamin supplements; here, the general features of vitamins and the benefits of vitamin-rich foods.

WHAT ARE VITAMINS?

Vitamins are organic (carbon-containing) molecules that are required for many of the body's metabolic processes. Because the body cannot manufacture them, vitamins must be consumed on a regular basis. All thirteen vitamins are essential nutrients. Only tiny amounts are needed to prevent vitamin-deficiency diseases, but slightly larger amounts of certain vitamins may provide additional benefits.

There are two basic groups of vitamins. The fat-soluble vitamins (A, D, E, and K) are absorbed into the body with dietary fat and are stored in the body's fatty tissues. You can store enough fat-soluble vitamins to last for months, but if you take excessive amounts you can build up toxic levels, especially of vitamins A and D. In contrast, the water-soluble vitamins (the B vitamins and vitamin C) are not stored in the body to any appreciable degree; extra amounts are passed into the urine, so toxic reactions occur only if very large amounts are ingested. But because the body has no storage depot for water soluble vitamins, you must consume them frequently, if not daily. Since these chemicals dissolve in water, excessive processing and cooking can remove them from food.

Table 4.8 reviews some important properties of the vitamins. Although all are important, certain groups of vitamins are of particular interest for men's health.

Folic Acid, B_6, and B_{12}

These three Bs reduce blood levels of *homocysteine,* the amino acid newly linked to atherosclerosis (see Chapter Three). The Physicians' Health Study found that men with low blood levels of folic acid and B_6 tend to have an increased risk of heart attacks. Looking at the other side of the coin, the Health Professionals Study found that a high consumption of folic acid and B_6 can help, reducing the risk of heart attack by 29 and 23 percent respectively. Folic acid may also reduce the risk of colon cancer, and the Health Professionals Study found that a high intake of vitamin-rich cruciferous (cabbage family) vegetables appears to reduce the risk of bladder cancer. It is a strong argument for an abundant consumption of vegetables, fruits, and fortified cereals and other whole grain products. It is also a good argument for multivitamins (see Chapter Six).

Antioxidants

Vitamin E, vitamin C, and vitamin A and the carotenoids are antioxidant vitamins. Diets high in these vitamins have been linked to a decreased risk of various cancers. The evidence is strongest for cancers of the lung, mouth, larynx (voice box), esophagus (food pipe), stomach, colon, and bladder. In general, individuals eating the smallest amounts of fruits and vegetables develop about twice as many malignancies as those who consume the largest quantities. Deep green and yellow-orange fruits and vegetables and cruciferous vegetables have been particularly helpful. For example, the Health Professionals Study found that men who eat lots of tomatoes, particularly cooked tomatoes, had a lowered risk of prostate cancer, possibly because tomatoes provide *lycopene,* one of the most potent antioxidants in the carotenoid family (see Chapter Twelve). Similarly, the study has demonstrated that men with a high intake of carotenoids had a substantially lower risk of lung cancer. Vitamin-rich foods, particularly broccoli and spinach, were also linked to a lower risk of cataracts. But while foods rich in antioxidant vitamins appear to protect against cancer, supplements have been disappointing. Vitamin E's potential ability to reduce the risk of prostate cancer may be an exception, at least in smokers (see Chapters Six and Twelve); the Health Professionals Study also reported that vitamin E may reduce a man's risk of bladder cancer (see Chapter Thirteen).

Early research held out great hope that antioxidants might reduce the risk of atherosclerosis. The Health Professionals Study helped raise those hopes when it reported that a high intake of vitamin E, mostly from supplements, appeared to reduce the risk of heart disease—but that antioxidants did not protect against stroke. More recently, however, three major studies reported no cardiac benefit from vitamin E supplements. As for beta-carotene, the Physicians' Health Study found no cardiac protection from supplements (see Chapter Six) and two other major studies suggested that beta-carotene might do more harm than good, at least in smokers.

VITAMIN D

Since it was first discovered about eighty years ago, vitamin D has been firmly enshrined as one of the four fat-soluble vitamins. Strictly speaking, however, vitamin D is not actually a vitamin. Vitamins are defined as organic chemicals that must be obtained from dietary sources because they are not produced by the body itself. Although only tiny amounts are needed, a healthy metabolism depends on getting these essential substances on a regular basis. Vitamin D is essential for health, and only minuscule amounts are required. In these respects it sure sounds like a vitamin—but unlike other vitamins, vitamin D is virtually absent from man's natural foods other than fish. Instead, it is produced right in the human body. But as habits change, people can no longer rely on their bodies to produce vitamin D in the old-fashioned way, by the action of sunlight on the skin. Instead, new evidence underlines the importance of getting vitamin D from artificially fortified foods and pills.

Vitamin D's major role is to keep bones healthy. It acts by increasing the intestinal absorption of calcium; without enough vitamin D, the body cannot absorb the calcium it needs. Over time, that can lead to *osteoporosis*, the "thin bone" disease caused by low bone-calcium levels.

If vitamin D did nothing beyond promoting calcium absorption, it would still be essential for health. But researchers have begun to suspect that vitamin D may do even more. That is because many of the body's tissues contain pro-

Table 4.8: THE VITAMINS

Vitamin	Functions	Deficiency Effects	Toxic Effects	Sources	Dietary Reference Intake for Adult Men	Daily Upper Limit Considered Safe for Adult Men
A (retinol, retinoic acid)	Vision, healthy skin; possible protection against skin cancers and atherosclerosis	Night blindness; increased susceptibility to infection	Birth defects, brain swelling, liver damage; yellowish skin discoloration by carotenoids	Liver, dairy products, eggs; dark-green and yellow-orange vegetables (carotenoids)	900 mcg	3,000 mcg
B_1 (thiamin)	Metabolism of carbohydrates, alcohol, and amino acids	Heart failure, mental abnormalities	None	Grains, legumes, nuts, poultry, meat	1.2 mg	ND
B_2 (riboflavin)	Cellular metabolism	Inflammation of skin and mouth; anemia	None	Grains, dairy products, meat, eggs, dark-green vegetables	1.3 mg	ND
B_3 (niacin, nicotinic acid)	Metabolism; in high doses, reduces LDL cholesterol and increases HDL cholesterol	Pellagra	Flushing, headaches, itching, liver damage, diabetes, and gout	Meat, poultry, fish, grains, peanuts, synthesized from tryptophan in foods	16 mg	35 mg
B_6 (pyridoxine)	Red blood cell production; nerve function; reduces blood homocysteine levels	Anemia, skin inflammation	Nerve damage	Meat, poultry, fish, grains, soybeans, bananas, nuts	19–50 yr, 1.3 mg; above 50 yr, 1.7 mg	100 mg

B_{12} (cobalamin)	Blood cell production; nerve function; reduces blood homocystein levels	Anemia, nerve damage	None	Meat (especially liver), poultry, fish, dairy products	2.4 mcg	ND
Folic acid	DNA synthesis (with B_{12}); reduces blood homocysteine	Anemia, birth defects	None	Vegetables, legumes, grains, fruit, poultry, meat	400 mcg	1,000 mcg
Biotin	Metabolic processes	Rare	None	Many foods	30–100 mcg	ND
Pantothenic acid	Metabolic processes	Rare	None	Many foods	5 mg	ND
C (ascorbic acid)	Production of collagen (a protein in tissue); possible protection against certain tumors	Scurvy	Kidney stones; diarrhea	Fruits, green vegetables, potatoes, cereals	90 mg	2,000 mg
D (calciferol)	Intestinal calcium absorption	Rickets	High blood calcium	Fortified dairy products, fatty fish, egg yolks, liver	Below 50 yrs, 200 IU; 51–70 yrs, 400 IU; above 70 yrs, 600 IU	2,000 IU
E (α-tocopherol)	Reduces peroxidation of fatty acids: possible protection against atherosclerosis and cancer	Rare	Antagonism of vitamin K, possible headaches	Vegetable oils, wheat germ, nuts, broccoli	15 mg	1,000 mg
K	Synthesis of clotting factors VII, IX, X, and possibly V	Bleeding	None	Leafy green vegetables (K_1), intestinal bacteria (K_2)	120 mcg	ND

HDL—high-density lipoprotein cholesterol, LDL—low-density lipoprotein cholesterol, IU—international units, mg—milligrams, mcg—micrograms, ND—not determined teins that bind vitamin D. In the intestines, the binding proteins capture vitamin D to trigger calcium absorption, but their role in the prostate, heart, muscles, endocrine glands, and other tissues is unknown. Still, when vitamin D is added to human cells being grown in the laboratory, it promotes normal cell maturation and reduces abnormal cell multiplication. That is what led doctors to wonder if vitamin D may have a role in preventing cancer. In particular, the Health Professionals Study raises the possibility that it may help reduce the risk of prostate cancer, at least in men who consume large amounts of calcium (see Calcium, page 121).

Until recently, the Dietary Reference Intake of vitamin D was just 200 International Units (IU). That modest amount is still considered adequate for people younger than fifty, but for fifty-one to seventy-year-olds, the adequate daily amount is now pegged at 400 IU, and for older people it is 600 IU. Some experts go even further, recommending 800 IU per day, especially for older individuals and for those with chronic illnesses, although large amounts can raise blood calcium to dangerous levels that may produce constipation, kidney stones, grogginess, and even death; however, doses below 2,000 IU per day are unlikely to be harmful.

The only meaningful dietary sources of vitamin D are milk and fish. Government regulations require manufacturers to add vitamin D to milk. Each eight-ounce serving should contain 100 IU, but many brands contain less. Even with full fortification, you would have to drink a quart of milk to get 400 IU of vitamin D. Although fish also provides vitamin D, you would have to eat five ounces of salmon, seven ounces of halibut, thirty ounces of cod, or nearly two cans of tuna to get 400 IU.

Although it is possible to get enough vitamin D from your diet, it is quite difficult. Exposure to sunlight could make up the difference, but since it can also lead to deadly *melanoma* and other skin cancers, it is not the way to go. All in all, vitamin D is a part of the case for a daily multivitamin (see Chapter Six).

Minerals

Minerals are chemically the simplest of nutrients, but their roles in the body's metabolism are complex. At least sixteen minerals are essential for health; ten are classified as trace elements because only tiny amounts are required (see Table 4.9). Although all sixteen essential minerals are important for health, I will discuss only the five of particular interest to men.

Table 4.9: ESSENTIAL MINERALS AND TRACE ELEMENTS

MINERALS AND ELEMENTS	DRI/ESADDI FOR HEALTHY ADULT MEN
Minerals	
calcium	1,000 mg below age 50, 1,200 mg above age 50
phosphorus	700 mg
magnesium	420 mg
sodium	1,100–3,300 mg
potassium	1,875–5,625 mg
chloride	1,700–5,100 mg
Trace Elements	
iron	8 mg
zinc	11 mg
iodine	150 mg
copper	900 mcg
manganese	2.3 mg
fluoride	4.0 mg
chromium	Age 19–50: 35 mcg Over age 50: 30 mcg
molybdenum	45 mcg
selenium	55 mcg
cobalt	Required in small amount as a component of vitamin B_{12}

DRI—dietary reference intake; ESADDI—estimated safe and adequate dietary intake; mg—milligrams; mcg—micrograms.

SODIUM

Sodium is every bit as controversial as vitamins. In this case though, the controversy is even more intense in the scientific community than in the general public. That is because sodium is the key mineral in salt, and scientists are divided about the role of salt in causing high blood pressure. It is an example of the complexity of human biology, the intricacy of the human diet, and the need for more research to sort things out. It is also an example of the way that headline-hungry reporters can exaggerate the debate, and the way commercial interests, led by the prepared foods industry, can rub salt in the wounds of scientific uncertainty.

The controversy boils down to this: Over the past thirty years, a series of international observational studies has linked salt consumption with high blood pressure, particularly in older people. In addition, a number of clinical trials have shown that reducing salt consumption can lower blood pressure, particularly in hypertensive individuals. For example, the 2001 report of The Dietary Approaches to Stop Hypertension (DASH) research group headed by Dr. Frank Sachs of Harvard demonstrates that reducing dietary sodium can lower nearly everyone's blood pressure. Even people adhering to the current recommendations for a moderate sodium intake of 2,400 milligrams a day benefited from a further reduction to 1,500 milligrams a day. At the same time, though, other studies have exonerated sodium, showing only a small effect on blood pressure and/or suggesting that other minerals such as potassium and calcium, or other nutrients, such as fruits, vegetables, and fiber, are more important. To make matters even more confusing, scientists who review the same data on salt and blood pressure come up with opposite conclusions. As the old proverb explains, two people can sleep in the same bed but have different dreams.

The Harvard men's health studies cannot resolve the controversy. The Health Professionals Study found no relationship between dietary sodium and blood pressure over a four-year period. Perhaps the most important perspective comes from Dr. Charles Hennekens. When he was directing the Physicians' Health Study, Dr. Hennekens observed, "The problem with the field is that people have chosen sides. What we ought to do is let the science drive the system rather than opinion."

Clearly more research is needed. A large randomized clinical trial of varying levels of sodium intake would be particularly helpful, though difficult. But until new data is available you should take several points into account as you decide how much sodium is right for you.

1. If you have congestive heart failure, certain liver or kidney diseases, or other conditions that cause fluid retention, you must restrict your sodium consumption, and you will need your doctor's help to plan your diet.

2. If you are healthy and have an excellent blood pressure (see Table 3.5), you do not have to worry about sodium. But if your blood pressure is high, or even high normal, you should think about salt, particularly if you find your pressure creeping up as you grow older.

3. Some people are clearly very sensitive to sodium and can reduce their blood pressure significantly by reducing their salt consumption. Other people are less sensitive, but can improve their blood pressure with other dietary adjustments (increased potassium, calcium, and fiber from fruits, vegetables, and nonfat dairy products) and lifestyle changes (exercise, weight control, prudent alcohol use, and stress control).

4. The average American diet contains much, much more sodium than is necessary. The average person gets more than 4,000 mg of sodium a day, or about the amount in two teaspoons of table salt; that is more than four times the amount the body needs to keep its fluids in balance.

5. Salt is not part of natural human diet. Only small amounts are present in fresh foods, but large amounts are added to processed foods. The average American man gets only 10 percent of his dietary sodium from the natural content of his foods; another 15 percent tumbles from the salt shaker, while 75 percent is added to food during the commercial manufacturing process.

6. Salt is an acquired taste—and, over time, men can reacquire a natural taste for low-sodium foods. Slow change is the key; sodium-free seasonings such as pepper, lemon juice, and various herbs can help.

Taking all the data about sodium into account, the American Heart Association and the Food and Drug Administration suggest a target intake of 2,400 milligrams a day (about one and a quarter teaspoons of table salt); the National Academy of Sciences proposes a 2,000 milligrams maximum. Unless your blood pressure is optimal, and stays that way as you age, you should consider adjusting your diet to meet (or beat) these goals. In most cases, that will mean cutting down on salted snack foods, canned juices, canned and dried soups, prepared condiments, relishes, and sauces, soy and teriyaki sauces, canned, processed, smoked and cured meats and fish, frozen dinners, packaged mixes for sauces and baked goods, cheese, and of course, table salt.

A reduced sodium diet may seem drastic, but it is not. In fact, it is a return to the basics. Low-salt diets tend to be high in vitamin-and-fiber-rich fruits and vegetables, but low in animal fat. In the last analysis, then, if you follow the essentials of a healthful diet you can forget about the sodium controversy; in most cases, your salt intake will take care of itself.

POTASSIUM

In many aspects, potassium is the antithesis of sodium. The two minerals concentrate in different body compartments. Potassium is found in the fluids within cells, sodium in the fluids that bathes cells from the outside. Potassium is found in fresh produce, sodium in processed foods. Diets high in potassium are generally associated with a low blood pressure, while high sodium diets are sometimes associated with hypertension.

In 1992, the Health Professionals Study found that men who consume large amounts of potassium have lower blood pressures than men on low potassium diets, particularly if they also eat lots of fiber-rich foods. It is encouraging news from an observational study, and a 1997 clinical trial adds to the evidence that diet can help control blood pressure. In the Dietary Approaches to Stop Hypertension (DASH) trial, a diet high in fruits, vegetables, and low-fat dairy products produced a significant reduction in blood pressure in just eight weeks. The original DASH diet was high on potassium (4,700 milligrams a day) and fiber (31 grams a day), moderate in sodium (3,000 milligrams a day) and calcium (1,240 milligrams a day), and low in fat (27 percent of total calories). In 1999, the Health Professionals Study added to the evidence, reporting that a diet high in fruits and vegetables is associated with a reduced risk of ischemic strokes, and in 2001 it linked a fruit-and-vegetable-rich diet to a reduced risk of coronary artery disease.

The only controversy about potassium is whether supplements help with blood pressure control. At present, they are routinely recommended only for people taking diuretics, medications that often lower blood potassium levels as they control blood pressure by flushing sodium into the urine.

Unless you have kidney disease or certain other conditions that may raise your blood potassium levels, you should dash to the market to stock up on foods high in potassium and fiber; citrus fruits, dates, bananas, raisins, beets, beans, potatoes, broccoli, squash, spinach, and tomatoes are examples.

IRON

In 1992, Finnish scientists shocked cardiologists when they reported that a high intake of iron more than doubled the risk of heart attacks in men. It was a completely unexpected observation. But in 1994, the Health Professionals Study reported that dietary iron does not appear to be a cardiac risk factor in American men, except, perhaps, if the iron comes from red meat. It was reassuring news and in 2001 the study provided confirmation when it found that donating blood, which lowers a person's iron levels, does not promote any protection against heart disease. The Physicians' Health Study agreed, when it reported that a man's iron stores are not related to his risk of heart attack. Three other studies of Americans support the two Harvard studies.

Men do not need much iron (see Table 4.9) and excessive amounts can be harmful, not by causing heart attacks, but by aggravating the effects of *hemochromatosis,* a hereditary disorder in which excess iron builds up in tissues. Although hemochromatosis may turn out to be more common than once thought, most men really do not have to worry about their dietary iron.

CALCIUM

You may be hoping for a break here: a short section, at long last, on a noncontroversial element. Indeed, calcium is on nearly everyone's "good" list, which is why the newest guidelines recommend that men take in 1,000 milligrams a day until age fifty and 1,200 milligrams a day thereafter. Without challenging these guidelines, though, the Health Professionals Study has raised several important questions about calcium.

1. *Calcium and Bones.* Everyone "knows" that calcium builds strong bones and so it does—at least in women. To date, though, very few studies have been conducted in men, whose bones are protected by testosterone, which declines only gradually with advancing age. When the Health Professionals Study examined calcium intake in men, it could not detect a protective effect on fractures. At the same time, however, the study could not exclude slight to modest benefit, and a 1999 Tufts University study of 176 elderly men did report benefit from daily supplements of calcium (500 mg) and vitamin D (700 IU).
2. *Calcium and Kidney Stones.* Most kidney stones are made of calcium (see Chapter Thirteen). To prevent stones—particularly in people who had already experienced the excruciating pain of a stone—doctors usually advised a sharp reduction in dietary calcium. Then along came the 1993 report of the Health Professionals Study. It showed that a high intake of dietary calcium appears to *decrease* the risk of painful

kidney stones. A high intake of potassium and fluids also seem to decrease risk, while a high intake of animal protein predisposes men to stone formation.

3. *Calcium and Blood Pressure.* Nobody in the know even thinks they have the answer here, but the best evidence suggests that a high intake of calcium from foods, but not supplements, reduces the risk of hypertension. The Health Professionals Study of diet and blood pressure also suggests that calcium can help lower blood pressure, though the protective effect of calcium is not as strong as potassium or fiber.

4. *Calcium and Colon Cancer.* It is another area of conflicting research. Various test-tube and animal experiments suggest that calcium may reduce the risk of colon cancer. Some human studies agree, others do not. The Health Professionals Study found no protection from a high intake of calcium, vitamin D, or dairy foods, but it could not exclude a modest benefit.

5. *Calcium and Prostate Cancer.* There had been no controversy here, because scientists had not given it much thought. A 1998 report from the Health Professionals Study changed that. The study found that a high intake of calcium, whether from foods or supplements, was linked to an increased risk of advanced prostate cancer. The risk was greatest in men consuming very large amounts of calcium, above 2,000 milligrams per day. The study also provided some good news: a high intake of *fructose* (fruit sugar) was associated with a reduced risk of prostate cancer. The study also confirmed previous observations that dietary fat, especially animal fat, increases the risk of prostate cancer.

Calcium and fructose have little in common, and neither substance seems to act directly on the prostate. The Harvard scientists speculate, however, that vitamin D explains the apparent associations. High levels of calcium can reduce the body's production of active vitamin D (1, 25 $(OH)_2$ vitamin D, *calciferol*); low levels of fructose can have the same effect, in this case by first lowering blood *phosphate* concentration. According to this hypothesis, then, active vitamin D is protective, and dietary practices that lower it may be harmful.

Both the Physicians' Health Study and a smaller Swedish study echo these concerns about a high calcium intake. In contrast, new Italian research and two recent American studies do not; one U.S. report exonerated calcium supplements and the other cleared dietary calcium.

More research is needed to examine a possible link between calcium, fructose, vitamin D, and prostate cancer. In fact, more research is needed to evaluate the effect of calcium on men's bones. Until new data are available, men should continue to follow current guidelines for healthy eating: reduce dietary fat (especially animal fat), eat plenty of fruits (and vegetables), and get enough vitamin D and calcium (but not too much).

SELENIUM

Because selenium is a trace element that functions as an antioxidant, scientists have wondered if it might help fight heart disease or cancer (see Chapters Six and Twelve). The Physicians' Health Study found no link between selenium and heart disease, but the Health Professionals Study found that men with high selenium levels have a low risk of prostate cancer. Indeed, selenium has antitumor activity in the test tube, and researchers from Arizona have demonstrated that selenium supplements appear to decrease the risk of several major malignancies, including prostate cancer. The mineral is present in vegetables and grains grown in selenium-rich soil. Its concentration varies greatly in different parts of the world. In the United States, selenium levels tend to be highest in soil west of the Mississippi. Fish is also an excellent source of the mineral. It is also present in shellfish, meat, poultry, egg yolks, garlic, and Brazil nuts.

Many experts still believe that food is the best source of selenium and that it is too early to recommend supplements for widespread use. Indeed, our hopes for supplements have often been dashed by medical research. Still, men who are concerned about prostate cancer might reasonably decide to take selenium while awaiting the results of additional research (see Chapters Six and Twelve).

I hope you will consider these guidelines carefully and that you will decide to adopt them. Remember, though, that they are guidelines written on paper, not commandments etched in stone; the fine print is likely to change as doctors learn more about nutrition and health. Remember, too, that they are intended for healthy men; people with medical problems should consult their doctors to develop individualized nutritional plans.

Even if you decide to change your diet, don't try to change everything at once. By age fifty, the average man will have more than 50,000 meals under his belt—to say nothing of all those snacks. It is hard to sweep away a lifetime of

The Best Diet

Men do not dine on polyunsaturated fats, carbohydrates with a low glycemic index, or trace elements—they eat food. Here are twenty guidelines for healthful and enjoyable eating:

1. Eat a variety of foods. Since no single food is perfect, you need a balanced mix of foods to get all the nutrients you need.
2. Eat more vegetable products and fewer animal products.
3. Eat more fresh and homemade foods and fewer processed foods.
4. Eat less fat and cholesterol. Fat should provide 20 to 30 percent of the calories in your diet. Restrict saturated fat to less than one-third of your total fat intake by reducing your consumption of meat, whole dairy products, and the skin of poultry. Limit your intake of trans fatty acids by reducing your consumption of partially hydrogenated vegetable oils found in stick margarine, fried foods, and many commercially baked goods. Favor monounsaturated and omega-3 fats that are found in olive oil, fish, nuts and possibly canola oil. Restrict your cholesterol intake to less than 300 milligrams per day by limiting your intake of egg yolks and other animal products.
5. Eat at least 25 to 30 grams of fiber per day by increasing your consumption of bran cereal, whole grains, vegetables, and fruit. Favor oats, barley, beans, and other sources of soluble fiber. Consider fiber supplements if you cannot obtain enough fiber from foods.
6. Eat more complex carbohydrates and less sugar by eating more grain products, starchy vegetables, and pasta. Complex carbohydrates should provide 55 to 65 percent of the calories in your diet. Favor foods with a low glycemic index.
7. Eat protein in moderation. Protein should provide 10 to 15 percent of the calories in your diet. Favor fish, legumes, and skinless poultry as protein sources. Experiment with soy as a protein source.
8. Restrict your sodium intake to less than 2,400 milligrams per day, particularly if your blood pressure is borderline or high, by reducing your use of table salt and processed foods such as canned soup and juices, luncheon meats, condiments, frozen dinners, cheese, tomato sauce, and snack foods.
9. Eat more potassium-rich foods, such as citrus fruits, bananas, and other fruits and vegetables. Eat more calcium-rich foods such as low-fat dairy products, broccoli, spinach, and tofu. Stay alert for new information about calcium and men's health.

10. Eat more grain products, especially whole grain products, aiming for six or more servings per day.
11. Eat more vegetables and legumes, especially deep green and yellow-orange vegetables. Aim for at least three to five servings of vegetables each day.
12. Eat more fruits, aiming for at least two to four servings each day.
13. Eat more fish, aiming for at least two 4-ounce servings per week.
14. If you choose to eat red meats, reduce your intake to about two 4-ounce servings per week. Avoid "prime" and other fatty meats, processed meats, and liver.
15. Eat chicken and turkey in moderation, always removing the skin.
16. Eat eggs sparingly; aim for an average of no more than one egg yolk per day, including those used in cooking and baking. Use egg substitutes whenever possible.
17. Use vegetable oils in moderation, favoring olive oil. Reduce your intake of partially hydrogenated vegetable oils, palm oil, coconut milk, and cocoa butter.
18. If you can use alcohol safely and choose to drink, drink sparingly. Do not average more than two drinks per day, and never drive or operate machinery after drinking.
19. Adjust your caloric intake and exercise level to maintain a desirable body weight. If you need to lose weight, aim for gradual weight loss by reducing your intake of calories and fat and increasing your aerobic exercise.
20. Avoid fad diets and extreme or unconventional nutritional schemes. If it is too good to be true, it's not true.

habits, so change slowly. Enlist the support and cooperation of your family and friends. Don't think of good nutrition as a punishment, but as an opportunity to explore new foods and recipes. Experiment creatively. Give your tastes time to change, and don't get down on yourself if you slip up from time to time. It is not the first day that counts—it is the lifetime of days that lie ahead.

As you plan your diet, remember to take your personal preferences into account. If roast beef is your favorite food, it is okay to eat it—but try to make it a Sunday treat instead of a daily staple. The choices are yours. If you take care of yourself you will have plenty of "wiggle room" to indulge your passions. And here is some more good news from the Harvard men's health studies: If you are a coffee lover, you will be glad to know that the Health Professionals Study found no link between coffee and heart attacks or strokes. In fact, it reported that drinking coffee appears to reduce a man's risk of painful gall bladder attacks and of Parkinson's disease. More good news: The Alumni Study reported that men who eat candy live almost a year longer than men who do not indulge (but only if their candy consumption is modest). Life is sweet when you are healthy.

The dietary plan outlined here is based on data from the Harvard men's health studies and many other sources. It is scientifically rational. But does it really work? Researchers in Europe think so; they recently reported a study of 3,045 men living in Italy, Finland, and the Netherlands.

When the study started in 1970, all the men were between fifty and seventy years of age. At that time, each volunteer provided a history of his tobacco and alcohol use, as well as detailed dietary information that allowed the investigators to estimate his food consumption for a six to twelve month period. Each man's diet was graded for its healthfulness, and men were followed for twenty years to see if there was any link between eating well and living long.

What diet was considered healthful? The study evaluated nine nutritional standards:

FOOD OR NUTRIENT	HEALTHY STANDARD (DAILY INTAKE)
Cholesterol	Less than 300 mg
Saturated fat	Less than 10 percent of calories
Polyunsaturated fat	3–7 percent of calories
Dietary fiber	27–40 grams
Simple carbohydrates	Less than 10 percent of calories
Complex carbohydrates	50–70 percent of calories
Protein	10–15 percent of calories
Fruits and vegetables	More than 400 grams
Legumes, nuts, and seeds	More than 30 grams

Although these benchmarks were developed in Europe more than twenty years ago, they are remarkably similar to the diet that is considered best for Americans today: a low intake of cholesterol, saturated fat, and simple sugars, a moderate amount of protein, and a high intake of dietary fiber, complex carbohydrates, fruits, and vegetables. Unfortunately, the researchers did not collect data about table salt, so there was no way to determine if their subjects complied with the healthful limit of 2,400 milligrams of sodium per day.

Did healthful eating pay off? Since all the men were fifty to seventy years old at the start of the study, it is no surprise that 59 percent died during the twenty years of observation. The men's dietary patterns were quite different in the three countries studied, but in all three, the men with the best diets lived the longest, even after accounting for the health impact of tobacco and alcohol. Good nutrition was particularly effective in reducing the risk of dying from heart disease and cancer, the two most common killers of American men today. All in all, the men with the most healthful diets were 13 percent less likely to die during the twenty years of the study than were the men with the worst diets.

Closer to home, two new reports from the Health Professionals Study also demonstrate that a healthful diet pays big dividends. Like the European researchers of the late twentieth century, the Harvard scientists of the early twenty-first evaluated dietary patterns rather than individual nutrients. They found that men who followed a "prudent pattern," characterized by a high intake of vegetables, fruits, legumes, whole grains, fish, and poultry had a much lower risk of heart disease and diabetes than men who followed a "Western pattern," characterized by a high intake of red meat, processed meat, refined grains, sweets and desserts, French fries, and high-fat dairy products. It is an important message, but it has not been heard in the United States. At present, whole grains contribute only 1 percent of the country's energy intake, while refined grains account for 22 percent. Similarly, only 3 percent of Americans above the age of two consume three or more servings of vegetables a day (even counting fries as veggies!), while just 28 percent consume at least three portions of fruit a day.

Your mother was right: You should watch what you eat. It may not be startling, but it is very good to know that healthful eating really does work.

A good diet is necessary for good health, but not altogether sufficient to prevent disease. In the next chapter, we will turn to nutrition's natural partner, exercise, and in the chapter that follows, I will discuss the possible benefits and drawbacks of nutritional supplements.

CHAPTER FIVE

The Answers: Exercise

EXERCISE AND DIET are the hand and glove of healthful living; more than 2,400 years ago, Hippocrates explained that "eating alone will not keep a man well, he must also take exercise. For food and exercise, while possessing opposite qualities, yet work together to produce health." The great Greek physician was the founder of medicine, and his advice should be the foundation of every man's program for health.

The Harvard Alumni Study has had a particularly important role in demonstrating the health benefits of regular exercise. By now, the evidence is incontrovertible, yet only 23 percent of American adults meet the Surgeon General's recommended standard of thirty minutes of moderate physical activity, like brisk walking, biking, or gardening, on at least five days each week.

The Effects of Exercise

Exercise puts all parts of the body to work, and it works to promote health by producing improvements in nearly all bodily functions.

The Types of Exercise

In physiologic terms, there are two basic types of exercise:

In *aerobic* or *dynamic* exercise, muscle fibers shorten without a substantial increase in their tension. As fibers shorten, they move joints through their range of motion, propelling you along a trail, through the water, or across the dance floor. Blood vessels widen, reducing their resistance and lowering the blood pressure. But to keep the widened blood vessels full, the heart must pump more blood; the heart rate increases, as does the amount of blood pumped with each beat. The activities that doctors recommend for aerobic conditioning and cardiovascular fitness rely on endurance exercise; examples include walking, jogging, swimming, and biking.

In *resistance* or *static* exercise, muscle fibers do not shorten, but muscle tension increases. As a result, blood vessels narrow, increasing their resistance to the flow of blood. High resistance means higher blood pressure. The heart has to work hard against the increased vascular resistance, but the heart rate does not increase substantially and the heart does not pump much more blood than it does at rest. Although resistance exercise boosts blood pressure, the pressure returns to normal between exercise sessions. Weight lifting neither increases nor decreases a person's chance of developing sustained hypertension. Resistance exercise may do less for the circulation and metabolism than dynamic exercise, but it does much more for the musculoskeletal system, building muscle bulk and strength and increasing bone mineral density, which reduces the risk of osteoporosis and fractures.

EFFECTS ON HEALTH

How do these two types of exercise affect health?

Exercise improves the metabolism. In this respect, dynamic or aerobic exercise is best. When performed regularly, it lowers the LDL ("bad") cholesterol and raises the HDL ("good") cholesterol; it also lowers triglycerides, another blood lipid linked to heart disease risk. More visibly, regular physical activity burns away body fat. The Health Professionals Study is one of the many research efforts that demonstrate that active men are less likely to gain weight than sedentary men.

Endurance exercise improves the way the body's tissues respond to insulin. That results in lower blood insulin levels and lower blood sugar levels. The Physicians' Health Study found that men who exercise at least five times a week are 42 percent less likely to develop diabetes than sedentary men; even once-a-week exercise helps, reducing the risk of diabetes by 36 percent. Similarly, when the Harvard Alumni Study's Dr. Ralph Paffenbarger turned his attention to 5,990 male graduates of the University of Pennsylvania in 1991, he and his colleagues found that for each 500 calories of weekly exercise, men can reduce their risk of diabetes by 6 percent. TV watching is the opposite of exercise, the Health Professionals study agreed in 2001, when it reported that men who spend the most time in front of the tube are nearly three times more likely to develop diabetes than men who watch TV the least. Best of all, regular exercise is most effective in people who need the most help. It reduces the chances of diabetes most dramatically in men who are at high risk for it, meaning those who are overweight, have high blood pressure, or who have a family history of diabetes. Studies from far beyond the Ivy League show that these benefits of physical activity are not confined to the men of Harvard and the University of Pennsylvania.

The hormonal effects of exercise are not confined to insulin. Regular exercise tends to reduce the effects of stress hormones such as adrenaline and cortisone. In women, intense exercise training can affect sex hormones, temporarily interfering with menstrual function and fertility. In men, bursts of exercise boost testosterone levels, but the effect is brief. In fact, very intense exercise training produces an overall lowering of testosterone; a few marathon runners have experienced impaired potency and fertility, but their reproductive function returns to normal when they reduce the intensity of their training.

Exercise lowers blood pressure. Here, too, endurance exercise is best. In the Alumni Study, for example, active men were 26 percent less likely to develop hypertension than sedentary men. As in the case of diabetes, the benefit was greatest for men at highest risk; exercise proved particularly effective in reducing blood pressure in overweight men and in those with hypertensive parents.

Exercise also affects the blood itself. It lowers the clotting protein fibrinogen and reduces clot formation while also boosting the body's ability to dissolve clots. Some highly trained athletes develop "sports anemia," not because they actually have fewer red blood cells but because they have an increased amount of fluid in the circulation.

Exercise strengthens bones. Here, though, resistance exercise is more effective than dynamic exercise. Although most studies have been conducted in women, observations of male athletes indicate that exercise enhances bone calcium content in both sexes, reducing the risk of osteoporosis and fractures. Weight-bearing or resistance exercise is best, but it helps only the bones that are actually stressed by a particular form of exercise.

Both types of exercise strengthen muscles. Aerobic exercise improves muscle endurance; while resistance exercise enhances muscle bulk and power; both can be beneficial for health. The muscular effects of exercise are confined to the specific muscles that are being used; walking will improve muscles in the legs, but not the arms.

The most important muscle in the body is the heart, and it, too, improves with exercise. Here aerobic exercise gets the nod. It improves the efficiency and pumping ability of the heart muscle, enabling it to pump more blood at a slower rate. It is one of the main ways that aerobic training improves physical work capacity, enabling men who are in shape to do much more exercise with much less effort. Aerobic exercise training also improves the way blood vessels function; a benefit that extends to vessels throughout the body, including the all-important coronary arteries.

MENTAL EFFECTS

The mind is not a muscle, but it is certainly vital for health and happiness. Exercise helps dissipate anxiety. It improves self-confidence and mood. It also fights depression. The Alumni Study, for example, found that physically active men had a lower risk of depression than sedentary men. A 1999 study from the University of Illinois suggests that endurance exercise may actually improve cognitive function. The scientists studied 124 healthy but previously sedentary adults between the ages of sixty and seventy-five. Half were assigned to a walking program, the others to a stretching and toning regimen. As expected, at the end of six months the walkers demonstrated improved cardiopulmonary fitness but the stretchers did not. Surprisingly, perhaps, the walkers also improved their scores on a battery of cognitive function tests, but the others did not.

It is an impressive array. Exercise improves cholesterol and blood sugar levels; it decreases body fat; it lowers blood pressure and improves cardiac function; it reduces blood clotting; it strengthens muscles and bones; and it improves emotional status and mental function. All this should add up to fewer heart attacks, better health, and longer life—and it does.

Exercise, Heart Disease, and Longevity

It was big news in 1978, and it is every bit as important in the new millennium as it was then. Although research was beginning to demonstrate the value of exercise as far back as 1953, the 1970s witnessed the first conclusive evidence of benefit—and the Alumni Study was one of the first to show that exercise prolongs life. Even today, it is one of the few studies that tells us how much exercise is best.

As you may recall from Chapter Two, the Alumni Study is an ongoing evaluation of men who entered Harvard College between 1916 and 1950. From the total of some 36,500 alumni, 16,936 were evaluated in 1962, 1966, and 1972. The men provided detailed information about their exercise patterns during college and in subsequent years. They also supplied facts about their height, weight, smoking habits, hypertension, diabetes, and their family histories. With the help of the Harvard Alumni Office (which is notorious for its ability to keep track of graduates, particularly during endowment drives), the researchers were able to follow the subjects over the years, collecting information on the occurrence of heart attacks, high blood pressure, diabetes, obesity, and other health problems. Finally, the scientists examined the death certificates of men who succumbed during the study.

When the results were first published in 1978, they demonstrated clearly the health benefits of exercise. The more men exercised, the lower their risk of heart attack and death; men who exercised enough to burn at least 2,000 calories per week were 39 percent less likely to suffer heart attacks than their sedentary classmates.

Even in its initial report, the Alumni Study provided additional details about exercise and health. Until then, some doctors argued that people exercise because they are healthy, not the other way around. But the study showed that the benefits of physical activity are not explained by genetic endowment or self-selection: men who were varsity athletes in college were no better off than their sedentary peers unless they continued to exercise in subsequent years. The research also showed that people of all ages benefit; men as young as thirty-five and as old as seventy-four were included in the analysis, and all were protected by exercise. And in a follow-up study fifteen years later, the scientists demonstrated that it is never too late to start. Previously sedentary men who did not exercise until after age forty-five clearly benefited, enjoying a 23 percent lower risk of death than their classmates who remained inactive. Substantial benefits were linked to amounts of exercise equivalent to walking for about forty-five minutes a day at a pace of about seventeen minutes per mile. Not surprisingly, the Alumni Study found that other lifestyle changes also helped, even if they did not occur until after age forty-five. Giving up cigarettes, maintaining a normal blood pressure, and avoiding obesity were all associated with less heart disease and longer life.

Which changes matter most? In 1994 the Alumni Study found that sedentary men gained 1.6 years of life expectancy from becoming active, smokers gained 1.8 years from quitting, and men gained 1.1 years from maintaining normal blood pressures. Best of all was a combination of changes; sedentary smokers gained 3.7 years from quitting and becoming active.

The original 1978 report of the Alumni Study also provided important insights into the "dose" of exercise that is best for health. Death rates declined steadily as physical activity increased from 500 to 3,000 calories per week, but at very high levels, the rewards of exercise leveled off in a plateau-like fashion. Figure 5.1 shows a graph from the original publication; based on this information, doctors have concluded that about 2,000 calories of exercise a week would provide optimal benefits for longevity. Finally, although the Alumni Study demonstrated that the total amount of exercise was the main determi-

FIGURE 5.1. BENEFITS OF EXERCISE

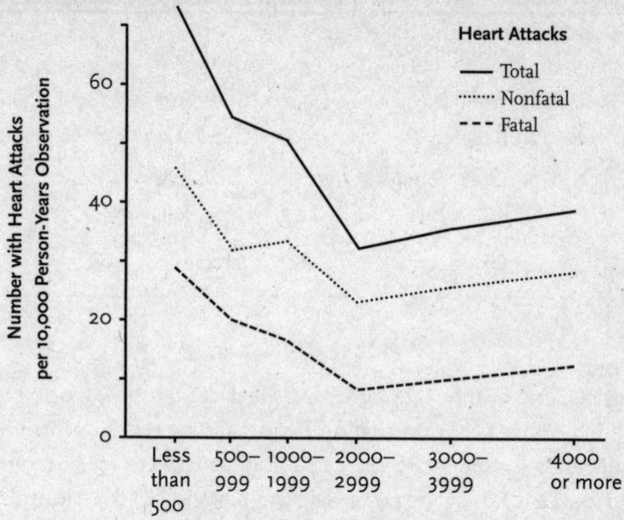

Age-adjusted first heart attack rates, by physical activity index in a 6–10-year followup of Harvard male alumni.

nant of benefit, it also found that vigorous exercise produced greater rewards than less intense activities. Table 5.1 illustrates some ways you can get 2,000 calories of exercise.

Although it established the basics back in 1978, the Alumni Study has continued to track its group of Harvard men, and a series of reports published in 2000 provides some additional insights. For one thing, the study found that the duration of individual exercise sessions is less important than the total amount of exercise performed in a week. That means you can do about as well with three 10-minute sessions a day as with a single thirty-minute work-out. For another thing, the study found that the intensity of exercise does matter. Light exercises such as bowling, boating, and household chores do not reduce mortality rates. Moderate exercises such as golfing, dancing, and gardening do help, but more vigorous activities such as jogging and swimming laps are even more beneficial. Finally, the combined impact of the duration, intensity, and frequency of exercise can be summarized in terms of the amount of exercise energy expended in a week. By using this standard, the study found that exercise that burns a total of 1,000 calories a week can reduce a man's cardiac risk

Table 5.1: TYPICAL DISTANCES REQUIRED TO BURN 2,000 CALORIES:

Swimming	5 miles
Walking	20 miles
Running	20 miles
Cross-Country Skiing	20 miles
Skating	60 miles
Biking	100 miles

by about 20 percent. Without contradicting the data that show 2,000 calories a week is optimal, this new information helps validate the Surgeon General's current guidelines for moderate exercise for all Americans (see Second Opinions, page 138). That's the good news. The bad news is that the Alumni Study's 2000 report also found that lesser amounts of exercise produce much less benefit, particularly in terms of extending life expectancy.

Exercise and Health

The Alumni Study was one of the first to show that exercise prolongs life, and it has been joined by well over 100 studies that agree. The data show that longevity improves chiefly because of exercise's dramatic impact on heart disease. It is no surprise, since physical activity improves major cardiac risk factors such as cholesterol, blood pressure, blood sugar, and body fat.

Although the heart is the major beneficiary of regular exercise, the gains do not stop there. In fact, exercise can also help in a number of other areas:

- *Stroke.* In a 1998 report, the Alumni Study found that exercise reduces the risk of stroke. Benefit was evident in men who exercised to the tune of 1,000–1,999 calories a week. They enjoyed a 24 percent reduction in stroke as compared with sedentary men. As in the case of heart disease, maximum gain required 2,000–3,000 exercise calories a week, which cut the risk of stroke by 46 percent.
- *Cancer.* Exercise protects against the first and third leading causes of death in the United States, heart disease and stroke, but can it also reduce the risk of our second leading killer, cancer?

The answer depends in part on who you ask. It is actually one of the few areas of disagreement among the Harvard men's health studies. The Health Professionals Study found that exercise is linked to a reduced risk of cancer of the pancreas, particularly in men who are overweight. Although pancreatic cancer is deadly, it is relatively rare. But colon cancer is the third most common malignancy in men, and the study demonstrated an impressive benefit of exercise: The most active men had a 47 percent lower risk of developing colon cancer than the men who exercised the least. The Alumni Study agreed; it found that men who burn more than 1,000 calories a week in exercise have only half the risk of colon cancer as men who expend less than 1,000 exercise calories a week. The protection is most evident in men who stay very active over the years, and it is particularly effective in men who are obese. In contrast, the Physicians' Health Study found no link between exercise and colon cancer, either in men who are obese or in those who are lean.

There is no ready explanation for the different results. Fortunately, I do not have to take sides in a disagreement among excellent studies conducted by my Harvard colleagues. That is because the U.S. Surgeon General's report on physical activity and health has made the decision for me. After evaluating nearly thirty studies of exercise and colon cancer, the review concluded that exercise reduces the risk of colon cancer, and that the impact is substantial.

The data for prostate cancer are less conclusive. The Alumni Study reported that very large amounts of exercise may reduce risk, but benefit was restricted to men who burn more than 4,000 calories a week. The Health Professionals Study found no overall protection, but its data raise the possibility that high levels of vigorous activity may reduce the risk of advanced disease. Other research is divided, sometimes reporting benefit from exercise as modest as walking, but sometimes finding no protection at all. After reviewing nineteen studies of exercise and prostate cancer, the Surgeon General could conclude only that further research is needed.

- *Other Diseases:* Exercise helps prevent three major killers: heart disease, stroke, and colon cancer. It also protects against chronic disorders that are major causes of disability, including hypertension, diabetes, obesity, and fractures from osteoporosis. Regular exercise helps counter depression and anxiety, and two 2001 studies suggest it may do even more for the mind, reducing the risk of Alzheimer's disease and other forms of cognitive impairment by up to 50 percent (see Chapter Eight). If that's not enough to get you moving, new results from the Health Professionals Study suggest that exercise also helps with some minor ailments—minor, that is, unless they strike you. The study found that exercise reduces the risk of painful gallbladder attacks and of bothersome urinary symptoms of *benign prostatic hyperplasia,* or BPH (see Chapter Eleven). The study also reports that regular exercise protects men against erectile dysfunction (see Chapter Ten). Thirty minutes of daily exercise reduces the risk of impotence by an impressive 41 percent. It is more good news about exercise and health.

- *Aging*. Exercise will not turn back the clock, but it really can slow its tick. Consider the bodily changes that occur with advancing years: blood pressure, cholesterol, blood sugar, and body fat all increase. Muscle mass and bone calcium decrease. The heart's pumping capacity decreases, and the nervous system's reflexes slow. Every one of these changes can be duplicated by prolonged bed rest, and every one can be reversed by regular exercise. Many of the disabilities that occur with advancing years are not the product of aging itself, but of disease. The poet John Gay got it right some 300 years ago: "Exercise thy lasting youth defends." If you keep your body active, you will help it stay young. You will do even better if you add a good diet to your anti-aging program. As the Roman poet Cicero explained: "Exercise and temperance will preserve something of thy youthful vigor, even into old age."

The Fitness Revolution

Along with investigations by Dr. Kenneth Cooper's Aerobic Institute in Dallas and other research of the 1970s and 1980s, the Alumni Study helped establish a gold standard for exercise. It was, and is, a high benchmark, calling for three to four hours of moderate to vigorous exercise each week. The aerobics revolution was underway.

The doctrine of aerobics is based on the observation that cardiovascular function improves most when large muscle groups are used in a rhythmic, repetitive fashion for prolonged periods of time. The theory of aerobics emphasizes the importance of elevating the heart rate to 70 to 85 percent of maximum, then maintaining that pace for twenty to sixty minutes or more. The practice of aerobics calls for three to five sessions a week; each workout consists of twenty to sixty minutes of aerobic-intensity exercise preceded by a five to ten minute warm-up and followed by a five to ten minute cool-down.

How can you tell if you are exercising in the aerobic range? The simplest way is to set a "talking pace." Work hard enough so that you will break into a sweat and breathe a bit faster, but not so hard that you are out of breath and unable to talk to a companion (real or imaginary). Even better, check your heart rate to see if you are in range. It is the best way to gauge the intensity of exercise.

The first step is to learn how to take your pulse. You can use the carotid artery in your neck or the radial artery in your wrist. Practice while you are resting comfortably; because your heart rate will be slower at rest, it will be easier to take your pulse. After you have mastered the technique, begin checking your pulse during exercise. Count the beats during ten seconds, then multiply by six to find your heart rate.

Once you know how to count your heart rate, you can adjust your pace to keep your heart rate in the target range of 70 to 85 percent of maximum. If you have had a stress test, you will have been told your maximum rate and can determine your target range with precision. Stress tests are important for people with known or suspected heart disease or major cardiac risk factors, but they are not necessary for most other people.

Fortunately, even without a stress test you can use your age to calculate your maximum rate. For more than three decades, doctors have relied on a formula designed by Doctors William Haskell and Samuel Fox. After reviewing the results of ten earlier exercise studies, they noticed that the maximum heart rate declines in a predictable fashion as people age. When they constructed a graph comparing maximum heart rate with age, they came up with a simple equation to explain the relationship:

Maximum Heart Rate = 220 – (age in years).

The formula has been so useful that it has been applied to virtually all healthy men and women without a critical reappraisal—until now. When a team of Colorado scientists reviewed 351 publications that reported the results of exercise tests on 18,712 subjects of all ages and both sexes, they found that the old formula overestimates the actual maximum heart rate in young adults but underestimates the maximum heart rate in people above forty-five. Based on this analysis, the researchers devised a new formula, and then validated it by testing it on 514 men and women between the ages of eighteen and eighty-one. Although the new formula involves a bit more math than the original equation, it appears to be more accurate:

$$\text{Maximum Heart Rate} = 208 - 0.7 \times (\text{age in years}).$$

You can use either the old formula or the new equation to estimate your maximum heart rate. To make it easier, Table 5.2 compares the two and gives you training targets for each.

If you are just getting started, aim for the low end of your target range. If that seems tough, exercise at 50 to 60 percent of maximum. You will still get plenty of help for your health and you'll be able to build up gradually as you get in shape.

You can choose among many activities to exercise in the aerobic range; brisk walking, jogging, swimming, stair climbing, aerobic dance, cross-country skiing, rowing, and singles racquet sports are examples. Best of all is a mixed program; variety will keep your muscles vigorous and your mind fresh. Remember to warm up before you exercise and to cool down afterward; walking, stretching, and calisthenics are ideal. Remember, too, to get a medical checkup before you start a serious exercise program (see Epilogue). Men with health problems require individualized exercise guidelines from their doctors, and men with heart disease may need to begin their program under direct medical supervision.

Second Opinions

In their rush to get Americans into shape, doctors nearly overlooked some fine print in the major exercise reports of the 1970s and 1980s. For example, while the Alumni Study demonstrated maximal benefit from 2,000 to 3,000 calories of exercise per week, it also documented important gains for 1,000 calories a week. While it reported best results from vigorous sports, it also recorded real improvements from climbing stairs and other daily activities. Similarly, the Cooper Institute found that while three or more hours of weekly exercise produced optimal fitness and health, the first hour was the most important of all. Despite years of derision from sports physiologists and marathoners, it turns out that moderate exercise is good for health—very good, in fact.

Table 5.2: YOUR TARGET HEART RATE FOR AEROBIC EXERCISE: COMPARING THE FORMULAS

Age	Maximum Heart Rate		Target Range (Beats per minute) Low (70% max)		Target Range (Beats per minute) High (85% max)		10-Second Pulse Count Low		10-Second Pulse Count High	
	Old Formula	**New Formula**	Old Formula	**New Formula**	Old Formula	**New Formula**	Old Formula	**New Formula**	Old Formula	**New Formula**
20	200	**194**	140	**136**	170	**165**	23	**23**	28	**28**
25	200	**191**	140	**134**	170	**162**	23	**22**	28	**27**
30	194	**187**	136	**131**	165	**159**	22	**22**	27	**27**
35	188	**184**	132	**129**	160	**156**	22	**21**	26	**26**
40	182	**180**	128	**126**	155	**153**	21	**21**	26	**26**
45	176	**177**	124	**124**	150	**150**	20	**21**	25	**25**
50	171	**173**	119	**121**	145	**147**	20	**20**	24	**25**
55	165	**170**	115	**119**	140	**145**	19	**20**	23	**24**
60	159	**166**	111	**116**	135	**141**	18	**19**	23	**24**
65	153	**163**	107	**114**	130	**139**	17	**19**	22	**23**

WALKING TO HEALTH

In the seventies and eighties, Americans were told to run; in the nineties, they were asked to walk. Walking can be quite an intense aerobic activity; a glance at race walkers proves the point. But even at a more relaxed pace, walking has enormous benefits. For longevity and health, the distance seems more important than the pace, and it does not take heroic distances to get real benefit. In 1993, fifteen years after its original report, the Alumni Study demonstrated that men who walk just 1.3 miles a day have a 22 percent lower rate of death than those who walk less than 0.4 miles a day. A 1996 study from Washington State provided confirmation. Researchers evaluated 1,645 men and women over age sixty-five who were free of heart disease and serious disability at the start of the investigation. After four years, people who walked at least four hours a week enjoyed a 31 percent lower risk of hospitalization for heart disease and a 27 percent lower rate of death than people who walked less than one hour a week. Similarly, a twelve-year study of 707 retired men in Hawaii found that the death rate of men who walked at least two miles a day was more than 50 percent lower than the death rate of men who walked less than one mile a day. Men who walked an intermediate distance of one to two miles a day had an intermediate risk. Although walking was the main focus of the investigation, other forms of moderate exercise were also protective. As in the other studies, the benefits of physical activity held up even after age, diet, blood pressure, diabetes, and cholesterol were taken into account.

Walking is excellent for health; it is natural, convenient, easy, and inexpensive, yet it reduces substantially the risk of heart disease and death. But for all its advantages, walking is not unique. In fact, other daily activities can have excellent effects. Among Harvard alumni, climbing fifty-five flights of stairs a week reduced the rate of death by 25 percent, even more than the 22 percent reduction associated with walking more than nine miles a week. Participating in moderately intensive sports activity was even more helpful. It was linked to a 37 percent lower rate of death, and playing moderate sports for more than three hours a week was associated with a 50 percent lower death rate.

The Benefits of Daily Activity

Although moderately intense sports and other vigorous workouts may have a statistical edge over walking and other activities of daily life, it is hard to get most people to participate in structured exercise. But five studies published between 1999 and 2001 show that even without formal workouts, lifestyle activities work very well.

Scientists at the Cooper Institute for Aerobics Research conducted the first trial. They studied 235 healthy but sedentary individuals over a two-year span. Half the participants were placed on a structured exercise program stressing aerobic-intensity exercise for twenty to sixty minutes three to five times a week. Instead of this traditional type of regimen, the other people were encouraged to accumulate at least thirty minutes of moderate intensity physical activity on most, or preferably all, days of the week. At the end of the study, both groups improved, and they achieved similar reductions in their blood pressures and body fat and similar improvements in their cardiopulmonary fitness.

A smaller, briefer study of forty obese women found much the same thing: in conjunction with a 1,200 calorie low-fat diet, both structured aerobic exercise and moderate lifestyle activity produced similar reductions in body weight and blood cholesterol levels.

Another 1999 study took a different approach. It examined the risk of sudden death in King County, Washington, in relation to the amount of exercise performed during an average week. The results provide an impressive endorsement for daily activity. In comparison with sedentary individuals, people who gardened for at least one hour a week had a 66 percent lower rate of death, and people who walked at least an hour a week had a 73 percent lower death rate. The results held up even after age, smoking, diabetes, high blood pressure, chronic illness, and educational levels were taken into account. As in the other studies, benefits of daily activity were at least as good as high intensity exercise, which was associated with a 66 percent reduction in the risk of sudden death.

The most recent endorsements of moderate exercise came from Harvard, but were investigations of women, not men. Still, men should note the results: a study of 72,448 nurses found that walking for three hours a week reduced the risk of heart attacks by about one-third, or exactly as much as one-and-a-half hours of intense exercise. A study of 39,372 professional women was even more optimistic, reporting that walking for just an hour a week cut the risk of heart attack in half. Women who increased their weekly mileage enjoyed extra benefits, but women who accelerated their pace did not.

GUIDELINES FOR MODERATE EXERCISE

It's one of the few things that has gotten easier: Instead of counting your pulse and working up a sweat for two to four hours a week, all you have to do is to accumulate at least thirty minutes of moderate physical activity a day. But to get best results, you have to do it every day, or nearly every day.

The U.S. Surgeon General, The Centers for Disease Control and Prevention, The National Institutes of Health, and The American College of Sports Medicine all agree on the basic theme. The goal is to burn at least 150 calories a day with exercise. You can do it in less than 30 minutes by exercising more intensely, but it will take longer if your activity is less demanding. The list on page 142 gives some examples of physical activities that consume about 150 calories.

Exercising Your Options

Will the new guidelines make pulse counting obsolete and put gyms and health clubs out of business? Not at all. The latest research shows that mild exercise is better than no exercise and that moderate exercise is better still, but it

Ways to Burn About 150 Calories

Washing and waxing a car for 45–60 minutes	(Less vigorous, more time.)
Washing windows or floors for 45–60 minutes	
Playing volleyball for 45 minutes	
Playing touch football for 30–45 minutes	
Gardening for 30–45 minutes	
Wheeling self in wheelchair for 30–40 minutes	
Walking 1 3/4 miles in 35 minutes (20 min/mile)	
Basketball (shooting baskets) for 30 minutes	
Bicycling 5 miles in 30 minutes	
Dancing fast (social) for 30 minutes	
Pushing a stroller 1 1/2 miles for 30 minutes	
Raking leaves for 30 minutes	
Walking 2 miles in 30 minutes (15 min/mile)	
Water aerobics for 30 minutes	
Swimming laps for 20 minutes	
Wheelchair basketball for 20 minutes	
Basketball (playing a game) for 15–20 minutes	
Bicycling 4 miles in 15 minutes	
Jumping rope for 15 minutes	
Running 1 1/2 miles in 15 minutes (10 min/mile)	
Shoveling snow for 15 minutes	
Stairwalking for 15 minutes	(More vigorous, less time.)

Source: *Physical Activity and Health*. A Report of the U.S. Surgeon General.

does not contradict the Alumni Study's findings that vigorous exercise is best of all.

Taken together, the exercise research of the past twenty years shows that you have options and choices. Instead of following a rigid protocol, you can be flexible, choosing the plan that is best for you. The only rule is that to be healthy, you should be physically active.

The U.S. Surgeon General recommends that you exercise enough to burn 1,000 calories a week, but the Alumni Study suggests that you will gain even more from two or three times as much exercise. The choice is yours. Start gradually and build up to the 1,000 calorie target. If you are satisfied with your results or if age, medical problems, or personal considerations make it hard for you to do more, stay at that level. But if you still need more help with your weight, cholesterol, or blood pressure, push on toward the higher goal. You may even find that you enjoy exercise so much that you want to explore new activities and develop new abilities, just for the pleasure of it.

Exercise Precautions

Exercise is great for health—but to get gain without pain, you must do it wisely, exercising restraint and judgment at every step of the way. Here are a few tips:

- Get a medical check-up before you begin a moderate to vigorous exercise program, particularly if you are older than forty, if you have medical problems, or if you have not exercised previously (see the Epilogue). Although treadmill stress tests were once considered an important precaution, they are not necessary for most people. The best evidence comes from a study of 3,617 men aged thirty-five to fifty-nine who were at high risk for heart disease because of elevated cholesterol levels. Even in these at-risk men, annual stress tests were not able to predict exercise-induced cardiac problems before they developed. The good news, though, is that such problems were rare, occurring in only 2 percent of men during seven years of exercise. But even if preexercise stress tests are not useful for healthy men, they are mandatory for anyone with heart disease or symptoms that suggest problems.
- Eat and drink appropriately. Do not eat during the two hours before you exercise, but drink plenty of water before, during, and after exercise, particularly in warm weather.
- Warm up before each aerobic exercise activity and cool down afterward. Stroll before you walk, and walk before you jog. Stretches and light calisthenics are ideal warm-up and cool-down activities.
- Dress comfortably, aiming for comfort, convenience, and safety rather than style.
- Use good equipment, especially good shoes.
- Exercise regularly. Unless you are ill or injured, try to exercise nearly every day, but alternate harder workouts with easier ones.

- Explore a variety of activities to find what suits you best. If you master different forms of exercise you will be able to adjust to constraints imposed by climate, travel, and injury. Variety will keep your muscles fresh and will keep you from getting stale or bored. Build a balanced program. Add strength training, stretches, and exercises for balance to your basic aerobic regimen (see below). Consider getting instruction or joining a health club (see below).
- Exercise safely. Avoid heavy traffic, and be cautious about remote areas, especially if you are alone. Walk or jog facing the traffic. Bike with the traffic, always wearing a helmet. Wear bright clothing and reflective gear after dark. It makes little sense to reduce your risk of heart attack or stroke by increasing your risk of accidental injury or death. Adjust your routine in weather that is hot, cold, or wet.
- Listen to your body. Learn warning signals of heart disease, including chest pain or pressure, disproportionate shortness of breath, fatigue, or sweating, erratic pulse, lightheadedness, or even indigestion. Do not ignore aches and pains that may signify injury; early treatment can often prevent more serious problems. Do not exercise if you are feverish or ill. Work yourself back into shape gradually after a layoff, particularly after illness or injury.

Your Exercise Menu

Men who understand how to eat for both health and pleasure know how to make the choices that suit them best. To plan your fitness program, consider the many options on your exercise menu:

- Daily Activities. In today's high-tech world, it's possible to get through a day—or year—with hardly any physical activity. In fact, 60 percent of Americans seem to be doing their best to avoid all forms of exercise, and most succeed. Do not join them. Instead, build activity into your daily life; each little bit of exercise may not seem like much, but they can add up to an important benefit. Walk for transportation, or at least get off the bus or train one stop early, then walk to your destination. Park a few blocks from your home or office. Climb stairs. Carry your own bundles. Wash your car yourself. Walk the golf course. Do your own yard work and use a hand mower on your lawn. Use your body whenever you can; it will reward you with good health.

- Walking. In many ways, it's the ideal exercise. It's easy and convenient, requiring only good shoes and appropriate clothing. It can be solitary or social, and it is adaptable to nearly any climate. Walking can be a mild to moderate exercise or it can be quite intense. Best of all, walking is nearly injury-free. As Charles Dickens put it: "Walk and be happy, walk and be healthy."
- Jogging and running share many features of walking with two major exceptions. They are more intense, enabling you to get a better workout in less time. But they also subject your body to much more impact, increasing the risk of injury. Still, jogging and running are excellent forms of exercise, though they do require extra care to avoid injuries.
- Swimming and aquatic exercises are the easiest on your muscles and joints. That's because the water absorbs 90 percent of the force of gravity, providing cushioning and protection. Swimming also has the advantage of exercising your arms and trunk as well as your legs. But it's much less convenient than walking or jogging, and it requires much more expertise. Swimming is also less effective for weight loss and for strengthening your bones.
- Biking is another excellent activity that can be gentle or vigorous, solitary or shared. Although it is a low-impact activity, accidents and falls greatly increase the risk of injury. Prolonged biking can also cause erectile dysfunction in some men.
- Racquet sports can be wonderful conditioning activities if you play them hard. Singles are best, but doubles will serve nicely if you spend enough of your time on the move.
- Golf is splendid recreation but it will not give you much exercise unless you walk the course. But if you do walk, you can give yourself credit for four miles for each eighteen-hole game.
- Home exercise machines are a big business. Americans shell out $2.5 billion each year to purchase them. With so much money at stake, it's no surprise that men are subjected to relentless sales pitches from manufacturers and retailers: Buy my machine and you will lose

weight, improve your physique, and live longer. The funny thing is that these claims are accurate, with just one proviso. Exercise machines can do great things for you, but only if you use them regularly.

Like the human body itself, exercise machines are subject to a major problem: disuse. The stationary bike is an example. It is an excellent tool for cardiovascular fitness, but too often it features two pedals, one seat, and no rider. Good intentions alone will not get you good health; for that, you'll have to sweat. Boredom is the main lament. To help maintain your motivation, listen to music or watch TV or videos while you exercise. You can read while pedaling a bike and you can read with your ears while using any machine. Recorded books are great for motivation—particularly if you resist the temptation to finish the tape in your car or den, so you will have to get on your treadmill or climber to find out how the story ends.

Exercise machines have two other drawbacks: They can take up lots of space and they can be very expensive. To conserve space, some men buy machines that fold for storage. A fine idea, but it usually does not work. Folding machines are often less sturdy than stationary models, and the extra effort of hauling a machine out of storage is the dagger in the heart of motivation. Another common solution to the space dilemma is to set up the machine in an out-of-the-way place, such as a basement, attic, or garage—another bad idea. Out of sight is out of mind. Put your machine in a convenient, pleasant location that will help make exercise enjoyable. If your space is limited, choose a compact device such as a climber or bike instead of a larger machine such as a treadmill or rower.

The expense factor can also be overcome. Except for treadmills, which cost two to three times more, you can get many excellent machines for $400 to $600. The trick is to favor function over form. Look for a sturdy machine with adjustable intensity settings, one that fits you comfortably. The electronic bells and whistles run up the bill, but unless you need them for motivation, they are entirely optional. In general, it is better to choose a stripped-down utilitarian machine made by a reputable manufacturer specializing in fitness equipment.

Which machine is best for you? Don't let infomercials choose for you. Instead, try out various types at a fitness store, health club, or "Y," remembering that the machines you test in clubs are likely to be high-end models, costing far more than you would like to spend for a home exerciser. If possible, use a machine several times before you write a check. Look for one that is easy to use but still challenging and enjoyable. For many men, a treadmill is best, but if you already walk or jog outdoors, you might decide to diversify by buying a stationary bike, elliptical trainer or stair climber. On the other hand, if your passion is cross-country skiing or rowing, you might pick a machine that simulates these sports so you can extend your short season and stay in shape the year around.

Strength Training

Even if you walk, jog, bike, or swim nearly every day, you should set aside an extra ten to twenty minutes two or three times a week to do some strength training. It will help your sports performance and it will improve your physique. Both are nice benefits, but they are not the main reason to pump iron. In fact, you should do strength training to preserve your muscles and bones.

Without resistance exercise, bones lose calcium during the aging process; weight bearing exercises such as walking will protect your legs and hips, but not your arms and wrists. Muscles also become smaller and weaker as the years go by; tissue loss begins at age thirty to forty and it accelerates beyond age sixty. In all, the average thirty-year-old will lose about 25 percent of his muscle mass and strength by age seventy and another 25 percent by age ninety.

What accounts for weakening bones and muscles? Dietary deficiencies of calcium and vitamin D often contribute (see Chapter Four), and the slow decline in testosterone levels that begins at age forty also plays a role (see Chapters One and Ten). But the major culprit is disuse. The boys in the locker room were right; when it comes to your muscles and bones, use them or lose them. To maintain their strength, muscles and bones need work. However, not all types of work will do the trick. The endurance exercises that improve the heart and circulation, lower blood pressure, burn body fat, and improve the cholesterol and blood sugar will not do much for strength. For cardiovascular health and optimal longevity, endurance exercise such as walking, jogging, or biking are essential, but for muscles and bones, resistance exercise is the key.

Unlike endurance exercise, which should be done nearly every day, resistance exercises should be performed only two or three times a week, so that muscles can recover fully between sessions. It is important to warm up before and cool down after each session. Five or ten minutes of stretching or light calisthenics are ideal.

High-repetition, low-resistance exercise is best. That means picking an exercise that does not seem difficult when it is performed once or twice but that causes fatigue without exhaustion when it is repeated eight to twelve times over thirty to ninety seconds. As you improve, you will be able to gradually increase the resistance until you reach a sustainable plateau. In general, each exercise should be performed in a set of eight to twelve repetitions that is repeated after a one or two minute rest.

Resistance training will strengthen only the specific muscles that are being exercised. For optimal benefit, that means constructing a program that exercises each of your major muscle groups in turn.

As with all forms of exercise, strength training requires care. Older men and those with hypertension, heart disease, arthritis, muscle disease, neurologic problems, or other disabilities should get specific medical clearance and guidance. No one should exercise when ill or injured; after recovering from an illness, strength training should be resumed gradually and built up slowly.

Above all, use common sense and listen to your body. Most often, you will hear sounds of harmony and improvement, but if you hear sounds of distress you should back off and get help. Fatigue and mild muscle aches and stiffness usually resolve with rest and simple self-help measures, but chest pressure or pain, undue breathlessness, and lightheadedness head the list of symptoms that warrant medical attention.

Practicalities

Because each person has a different starting point and unique goals, strength training must be individualized. Technique is important, and special equipment can help. That's why health clubs, "Y's," and personal trainers can be a big asset, particularly when you are just getting started.

Resistance training can be achieved in many ways. Machines such as the Cybex, Universal, or Nautilus systems provide the most precise programs, but you will need a gym and instruction for these. Fortunately, you can do very well at home using your body weight (calisthenics), elastic bands ("stretchies"), or free weights (dumbbells and ankle weights).

Weight training requires special care. Start with weights that are comfortable; for some men it is as little as two to five pounds, for others it is ten to fifteen pounds or more, but it should never be more than 50 percent of the heaviest weight you can lift comfortably at one time. Be sure your body mechanics are good; keep your feet ten to twelve inches apart, your knees slightly bent and your back straight. Do not rock or sway; move only the part of your body that you are trying to exercise. Lift slowly, giving yourself two seconds to lift and another two to four to return to your starting position. Breathe slowly, but never hold your breath. If you find yourself grunting with exertion, the weight is too heavy.

Figure 5.2 suggests a representative program that you can do at home using just a set of dumbbells, and ankle weights, sturdy chair, and a towel or exercise mat plus, of course, your body. Start with the standing exercises then move to the chair and finally the floor. Do each exercise eight to twelve times, rest for a minute or two, then repeat a second set of eight to twelve repetitions.

Exercises for Flexibility

As muscles and tendons become stronger, they also become tighter and shorter. It is recipe for injury, but a stretching program can minimize risk. Since many stretching exercises are based on yoga, they may help reduce mental tension as well as muscle tension.

Plan a routine that fits your body's needs, concentrating on your stiffest muscles. Give yourself time to improve. Restoring flexibility is a slow process, and if you are impatient and push too hard, you can produce the very injury you are trying to prevent. Never stretch to the point of pain; there is no point in trying to stretch the limits of your own body. A physical therapist, personal trainer, or yoga instructor can be a great help, especially when you are getting started. Figure 5.3 demonstrates a basic stretching routine.

A good stretching routine should take about ten minutes. That makes it an excellent way to warm up before exercise and to cool down afterward. Many people also like to do some stretches as they start the day, before bed, or at times of stress. Stretching can make a long car trip tolerable, and it can make gardening and household chores easier on your body. Work out a routine that is best for you, but try to stretch at least two to three times a week.

Exercise for Balance

I have urged you to construct a balanced exercise program. In order to do so, you should incorporate a few additional exercises to improve your balance. Balance is a highly specialized skill that requires the combined efforts of nerve cells that access the body's orientation in space, the eyes, the vestibular apparatus in the inner ear that functions as the body's gyroscope, and the spinal cord and brain, which coordinate all the information. These skills tend to dete-

FIGURE 5.2.
STRENGTH TRAINING EXERCISES

When it comes to exercise, one plan will not fit all. Although a supervised individual exercise prescription is best, it's not always available. Here is a set of ten basic exercises that can help most men build strong bones and muscles. Start slowly and cautiously, but build up steadily as you improve. Be sure to read the text carefully for instructions and precautions.

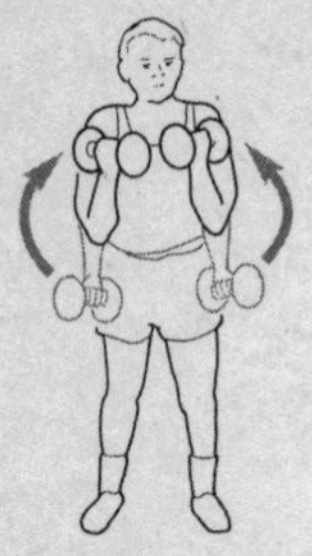

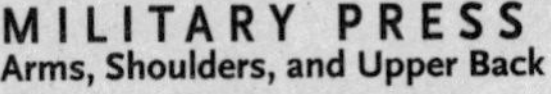

MILITARY PRESS
Arms, Shoulders, and Upper Back

Stand with your feet slightly apart. Hold a dumbbell in each hand at shoulder height. With your palms facing away from your body, slowly lift upward until your arms are fully extended, then slowly lower the dumbbells to chest level. Repeat 8–15 times; rest and repeat the set.

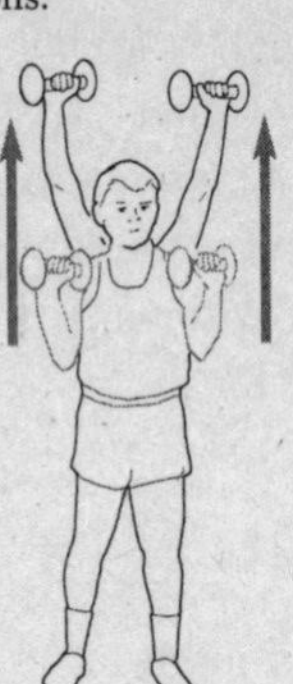

CURLS
Arms, Shoulders, and Upper Back

Stand or sit comfortably with your arms at your sides. Hold a dumbbell in each hand and slowly lift them to the level of your upper chest, keeping your arms close to your sides. Lower the weights slowly, then repeat. Alternate the position of your hands, first facing your palms forward, then backward (reverse curls). Repeat 8–15 times; rest and repeat the set.

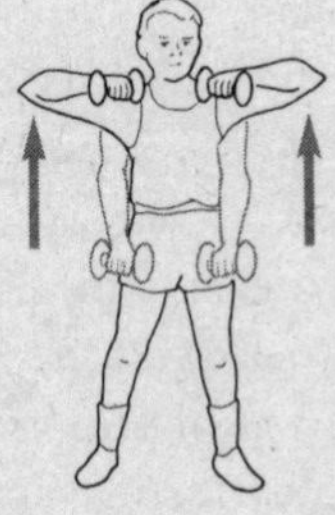

UPRIGHT ROW
Arms, Shoulders, and Upper Back

Stand with your feet at shoulder width. Hold a dumbbell in each hand with your palms facing your thighs. Slowly lift the dumbbells to shoulder level, keeping them close together by allowing your elbows to point outward. Slowly lower the dumbbells to your thighs. Repeat 8–15 times; rest and repeat the set.

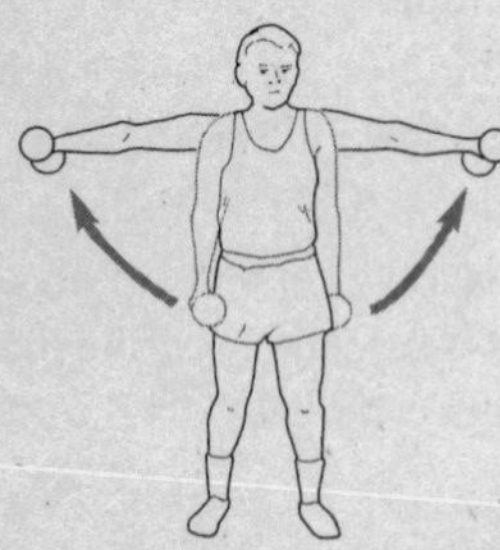

LATERAL RAISE
Arms, Shoulders, and Upper Back

With your feet slightly apart, hold a dumbbell in each hand at your side. Keeping your arms straight, slowly lift the dumbbells until they are slightly above your shoulders. Slowly lower the dumbbells to your side. Repeat 8–15 times; rest and repeat the set.

BENT-KNEE CURL-UPS
Abdomen and Trunk

Lie on your back with your knees bent, your feet flat on the floor, and your arms folded across your chest. Raise your torso until your elbows touch your knees. Slowly lower yourself to the floor. Repeat 8–15 times; rest and repeat the set.

FIGURE 5.2.
STRENGTH TRAINING EXERCISES

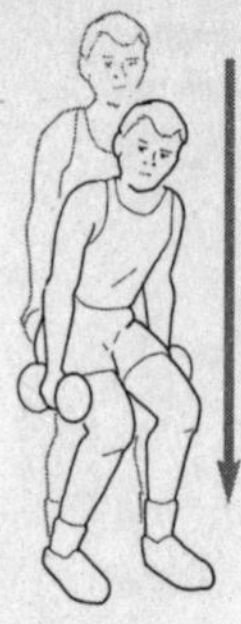

PARTIAL SQUATS
Hips and Legs

Stand with your feet at shoulder width. Hold a dumbbell in each hand with your arms at your sides and your palms facing inward. Slowly bend your knees, lowering your buttocks about 8 inches while keeping your arms down straight. Slowly rise to an upright position. Repeat 8–15 times; rest and repeat the set.

KNEE EXTENSION
Hips and Legs

Wearing an ankle weight, sit in a firm straight-backed chair, with your knees 6 inches apart and a small towel folded under your lower thigh. Slowly lift your right foot until your leg is straight out in front of you. Lower your foot slowly to the floor. Repeat 8–15 times with each leg; rest and repeat the set.

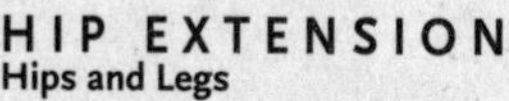

HIP EXTENSION
Hips and Legs

Wearing an ankle weight, stand 8 inches behind a sturdy chair. Using its back for balance, bend your trunk forward 45 degrees, then extend your right leg straight behind you. Slowly lower your foot to the floor. Repeat with each leg 8–15 times; rest and repeat the set.

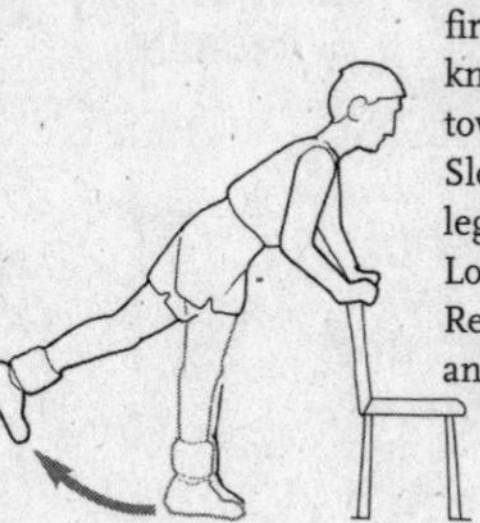

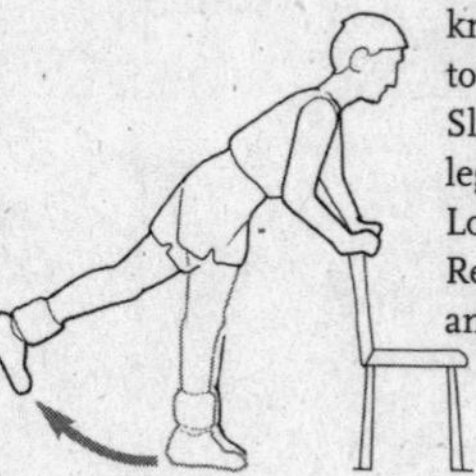

LATERAL LEG RAISES
Hips and Legs

Wearing an ankle weight, stand behind a sturdy chair, using the back for balance. Slowly raise your right leg to the side until your foot is 8 inches off the floor. Keep your knee straight and slowly lower your foot to the floor. Repeat with each leg 8–15 times; rest and repeat the set.

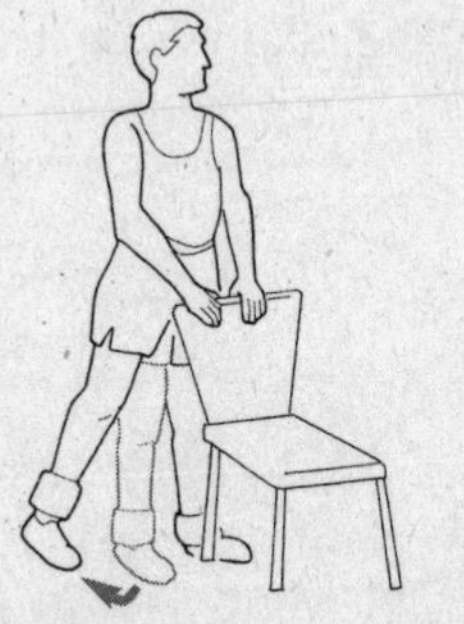

HEEL RAISES AND DIPS
Hips and Legs

Stand on the bottom step of a staircase, holding on to a handrail for balance. Place the balls of your feet on the step with your heels projecting out. Slowly raise your heels, shifting your weight to your toes. Slowly lower your heels as far as you can, shifting your weight to your heels. Return to the starting position. Repeat 8–15 times; rest and repeat the set.

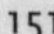

FIGURE 5.3. STRETCHING EXERCISES

Plan a routine that fits your body's needs, concentrating on your stiffest muscles. Give yourself time to improve. Restoring flexibility is a slow process and if you are impatient and push too hard, you can produce the very injury you are trying to prevent. Never stretch to the point of pain. There is no point in trying to stretch the limits of your own body. A physical therapist, personal trainer, or yoga instructor can be a great help, especially when you are getting started. These drawings demonstrate a basic stretching routine.

1. Shoulder blade stretch
2. Towel stretch
3. Wall lean
4. Hamstring stretch
5. Thigh stretch
6. Hip stretch
7. Groin stretch
8. Starter's stretch
9. Williams stretch
10. Cat's stretch

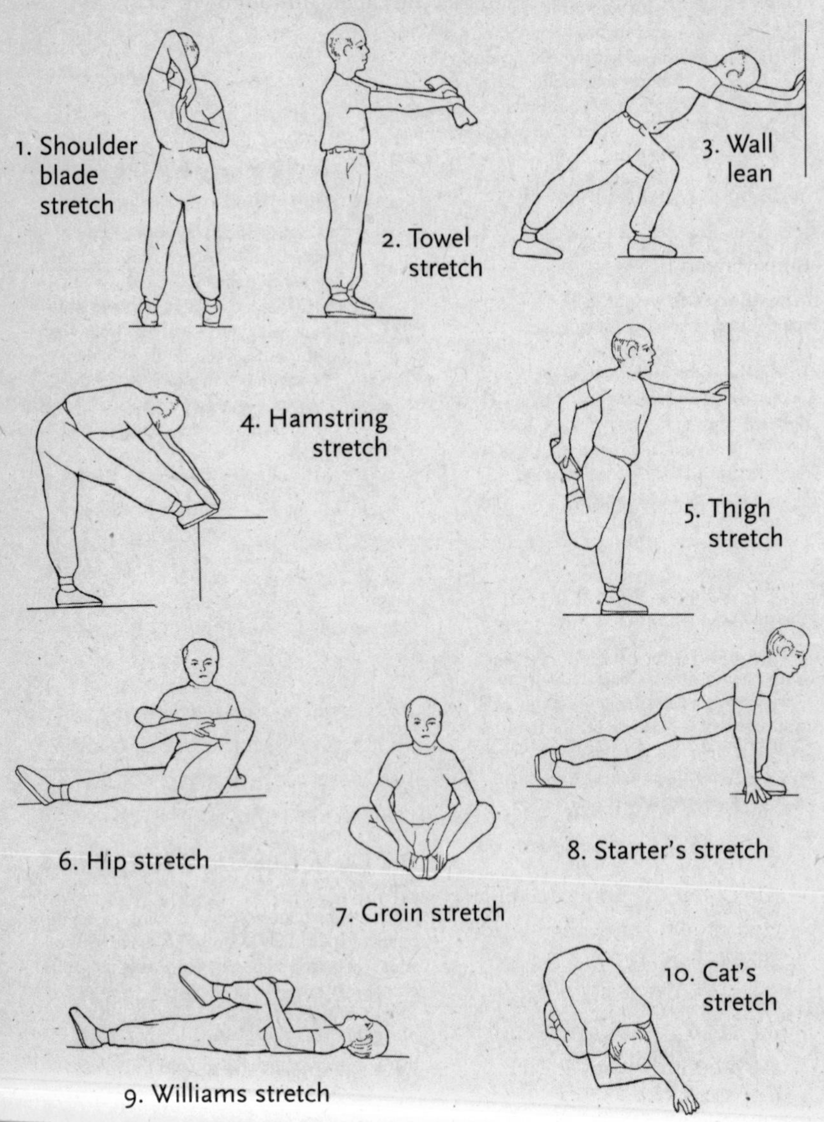

riorate with age, contributing to the falls that plague one out of every three men older than sixty-five. Walking, climbing stairs, resistance exercises, and stretching will all help, but Tai Chi exercises and the special balance classes offered by many health clubs and senior centers can help everyone. Figure 5.4 demonstrates some simple balance exercises you can do on your own.

Health Clubs and Trainers

With more than 20 million members in the United States, health clubs are riding the crest of the fitness wave. A club can provide three major benefits: instruction and supervision, equipment and facilities, and motivation and companionship. But many clubs are expensive, some are inconvenient, and more than a few go out of business without refunding all fees. In a sense, a club is just a big, expensive piece of exercise equipment. If you use it you will enjoy many health benefits, but if not, you will just feel guilty and wasteful.

Here are some tips to help you find the club that's best for you:

- Find a club that is convenient. A long commute is a short way to finding excuses for staying away. If at all possible, pick a club within ten to fifteen minutes of your home or work. Location is everything, or nearly everything.
- Be sure the club is open when you want to use it, and that it is not too crowded at your favorite times.
- Be sure the club has what you want, but do not pay for more than you need. If you are a treadmill, bike, and Nautilus guy, you can save big bucks by staying away from clubs that have racquetball courts and steam rooms. On the other hand, if your stroke is the crawl, seek out a club with a lap pool.
- Check out the atmosphere. Intangibles can make or break a club. A club should be inviting—clean, bright, and upbeat. That goes for the showers and lockers, too. If television or music will help you work up a sweat, be sure the club has what you need. If you prefer Schubert to the Stones, steer clear of high-decibel rock music. Be sure, too, that the other members are compatible with your personality and style. If you like to jog in your old T-shirt and shorts, you may feel out of place in a Spandex crowd.

FIGURE 5.4. BALANCE EXERCISES

Although group classes and individual instruction are the best ways to improve balance, you can do some simple work on your own. Walking and climbing stairs will help. And here are three exercises to consider:

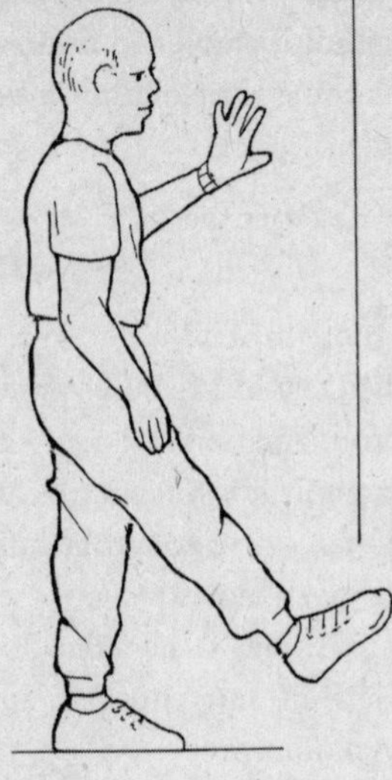

Stand about 2 feet from a wall so you can use your hand for support if necessary. Keeping both knees straight, lift one leg forward until your toe points 30–45 degrees upward. Hold the position for 5–10 seconds, then relax. Repeat at least five times, then repeat with your other leg.

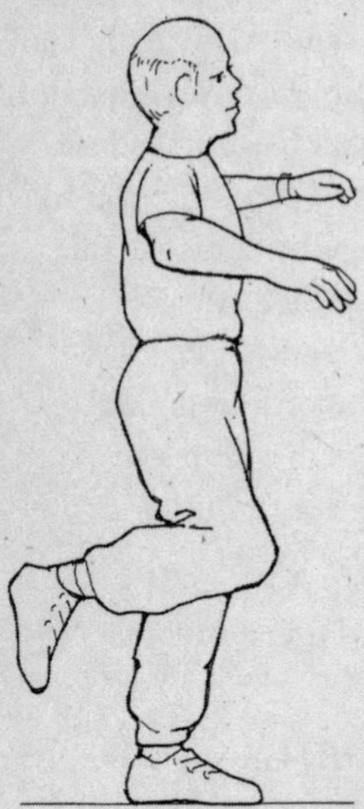

Balance on one foot while you bend your other leg up at the knee. Hold for 5–10 seconds, then relax. Repeat five to ten times, then switch to the other leg. At first you may need to touch a wall for balance, but as you improve you may be able to keep your arms out in front of you. As you improve, try to maintain the one-legged stance for longer periods of time. Your goal should be 1–2 minutes on each leg, first in shorter segments that are repeated, eventually in one to three continuous periods.

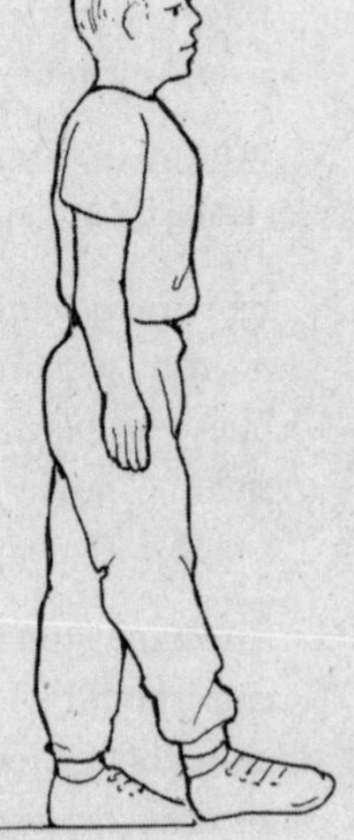

Practice heel-to-toe walking as if you were on a tightrope. Hold your arms out at your sides or touch a wall for balance if necessary. Walk the length of a long hallway, then turn around and walk back.

- Give the club a check-up. Choose a club that is appropriate for your age and health. A good club should ask you to fill out a medical questionnaire, possibly including an okay from your doctor. If you have medical problems, find a club that has the equipment and personnel to provide first aid. But be leery of a club that insists you take an expensive stress test from them, whether you need one or not.
- Check out the staff. Are they just body builders who look good, or are they well-trained fitness experts? A good credential is certification by an organization such as The American College of Sports Medicine, the American Council on Exercise, or the Aerobics and Fitness Association of America.
- Visit the club at the time of day when you will be using it to see what it is really like.
- Talk to club members to find out how they like it; be sure to ask if the club delivers on its promises.
- Ask for a free introductory workout or an inexpensive trial membership. It is the best way to see if the club works for you.
- If you travel often, try to find a club that offers reciprocal memberships with facilities in other cities.

Most health clubs offer the services of personal trainers, usually for an extra fee. Trainers are also available for individual help, either in your home or at a gym. A good trainer can help you in five ways: by assessing your needs and abilities, by establishing goals, by providing instruction, by monitoring your program, and, above all, by providing motivation.

Personal trainers are not physical therapists, and you should not rely on them to treat injuries. In fact, because they are not licensed, no standards assure quality. A personal recommendation is the best way to find a trainer, but remember to interview the trainer yourself before you sign up. Certification by organizations such as the American College of Sports Medicine, the National Academy of Sports Medicine, the Aerobics and Fitness Association of America, or the American Council on Exercise is important. It means that a trainer has attended a two-to-four-day course and has passed an exam. Finally, evaluate a trainer's personality and style. Since motivation is a primary reason for using a trainer, good chemistry is essential. Personal trainers are expensive. They can be a great help in shaping you up, but exercise books and videos, group classes, and even athletically experienced friends are less costly alternatives. In the last analysis, the only trainer who really matters is you. A personal trainer can push and prod, but your muscles have to do the work that will earn such rich rewards in fitness and health.

Complications of Exercise

It does not happen often, but in man-bites-dog fashion it usually makes the evening news; a few people die while they are exercising. In young athletes, the cause is usually an inborn abnormality of the coronary arteries, an abnormal thickening of the heart muscle (*hypertrophic myocardiopathy*), inflammation of the heart muscle (*myocarditis*), or a noncardiac problem such as drug abuse. In older men, the cause is usually coronary artery disease that triggers an abnormal heart rhythm (*ventricular fibrillation*) or a heart attack.

It does not happen often, and it does not change the fact that exercise reduces the risk of heart attacks and death. That is the message of the Alumni Study and much subsequent research. The Alumni Study evaluated overall health and survival, but did not separate problems that occurred during exercise from those that occurred at other times. Doctor Cooper's Aerobics Institute did check for exercise-related deaths, but found none in more than 375,000 hours of exercise, including 1.2 million miles of walking and jogging.

Researchers in Seattle provided additional perspectives. They found that "weekend warriors," people who engage in strenuous exercise without first working themselves into shape, are fifty-six times more likely to die during an hour of exercise than during a sedentary hour. People who exercise regularly also experience an increased risk during peak exertion, but that risk is small and—most important—their overall risk of sudden cardiac death is 60 percent lower than the risk of sedentary people. In a recent report, the Physicians' Health Study agreed. The risk of sudden death was almost seventeen times higher during and up to thirty minutes after a bout of vigorous exercise than during a similar time span with little or no exercise. As in the Seattle study, though, regular exercise substantially reduced the cardiac hazards of intense exertion. Best of all, the risks were extremely low, amounting to just one sudden death per 1.51 million bouts of exercise, even when out-of-shape men were included in the analysis.

It does not happen often, but it is a reminder that exercise is a serious business—and you can minimize your risk by taking it seriously.

First, be sure you have had a recent check-up before you start an exercise program, particularly if you are over forty or if you have never exercised before (see the Epilogue). Your check-up should include an evaluation of your family history and your health habits as well as a review of any symptoms you may have. Your physical should include a check of your blood pressure, your heart and lungs, your pulses, and your joints. Useful lab tests include a complete blood count, cholesterol profile, and blood sugar levels. An electrocardiogram (ECG) is reasonable, particularly if you have not had one within five years, but you probably will not benefit from a stress test unless the other results raise a question about your heart.

Second, get into shape gradually. Set reasonable goals and build up slowly as you improve.

Third, don't let your stomach compete with your heart. Do not eat within two hours of exercise, but be sure to stay well hydrated by drinking plenty of water before, during, and after exercising.

Fourth, avoid extremes of climate. Both the cold winds of January and the dog days of summer can stress your heart. It is another reason to have a home machine, a mall with a corridor for walking, or a health club so you can stay active the year round.

Fifth, warm up before you work out and cool down afterward. Your joints and tendons will thank you and so will your muscles, including the most important muscle, your heart.

Finally, and most important, listen to your body. Vigorous exercise will always make you breathe hard, but do not ignore disproportionately labored breathing or shortness of breath. Be alert for chest pressure, tightness, or pain. Do not try to play through excessive fatigue or sweating. Take note of dizziness, lightheadedness, fainting, or an irregular or unduly rapid heartbeat. Even "indigestion" warrants your attention. If you experience any of these symptoms during physical activity, stop exercising at once and be prepared to get help if you do not improve promptly. Be sure to let your doctor know about such symptoms, whether they come on during exercise or at rest.

Fortunately, cardiac complications of exercise are uncommon. Unfortunately, musculoskeletal complications are quite common, but they, too, can usually be prevented or, at least, treated with simple remedies at home.

The same regimen of warm-ups, cool-downs, and gradual progress that will protect your heart will also help prevent many musculoskeletal injuries. Stretching is particularly helpful, since exercise itself can make muscles tight and tense. It is also important to use good equipment, particularly well-fitting, supportive shoes. Good technique will also prevent many injuries. A few lessons that improve your mechanics will do as much for your health as for your performance. Above all, don't overdo it. Fatigue and dehydration impair concentration, often leading to a misstep or fall. Overuse is the major cause of injuries. Give your body a chance to rest and recover after workouts, particularly when you are first getting into shape. Alternate hard sessions with easier ones. Vary your routine so that you use different parts of your body. Some men, for example, might walk one day, play golf the next, and bike the third. A day off now and then does not hurt, either.

Even with all this, injuries may occur. If you spot them early, you may be able to treat them yourself. A bit of soreness and stiffness is normal, but pain, swelling, diminished strength or mobility, and discoloration of the skin are not. If your problem seems small, treat it yourself. But if you do not improve, or if you have a major injury, get expert help.

PRICE: *Protection, Rest, Ice, Compression,* and *Elevation* is a five point program to handle injuries:

PRICE

- *Protection.* Injured tissues must be protected against further injury. Protect your small injuries by applying bandages, elastic wraps, or simple splints. Something as simple as taping an injured toe to its healthy neighbor can do the job. See your doctor for problems that require precision splints or casts.
- *Rest.* Injured tissues need time to heal. It is an obvious principle, but once you are hooked on exercise you may be tempted to ignore it. Do not give in to temptation—you will shortchange yourself with shortcuts. But you can rest *selectively;* you may have to give up tennis while your serving shoulder recovers from tendinitis, but you can still walk, jog, or bike. In a curious way, an injury is often a blessing in disguise, forcing you to diversify your workouts and acquire new skills.
- *Ice.* It is the cheapest, simplest, yet most effective way to manage many injuries. Ice is an excellent antiinflammatory, reducing swelling and pain. For best results, apply an ice pack for ten to fifteen minutes as soon as possible after an injury. Repeat the ice treatment each hour for the first four hours, then four times a day for the next two to three days. Protect your skin with a thin cloth, and do not allow your skin to become red, blistered, or numb. After forty-eight to seventy-two

hours, switch to heat treatments, using the same schedule and principles.

- *Compression.* Pressure will help reduce swelling and inflammation. In most cases, a simple elastic bandage will suffice; it should be snug but not too tight. Remember that swelling may develop slowly hours after your injury, so you may have to loosen your wrap. Another trick is to place a small piece of foam rubber directly on the injured area before you wrap it; this will allow you to put gentle pressure where it is needed without constricting an entire joint or limb.
- *Elevation.* It's a simple strategy that enlists the force of gravity to drain fluid away from injured tissues, reducing swelling, inflammation, and pain. Keep your sore foot up on a hassock or put a pillow under it in bed; elevating an injured area will help you get back to earth faster.

PRICE is the key to the early management of most kinds of injuries, but you may also need medication for pain or inflammation. *Acetaminophen* (Tylenol and other brands) may be the best choice for the first day, since it will reduce pain without increasing bleeding into the injured tissue. After the first day or two, consider *aspirin* or other *nonsteroidal antiinflammatories* (NSAIDs) such as *ibuprofen* (Advil and other brands) or *naproxen* (Aleve) to fight inflammation as well as pain. NSAIDs can irritate the stomach; as with all medications, use them carefully, always following directions.

Your pain is gone and your swelling is down—but your treatment is not yet over. Instead, plan your rehabilitation and return to exercise with the same care that you used to treat your injury. As a rule of thumb, give yourself two days of rehab for each day of inactivity due to injury. Start with gentle range of motion exercises, then gradually increase your weight-bearing exercises. When you are comfortable, consider building up your tissues with graded resistance training using calisthenics, light weights, or Nautilus equipment. If all goes well, you can be stronger than before your injury, thus reducing your risk of reinjury. Do not neglect stretching exercises to improve your flexibility. Use heat or massage to warm up your injured tissues before you start your rehab exercises; afterwards, apply ice to the area to reduce inflammation. The judicious use of aspirin or other NSAIDs may also facilitate your rehabilitation program.

You can manage many injuries yourself, but don't be stubborn. If you have a major injury—or if your nagging woes do not clear up—get help. An experienced exercise buddy who has been there and done that may be all the help you need. Primary care physicians should be able to handle 50 to 60 percent of exercise-induced problems, but more difficult issues require orthopedists, physical therapists, and sports podiatrists. In many centers, these specialists come together in sports medicine clinics.

More than being merely important for health, exercise is essential for optimal well-being. Minor aches and pains are inevitable but are worth the price. With care, you should be able to prevent most injuries and treat many others yourself. Expert help is available for major problems. It may sound formidable but it is all part of the game—the health game.

CHAPTER SIX

The Answers: Aspirin and Other Supplements

"IF ONLY THERE WERE A PILL."

Every man would like an easy way to stay healthy. Good nutrition and regular exercise are the keys for preventing illness, but diets take discipline and exercise takes time. Is there a shortcut? Can a few pills do the trick? Can "all-natural" supplements replace the physical activity and healthful eating that should be part of human nature?

If you look for the answer on the Internet or listen for it on TV or radio, you are likely to come away with a resounding "yes." That's mostly because vitamins, herbs, and other supplements are not subject to the jurisdiction of the Food and Drug Administration. Congress took care of that in 1994, when it passed the Dietary Supplement Health and Education Act. As a result, the supplement industry can tout its products without having to substantiate their claims for efficacy and safety. With billions of dollars at stake, the hype is relentless. In all, more than 50 percent of all Americans take supplements, spending upwards of $4 billion a year to buy health in a bottle.

Most doctors have been skeptical of supplements, pointing out correctly that anecdotes and testimonials can never be relied on in place of sound scientific studies. In the past few years, though, good studies have started to appear. While few herbs have been scrutinized, research by the Physicians' Health Study, the Health Professionals Study, and other investigations suggests that some supplements may be helpful while others are wasteful or even harmful. Surprisingly, perhaps, one of the most promising of all is not a vitamin or an herb, but an inexpensive, old-fashioned, medicine chest standby: aspirin.

Aspirin

Its name is more than a century old, but its parent compound has been in use for thousands of years. The ancient Assyrians, Egyptians, and Greeks all used willow leaves to treat inflammation, fever, and pain. The practice was popularized in England by Reverend Edward Stone in 1763. The active ingredient was purified from willow bark in Germany sixty-five years later. At the tail end of the nineteenth century, scientists at the Bayer Company succeeded in producing the modern derivative, *acetylsalicylic acid,* or aspirin. The very same drug has been used for fever and pain ever since. In the past thirty years, it has gained new importance in the management of heart disease and stroke, and current studies suggest it may someday assume a role in preventing colon cancer and possibly even Alzheimer's disease. And just as aspirin is finding new uses, scientists are finding out exactly how it works. It is important research that is likely to result in a new generation of even better drugs. But even in the dawning era of "super-aspirins," the original drug is certain to retain much of its value.

How It Works

Aspirin does its job by inhibiting the body's production of *prostaglandins.* Although you may never have heard of them, prostaglandins have a wide-ranging impact on human health. For example, they keep the stomach lining healthy, they regulate blood flow to the kidneys, and they enable platelets to trigger blood clotting. But prostaglandins also contribute to disease; in the brain they cause fever, and in joints and other tissues they can produce inflammation and pain.

Aspirin is not the only drug that inhibits prostaglandins. In fact all the *nonsteroidal antiinflammatory drugs* (NSAIDs) act in similar fashion (see Table 6.1, page 168). But although *acetaminophen* (Tylenol and other brands) fights fever and pain as well as aspirin, it does not inhibit prostaglandins. As a result, it does not share either the antiinflammatory benefits or the major side effects of aspirin and other NSAIDs.

Aspirin and Atherosclerosis

Aspirin does not prevent or even minimize atherosclerosis, but it can help prevent heart attacks and some strokes. It sounds like a paradox, but it is not. Aspirin cannot prevent cholesterol-laden plaques from building up in the wall of an artery, though it may be able to reduce the inflammation that perpetuates the damage (see Chapter Three and Figure 3.1). But while plaques narrow arteries, rarely do they produce the complete blockages that cause heart attacks. Instead, the culprit is a blood clot or *thrombus* that forms on the surface of a ruptured plaque. The clot completes the blockage, and aspirin exerts its protective effect by inhibiting clot formation.

Clots are triggered by platelets, fragmentary blood cells that are produced in the bone marrow, and then pour into the bloodstream. A man's blood contains a total of 100 million platelets, but because each platelet only lasts about ten days, the marrow must produce them continuously at a prodigious rate. Aspirin does not reduce the number of platelets in the blood, but it does inhibit their ability to trigger clots.

Platelets are extremely sensitive to aspirin. In some studies, doses as low as 10–30 milligrams can inhibit all the platelets in a man's body. Once platelets are inhibited by aspirin, they stay inhibited, but since new platelets are entering the blood continuously, the aspirin dose must be repeated every twenty-four to forty-eight hours to keep the majority of platelets under control.

PRIMARY PREVENTION OF HEART ATTACKS

You would probably call it staying healthy, but doctors call it primary prevention. By either name, it means heading off a problem before it makes its first appearance. Can aspirin prevent a first heart attack in men without diagnosed heart disease?

This is the question that the Physicians' Health Study set out to answer in 1982. A total of 22,071 male physicians volunteered to be subjects in a randomized clinical trial of low-dose aspirin. Half the men were assigned to take 325 milligrams of aspirin every other day, while the others each were given an identical-appearing placebo tablet every other day. To eliminate bias, the assignments were made randomly and neither the subjects nor the researchers knew which men were taking aspirin and which the placebo.

The researchers had planned to continue the trial until 1990, but it was terminated three years ahead of schedule. That was because an independent Data Monitoring Board that was tracking the results declared it would be unethical to continue the study since a clear winner was already evident. The winner was aspirin.

In the Physicians' Health Study, the men who took aspirin had a 44 percent reduction in the risk of suffering a heart attack. Benefit did not depend on a man's family history of heart disease or on his cholesterol, blood pressure, blood sugar, body fat, amount of exercise, or his drinking or smoking habits. But one risk factor did predict benefit: age. Aspirin was highly effective in men older than fifty, but not in younger individuals.

The results of the Physicians' Health Study were published in the same year as the report of the British Doctors Trial, which found no benefit from aspirin. Does that mean men should take aspirin in America but not in Europe?

Not at all. The British trial was much smaller than the U.S. study, involving just 5,139 men. It was also less carefully controlled. But the biggest difference was in the dose of aspirin; the British doctors took 500 milligrams every day, the Americans just 325 milligrams every other day.

When you have a headache or a fever, you are likely to take two 325 milligram aspirin tablets every four to six hours. Even the British doctors' dose is tiny in comparison, but it may still be too high to produce maximum protection against heart attacks. That is because tiny doses of aspirin will inhibit only *thromboxane* A_2, the enzyme in platelets that triggers the clotting process, but higher doses can also inhibit *prostacyclin,* an enzyme in blood vessels that reduces clotting. In theory, at least, low doses of aspirin will reduce clot formation, but even slightly higher doses might lessen that benefit. Two 1998 studies found that 75 milligrams of aspirin a day can reduce the risk of a first heart attack by about one-third, and a 2001 investigation found that 100 milligrams a day reduced the risk of cardiovascular death by 44 percent, but none of these reports investigated varying amounts of aspirin. However, a 1999 study from six European countries compared four aspirin doses and found that low amounts (81 or 325 milligrams a day) were actually better than higher doses (650 or 1,300 milligrams a day) in preventing strokes.

When it comes to aspirin for prevention, less is more.

Although the Physicians' Health Study demonstrated that low-dose aspirin could help prevent heart attacks in healthy men fifty or older, its 1989 report did not link aspirin use with a reduction in overall cardiovascular deaths. The aspirin trial was terminated early, and its five-year span may have been too short to discern an effect on mortality. But even after the randomized clinical trial was terminated, 11,010 of the subjects continued to take the drug on at least 180 days a year, while 3,849 took little or no aspirin. In 2000, the study reported that over a seven-year period, a low-dose aspirin was associated with a 35 percent reduction in cardiovascular deaths and a 36 percent drop in total mortality.

The Physicians' Health Study trial has provided additional information about aspirin's effect on the heart. The drug seems most effective in the early morning hours, when platelets are particularly likely to stick together and produce clots. It is a good thing, since that is when heart attacks are most likely to occur. Aspirin begins working rapidly and it remains effective as long as it is being taken. That is because the very first dose will inhibit all the platelets in a man's blood, but the body does not build up resistance to the drug. Aspirin was effective in preventing heart attacks in men who had angina, but it did not prevent healthy men from developing angina. That's because angina is caused by plaques that produce partial blockages, but heart attacks are the result of clots that form on plaques.

SECONDARY PREVENTION OF HEART ATTACKS

The Physicians' Health Study was the first to show aspirin can protect healthy men older than fifty against heart attacks, but it was not the first to show that aspirin can help the heart. In fact, dozens of studies dating back to 1971 have demonstrated that aspirin has an important role in secondary prevention, in preventing second or third heart attacks in patients who have survived a first attack. In all, aspirin reduced the risk of recurrent heart attacks by about 25 percent. It only takes low doses of aspirin, between 75 and 325 milligrams a day, to produce this major benefit. At present, up to 25 percent of American heart attack survivors fail to take aspirin. It is a shame, since if all the heart attack patients who could take aspirin did so, it could prevent another 20,000 deaths annually.

OTHER VASCULAR DISEASES

Atherosclerosis can strike any artery in the body; in addition to the heart, its most important targets are arteries in the legs and brain.

The Physicians' Health Study found that low-dose aspirin might protect the legs against severe blockages of peripheral artery disease. During an observation period that averaged about five years, men who took 325 milligrams of aspirin every other day were 46 percent less likely to require surgery for leg artery blockages than men who took placebos.

The issue of stroke is more complex because there are two types of strokes (see Chapter Three): *hemorrhagic strokes* occur when an artery in the brain ruptures, releasing blood into the tissue, but *ischemic strokes* result when clots block arteries in the brain. The Physicians' Health Study found that low-dose aspirin produces a slight increase in hemorrhagic strokes, but the heightened risk was too small to be statistically significant; other studies have reported similar results. At the same time, though, aspirin can help prevent ischemic strokes, which are four times more common than hemorrhagic strokes. In fact, two 1997 studies of more than 40,000 stroke patients found that low-dose aspirin (100 or 300 milligrams a day) produced a small but significant benefit, both by improving recovery and reducing the risk of a second stroke. More recently, a 1999 meta-analysis of eleven randomized, placebo-controlled trials found that low-dose aspirin reduced the risk of both types of stroke, combined, by 15 percent. But because high blood pressure increases the risk of hemorrhagic stroke, men with hypertension should not use low-dose aspirin until their blood pressures are brought under control (see Chapter Three).

Other Possible Benefits

Although the Physicians' Health Study was most interested in aspirin's effect on atherosclerosis, it also investigated other conditions. For example, it found that low-dose aspirin reduced the occurrence of migraine headaches by 20 percent. It also found a slight decrease in cataracts, but the difference was not statistically significant, and other research has failed to demonstrate protection against cataracts.

An area of much greater importance is the possibility that aspirin may reduce the risk of colon cancer. It is an unresolved question, and it is one of the few areas of disagreement among the Harvard men's health studies. The Physicians' Health Study found no reduction in colon cancer among the men who took 325 milligrams of aspirin every other day. In contrast, the Health Professionals Study found that men who used aspirin at least twice a week were 32 percent less likely to develop colon cancer than men who took it less often.

Although the issue is far from resolved, other research suggests that aspirin may help. In laboratory experiments, aspirin and other nonsteroidal anti-inflammatory drugs (NSAIDs) can influence *apoptosis,* programmed cell death that prevents the unchecked growth of cancer cells (see Chapter Three). In rodents exposed to cancer-causing chemicals, NSAIDs inhibit the development of tumors in the colon. In animals and humans with hereditary polyps, NSAIDs can reverse the formation of the benign polyps from which colon cancers develop. In ten of twelve observational studies in humans, aspirin or other NSAIDs seemed protective. For example, in a 1991 American Cancer Society study of 662,424 people, aspirin use was associated with a 40 percent lower risk of dying from colon cancer over a six-year period. In all, the majority of studies report that NSAIDs use is associated with a 40 to 50 percent reduction in the risk of colon cancer.

The effects of NSAIDs on cognitive function are also intriguing. A sixteen-year study of 1,686 people in Baltimore linked the use of various NSAIDs to a 50 percent reduction in Alzheimer's disease. Although various NSAIDs appeared effective, aspirin itself was not protective. Other research, also preliminary, suggests that aspirin may reduce the risk of another type of mental decline, *multi-infarct dementia,* perhaps by preventing "mini strokes" (see Chapter Eight).

More research is needed to learn if aspirin can reduce a man's risk of colon cancer or dementia. At present, neither possibility is strong enough to serve as the sole reason to take aspirin. But since low-dose aspirin has a proven role in preventing heart attacks and some strokes, at least in men over fifty and in patients of any age who have had cardiovascular events, another reason is not really necessary.

Side Effects

Although you can buy it in convenience stores and vending machines, aspirin is a medication—and a powerful one, at that. Like all medications, it can have side effects.

Bleeding is the most common adverse effect of aspirin and other NSAIDs. Even low-dose aspirin can prolong the oozing from a shaving nick or turn a small black and blue into a sizable bruise. Because aspirin inhibits platelets, it increases the risk of bleeding after injury, which is why no one should take NSAIDs within seven to ten days of elective surgery. More worrisome is stomach irritation and intestinal bleeding. In fact, about 41,000 Americans are hospitalized each year because of NSAID-induced intestinal bleeding. Other side effects can include ringing in the ears and elevated blood pressure, which is a particular concern for elderly patients or those with kidney disease. NSAIDs can cause temporary kidney dysfunction, especially in the elderly, and toxic doses of *acetaminophen* (Tylenol and other brands) and NSAIDs may produce permanent damage. In 2001, however, the Physicians Health Study found no evidence linking kidney disease to acetaminophen and NSAID use, even in men who had taken more than 2,500 pills during fourteen years of observation.

All of these aspirin side effects are dose-related; that is, they are much more common with higher doses than with the low dose used for prevention. In the Physicians' Health Study, aspirin was quite safe, though it did produce an increased risk of bleeding, which was usually minor. Still, men with histories of bleeding disorders, ulcers, hypertension, or kidney disease should not use aspirin without a doctor's okay, and the occasional man who is allergic to aspirin should not take it at all. Patients who take the anticoagulant *warfarin* (Coumadin) should not use aspirin or other NSAIDs unless they are specifically instructed to do so by their physicians; even then, close monitoring is mandatory.

Related Drugs

Americans consume some 385 tons of aspirin and spend about $18 billion on NSAIDs every year. Table 6.1 lists some of the many brands of NSAIDs.

Table 6.1: SELECTED NONSTEROIDAL ANTIINFLAMMATORY DRUGS

Generic Name	Brand Name
Aspirin*	Many
Diclofinac	Voltaren, Cataflam
Diflunisal	Dolobid
Etodolac	Lodine
Fenoprofen	Nalfon
Fluribrofen	Ansaid
Ibuprofen*	Advil, Motrin, and others
Indomethacin	Indocin
Ketoprofen	Orudis, Oruvail
Meloxicam	Mobic
Nabumetone	Relafen
Naproxen*	Aleve, Anaprox, Naprelan, Naprosyn
Oxaprozin	Daypro
Piroxicam	Feldene
Sulindac	Clinoril
Tolmetin	Tolectin

* Available without prescription.

All the NSAIDs inhibit prostaglandins, but they do not act on prostaglandins themselves. Instead, they inhibit *cyclo-oxygenase* (COX), the enzyme that generates prostaglandins. New research shows that there are actually two distinct forms of cyclo-oxygenase, COX-1, and COX-2. COX-1 is responsible for most of the "good" prostaglandins in the stomach and kidneys, while COX-2 is behind the "bad" prostaglandins that trigger inflammation, fever, and pain.

Aspirin and other NSAIDs produce many of their therapeutic effects by inhibiting COX-2, but because they also inhibit COX-1 they have unwanted side effects. New "super aspirin" including *celecoxib* (Celebrex), *rofecoxib* (Vioxx), and *valdecoxib* (Bextra) inhibit COX-2 but not COX-1. As a result, they can fight pain, inflammation, and fever, with a lower risk of stomach irritation and bleeding. Unfortunately, however, new research shows that the COX-2 inhibitors are far from perfect. They can trigger high blood pressure and kidney dysfunction, particularly in older people. The COX-2 inhibitors are also much more expensive than aspirin and most other NSAIDs, and because they are new, they may turn out to have additional side effects.

In terms of prevention, the COX-2 inhibitors may share aspirin's potential for inhibiting colon cancer, but they do not share low-dose aspirin's role in preventing heart attacks and strokes. To do that, a medication must block COX-1—or inhibit platelets in another way. Several drugs that inhibit platelets have been licensed for clinical use in the United States. *Dipyridamole* has long been available alone (Persantine), but is finding a new role in combination with aspirin (Aggrenox). For several years, cardiologists routinely prescribed *ticlopidine* (Ticlid) to prevent clots from reblocking coronary arteries newly opened by balloon angioplasty; it is effective but expensive. Although it spares the stomach, it has potentially serious side effects of its own, which is why it has been supplanted by a newer medication, *cloidoquel* (Plavix), which is safer but even more costly. In a 1996 study, cloidoquel proved slightly more effective than aspirin preventing cardiovascular events in 19,185 patients with atherosclerosis. Even more recently, the FDA approved *turbofan* (Aggrastat) and *ebtifibatide* (Intergrilin), injectable antiplatelet drugs modeled after viper venom, for early treatment of heart attacks. Attempts to develop oral forms of these drugs are underway, but have not yet been successful.

IS LOW-DOSE ASPIRIN RIGHT FOR YOU?

If you have had angina, a heart attack, a transient ischemic attack, or an ischemic stroke (see Chapter Three), you should be taking low-dose aspirin. Unless, of course, you have a specific reason to stay away from the drug.

If you are a healthy man older than fifty, you may also benefit from low-dose aspirin. The presence of cardiac risk factors (see Chapter Three) would tip the scales in favor of aspirin, but a history of bleeding, ulcers, or other aspirin-related problems would argue against routine aspirin use.

If you decide to take aspirin, you will have to pick a dose and a preparation. Low doses are best, but regimens of 81 milligrams or 160 milligrams a day or 325 milligrams a day or every other day are all reasonable. Many doctors recommend enteric-coated preparations to reduce the risk of stomach irritation, but it is not certain that coated or buffered formulations are really safer than plain aspirin. In any case, be alert for side effects, such as stomach irritation or bleeding, no matter which tablet you choose.

What if you develop a fever or pain while you are on preventive doses of aspirin? Since low doses are best, the logical step would be to use acetaminophen (Tylenol and other brands), which does not affect platelets at all. A COX-2 inhibitor would be another, more costly, prescription alternative. Remember, though, to continue your low-dose aspirin for prevention while you are taking acetaminophen or a COX-2 inhibitor for therapy. But if you need an NSAID or high-dose aspirin to treat arthritis or other problems, go ahead and use it while you have to, then get back to low-dose aspirin for prevention.

Aspirin is not a panacea, but low doses can substantially reduce the risk of heart attack and stroke. If aspirin is right for you, take a tablet every day or two, but call your doctor in the morning if you suspect side effects. Do not pin all your hopes on aspirin alone; instead, use it in conjunction with diet and exercise to keep your heart healthy. And read on to learn about other supplements that may help.

Multivitamins

The only way scientists can be sure if a supplement is beneficial is to conduct a randomized clinical trial. It is the way low-dose aspirin proved its worth, and the way beta-carotene and vitamin E lost their appeal (see Antioxidants, page 172). Multivitamins have not yet been subjected to this stern test, but even though proof of efficacy is lacking, many doctors are starting to recommend a daily multivitamin to nearly all their patients. I think it is the right thing to do. The cost is low, the risks are nil, and the potential benefits are substantial, depending largely on three B vitamins and vitamin D.

Folic acid, vitamin B_6 (*pyridoxine*), and vitamin B_{12} (*cobalamin*) may reduce the risk of heart attacks. These vitamins lower blood levels of *homocysteine,* a newly recognized cardiac risk factor (see Chapter Three). The evidence is best for folic acid and B_6; in 1996, the Health Professionals Study found that a high intake of folic acid was associated with a 29 percent reduction in heart attacks, and that a high intake of B_6 reduced risk by 23 percent. The Physicians' Health Study reported similar findings in the same year. And these benefits are not restricted to men. The Harvard-based Nurses' Health Study found women who had a high intake of folic acid and B_6 had risks of heart attacks that were 31 and

33 percent lower, respectively, than women with low intakes; women who consumed healthy amounts of both vitamins enjoyed a 45 percent reduction in risk. More good news: it does not take megadoses of vitamins to produce these gains. In fact, just 400 micrograms of folic acid and 3 milligrams of B_6 seem optimal. Both vitamins are found in leafy green vegetables and other foods, and folic acid is added to fortified breakfast cereals; still, many Americans do not get all they need (see Chapter Four).

Folic acid may also reduce the risk of colon cancer. In 1993, the Health Professionals Study and the Nurses' Health Study issued a combined report demonstrating that in both men and women a high intake of folic acid appeared to reduce the risk of the benign intestinal polyps from which cancers arise. In 1995, the Health Professionals Study found that a high intake of folic acid reduced the risk of colon cancer in men who drank alcohol, and in 1998, the Nurses' Health Study found that long-term use of folic-acid-containing multivitamins was associated with a substantial reduction in colon cancer.

Vitamin B_{12} is found naturally only in animal products, but is added to fortified cereals. Most American diets contain more than the 2.4 micrograms recommended each day, but strict vegetarian diets may provide less. Up to 30 percent of people over fifty do not absorb B_{12} well because they produce abnormally small amounts of stomach acid. A multivitamin can help by providing B_{12} in crystalline form, which is easier to absorb even without stomach acid.

The other important ingredient in a multivitamin is vitamin D (*calciferol*), which is essential for strong bones. It is hard to get enough vitamin D from your diet, and people who wisely avoid ultraviolet exposure in sunlight are often vitamin D-deficient (see Chapter Four).

Although multivitamins may be very beneficial, the gains depend on long-term use to reduce the risk of disease. If the Physicians' Health Study is right, you may even reduce your risk of cataracts as well as heart disease and colon cancer. In the short run, though, you cannot expect extra energy, improved sexuality, better sleep, less stress, or any of the other "benefits" hyped by the supplement industry. Look for a multivitamin that contains at least 400 micrograms of folic acid, 2–6 milligrams of B_6, at least 2.4 micrograms of B_{12}, and 400 International Units (IU) of vitamin D. Do not focus on other vitamins or minerals; most multivitamin tablets contain 50 to 100 percent of the recommended daily allowance of these chemicals, which is just fine (see Tables 4.8 and 4.9). Do not waste your money on designer vitamins that contain unnecessary herbs or other extras, megadoses, "all natural" preparations, or expensive brand names; generic multivitamins that contain the right amounts of the three B's and D will fill the bill. To assure quality, look for a formulation that meets the standards of the United States Pharmacopeia, a private rating organization; select a product that is fully labeled as to content, dosage, and expiration date. And remember that food is the best source of vitamins, minerals, and other nutrients. In particular, vegetables, fruits, and whole grain products supply dietary fiber and many other important nutrients as well as vitamins.

Antioxidants

Just a few short years ago, multivitamins were in eclipse and antioxidant vitamins were the rage. New research on B vitamins, homocysteine, and vitamin D has put the spotlight on multivitamins, while studies of beta-carotene and vitamin E have dampened the enthusiasm for antioxidants.

What are Antioxidants?

Antioxidants protect the body against free radicals—not the high-spirited youths of the Woodstock generation, but the high-energy molecules that are generated by the body's metabolism when it burns carbohydrates for energy. Free radicals are molecules that have extra, unpaired electrons; as a result, they are highly unstable. Oxygen free radicals are the most potent. In some circumstances, oxygen free radicals can be a boon to health; when they meet up with bacteria that have invaded the body, for example, they can use their extra energy to kill the microbes. But in other circumstances, oxygen free radicals are a bane; when they encounter LDL cholesterol, they turn it into the oxidized LDL that causes the inflammatory damage of atherosclerosis, and when oxygen free radicals attack DNA, they can contribute to defects that lead to unregulated cell growth, cancer (see Chapter Three). The damage caused by oxygen free radicals may also contribute to cataracts, dementia and other neurologic disorders, arthritis, and even the aging process itself.

The body produces oxygen free radicals continuously, but it also has an elaborate series of mechanisms to keep them in check. The food we eat can play a role in the struggle between oxygen free radicals and the antioxidants that neutralize them. Although oxygen free radicals are not present in natural foods, they can be produced when foods are processed or cooked. In particular, heating and frying can generate toxic oxidation products from polyunsaturated fatty acids. On the other side are the natural antioxidants in foods, including vitamin C, vitamin E, and vitamin A and its precursors in the carotenoid family.

ANTIOXIDANTS IN FOODS

One of the most important and consistent findings in nutritional research is that people who eat the most fruits, vegetables, and whole grains have the lowest risk of heart attacks, strokes, cancer, and premature death. It is tempting to think that the vitamins in these foods play an important role in protection. Indeed, several studies have reported that people with low blood or tissue levels of vitamin C, vitamin E, or carotenoids have a high risk of atherosclerosis. But nutrition is very complex. The same foods that provide antioxidant vitamins are also high in B vitamins, dietary fiber, and various minerals. Any of these ingredients could be the protective element. Or, perhaps, a combination of ingredients is necessary for protection. To carry the argument one step further, the protection afforded by a healthy diet may depend as much on the absence of animal fat as on the presence of vitamin-rich vegetable foods.

The best advice, of course, is to eat lots of vegetables, fruits, and whole grains. The multivitamins that I also suggest provide modest amounts of antioxidant vitamins—enough to prevent deficiency diseases, but much less than the amounts that some believe helpful for fighting heart disease and cancer. Should you take additional antioxidant supplements? In the case of beta-carotene the answer is no, in the case of vitamins E and C, maybe.

CAROTENOIDS AND VITAMIN A

The carotenoids are a family of more than 600 chemicals. Found only in plants, they are converted to vitamin A by the tissues of herbivorous animals. First discovered in 1909, vitamin A is essential for night vision and for healthy skin, hair, bones, and teeth. In addition, vitamin A is an antioxidant. The average American gets about two-thirds of his vitamin A from meat and dairy products, the remainder from carotenoids in vegetables that are converted into vitamin A.

The U.S. Dietary Reference Intake for vitamin A is 5,000 International Units a day. Because vitamin A is fat soluble, it is stored away in the body's tissue. Over time, daily doses of 10,000 units or more can build up to toxic levels that can result in liver damage, brain swelling, eye and skin problems, and an increased fracture risk.

The carotenoids, in contrast, seem to be nontoxic, even in very large doses. For years, scientists thought that carotenoids were important only as precursors of vitamin A, but it is now clear that they have important activities of their own, including potent antioxidant properties. Carotenoids are present in deep green and yellow-orange fruits and vegetables such as carrots, pumpkin, squash, sweet potatoes, apricots, cantaloupe, spinach, broccoli, turnip greens, and Brussels sprouts. Beta-carotene is the best-known member of the family, but *lycopene*, which is found particularly in tomatoes, is an even more potent antioxidant.

There can be little doubt that eating carotenoid-rich foods is good for you (see Chapter Four). The Health Professionals Study provides an important example: A high intake of lycopene from tomatoes (especially cooked tomatoes) was linked to a 20 to 30 percent decrease in the risk of prostate cancer, and it reduced the risk of the most aggressive prostate cancers by 50 percent. But can a beta-carotene pill provide the same benefit as carrots, cantaloupe, and broccoli?

To find out, the Physicians' Health Study conducted a randomized clinical trial in concert with its low-dose aspirin study. Starting in 1982, 11,036 men between the ages of forty and eighty-four took 50 milligrams of beta-carotene every other day, while 11,035 took a placebo. The men were randomly assigned to take the vitamin or the placebo, and neither the subjects nor the researchers knew who was taking beta-carotene and who was taking the inert tablet. When the study concluded in 1995, the scientists found no difference between the two groups, either in terms of heart disease, stroke, cancer, or overall mortality; in particular, the rate of lung cancer and prostate cancer was not influenced by beta-carotene. And in 1999, the Physicians' Health Study reported that the beta-carotene supplements had not reduced the risk of diabetes.

Dr. Charles Hennekens, who directed the study, termed it the greatest disappointment of his professional career, but he was not the only researcher disappointed by beta-carotene. Beta-carotene has been studied in four other randomized clinical trials. The Beta-carotene and Retinol Efficacy Trial (CARET) administered 30 milligrams of beta-carotene and 25,000 international units of vitamin A or a placebo to 18,314 men and women who were at high risk of lung cancer because of smoking or asbestos exposure. The trial began in 1985 and was scheduled to run until 1997, but it was terminated prematurely because a trend was emerging. Unfortunately, the trend was in the "wrong" direction: There were actually more cases of lung cancer and cardiovascular disease and more deaths in the vitamin-treated group. As in the Physicians' Health Study, beta-carotene supplements had no effect on prostate cancer.

The Alpha-Tocopherol, Beta-Carotene (ATBC) Cancer Prevention Trial compared a placebo with alpha-tocopherol (vitamin E, 50 milligrams) and beta-carotene (20 milligrams), either alone or in combination. The subjects were 29,133 Finnish male smokers. As in the CARET study, the men who took beta-carotene had an increased incidence of lung cancer and a slight increase in deaths from heart disease. Unlike the Physicians' Health Study and the CARET trial, however, the ATBC trial noted a slight increase in the risk of prostate cancer among the men who took beta-carotene. In contrast, vitamin E did appear to decrease the risk of prostate cancer (see vitamin E, below), but it did not affect the risk of lung cancer or cardiac deaths.

Another trial of beta-carotene was different in two respects. First, it did not test beta-carotene (15 milligrams) alone, but in a cocktail that also contained vitamin E (130 milligrams) and selenium (50 micrograms). Second, the subjects were not well-nourished Americans or Finns, but 29,584 poorly nourished residents of Linxian, China. In this population, the triple cocktail appeared to reduce the overall death rate, largely due to a decline in stomach cancer and other malignancies.

The final trial was much smaller, involving just 1,720 Americans, but it illustrates the dilemma of beta-carotene. When researchers measured beta-carotene blood levels before they administered the vitamin, they found that the people with the lowest blood levels had the highest risk of dying from cardiovascular disease and all other causes. But supplements of 50 milligrams of beta-carotene a day for more than four years did not change things, even for the people whose initial blood levels were low.

We do not yet know why beta-carotene supplements appear to increase the risk of lung cancer in smokers; part of the explanation may depend on the fact that smoking lowers vitamin C levels. Even though beta-carotene seems safe in nonsmokers, it is not beneficial.

It is an important message about beta-carotene and a cautionary tale for other supplements: Vitamin-rich foods are associated with better health but, in the case of beta-carotene at least, supplements are not.

VITAMIN E

Vitamin E is not a single compound but a family of chemicals called *tocopherols*. The most common member of the group is *alpha-tocopherol,* which is the form of vitamin E that is present in most supplements. Alpha-tocopherol was first discovered in 1922; despite our long familiarity with it, however, vitamin E is in many respects a mystery vitamin. Its precise function in the human metabolism is not known, and there is no clearly defined vitamin E deficiency disease. But it is clear that vitamin E is a potent antioxidant, and it appears to act as the first line of defense against oxygen free radicals. As a fat-soluble vitamin, in fact, vitamin E travels in the same package that carries LDL cholesterol, even entering the arterial wall with LDL. Vitamin E can also accumulate in the body's fat depots. There is concern that high doses might interfere with blood clotting or with the body's ability to fight infection, but actual toxic effects have not been documented.

For men, the Dietary Reference Intake of vitamin E is 15 milligrams, or about 22 International Units, a day. Vitamin E is present in many foods, including vegetable oils, wheat germ, nuts, butter, eggs, and margarine. In addition, most cereals are fortified with vitamin E. It's not hard to get the RDA of vitamin E from foods—a tablespoon of canola oil, for example, has about 12 international units—but it is very difficult to get the higher amounts that may help protect the heart without taking supplements.

In 1996, the Health Professionals Study provided some optimistic news about vitamin E; men who took at least 100 international units of vitamin E a day for two years or longer enjoyed a 37 percent lower risk of developing heart disease than men who did not take supplements. Similar results in women were reported by the Nurses' Health Study in the same year.

Although their findings were hopeful, these observational studies cannot establish a cause and effect relationship. Randomized clinical trials are the best way to do that, but for vitamin E and cardiovascular disease the latest evidence is discouraging. The ATBC trial found no benefit against heart disease in male smokers, but the dose of 50 milligrams, or about 75 international units, was low. However, a two-year Italian study of 11,324 heart attack survivors found that 300 milligrams of vitamin E did not protect against cardiac events. Similarly, the nineteen-nation HOPE trial of 9,541 patients failed to detect benefit from 400 international units of vitamin E over a four-and-a-half-year period. And in 2001, the Primary Prevention Project study of 4,495 people with cardiovascular risk factors found no benefit from 300 milligrams of vitamin E a day for nearly four years. Standing alone on the positive side of the ledger, the Cambridge Heart Antioxidant study (CHAOS) found that over a one-year period, a daily dose of 400 or 800 international units of vitamin E reduced the risk of heart attack in patients with known coronary artery disease. Even in this study, however, vitamin E did not reduce cardiovascular deaths.

Although scientists have been most interested in the possibility that vitamin E may reduce the risk of heart disease, they have evaluated other potential roles for the vitamin. The Health Professionals Study reported that vitamin E appeared to reduce a man's risk of bladder cancer, but it detected no protection against stroke. However, a small Rhode Island study of 100 patients with transient ischemic attacks ("mini-strokes") suggested that 400 international units of vitamin E could add to the protection afforded by aspirin. A 1994 study suggested that a very high dose of vitamin E, 2000 international units a day, might slow the progression of Alzheimer's disease, but there is no evidence that the vitamin will prevent healthy men from developing the disease. Although there is new evidence that a supplement containing zinc and multiple antioxidants can reduce the risk of visual loss due to macular degeneration, the Physicians' Health Study found no evidence of protection from vitamin E, vitamin C, or multivitamins.

Prostate cancer is a special concern for men, and here, too, vitamin E has had its ups and downs. The ATBC trial raised our hopes when it reported that supplements of vitamin E appeared to reduce the risk of dying from prostate cancer by 41 percent. But all 29,133 Finnish men in the trial were smokers. When the Health Professionals' Study evaluated the impact of vitamin E on prostate cancer, it found that apparent protection was confined to men who were smokers or recent quitters; nonsmokers did not benefit from vitamin E supplements.

The vitamin E story is complex, and its benefits for the prostate are far from certain. But even before the last chapter has been written, new research tells us that the situation is even more complex than it seemed.

The latest player is *gamma-tocopherol,* a form of vitamin E that is found in foods such as soybean and corn oil, but not in most supplements. A 2001 study of 10,456 residents of Maryland found that men with the highest blood levels of gamma-tocopherol were only one-fifth as likely to develop prostate cancer as men with the lowest levels. High levels of selenium and alpha-tocopherol also seemed to help, at least in men who also had high levels of gamma-tocopheral. And if this were not complex enough there is another wrinkle: vitamin E supplements that provide alpha-tocopherol (especially above 400 international units) may actually lower blood levels of gamma-tocopherol.

It will take time for scientists to sort this out. The Physicians' Health Study has begun a randomized clinical trial of vitamin E that may resolve the uncertainties. But until the results are available, soy is looking pretty good (see Chapter Twelve).

VITAMIN C

Vitamin C is one of the most popular supplements in America. Doctor Linus Pauling was responsible for much of its appeal; his stature as the winner of two Nobel Prizes—one for Chemistry and one for Peace—helped popularize his theory that megadoses of vitamin C prevent the common cold. Controlled clinical trials have disproved that theory, but vitamin C remains a best seller. Newer theories suggest that it may reduce the risk of heart disease and cancer, but the evidence is mixed at best.

Vitamin C (*ascorbic acid*) has an important role in the body's metabolism. It is a cofactor for at least eight enzymes involved in building proteins from amino acids and in the production of a stress hormone in the adrenaline family. Vitamin C is also an antioxidant. Research suggests that its main roles are to scavenge free radicals that have escaped vitamin E and beta-carotene, and to regenerate vitamin E. The Dietary Reference Intake for vitamin C is 90 milligrams a day. Vitamin C is found in many fruits and vegetables, including citrus fruits, potatoes, broccoli, melons, tomatoes, spinach, and cabbage; a cup of orange juice contains 120 milligrams. Dietary deficiencies of vitamin C cause scurvy, but that disease is now very rare in the United States.

Several studies suggest that people who eat large amounts of vitamin C-rich foods have a lower risk of heart disease and cancer. It is not clear, though, if the benefit depends on vitamin C itself or on other substances in fruits and vegetables. The Health Professionals Study found no evidence that a high intake of vitamin C reduces the risk of heart attack or stroke, and the Nurses' Health Study reported similar results. To date, no study has demonstrated benefit from vitamin C supplements. To clarify the issue, the Physicians' Health Study has embarked on a randomized clinical trial of vitamin C tablets in men.

Men should eat at least five servings of fruits and vegetables a day (see Chapter Four); meeting this goal will provide 200 to 300 milligrams of vitamin C a day. There is no evidence that additional doses are helpful, but men who wish to take more should not exceed 250 to 500 milligrams a day, since higher doses may be counterproductive.

Niacin (Vitamin B_3)

Niacin is a vitamin that goes by several names: nicotinic acid, niacinamide, and vitamin B_3. By any name, it is a water-soluble vitamin that has an important role in enabling the body to obtain energy from carbohydrates, fats, and proteins. People who don't get enough niacin develop *pellegra*, a deficiency disease characterized by diarrhea, fatigue, confusion, and a rash. Niacin deficiency is exceedingly rare in the developed world, since just 20 milligrams a day will maintain health. The vitamin is found in many foods, including legumes, peanuts, fish, poultry, meat, eggs, and products made from fortified grains.

Even though healthy men do not need extra niacin, it is present in multivitamins. However, niacin supplements are heavily promoted on their own to reduce cholesterol levels. They do work; niacin can lower LDL ("bad") cholesterol levels by 20 to 40 percent, making it as effective as many statin drugs. Niacin will also lower triglyceride levels by 40 to 60 percent, something most statins cannot do. Best of all, niacin is unrivaled in ability to boost HDL ("good") cholesterol levels, often by 10 to 30 percent.

An all-natural, inexpensive vitamin with wonderful effects on blood cholesterol levels—it sounds too good to be true. It is true, but there is an important catch: To improve blood cholesterol levels, niacin must be consumed in amounts 25 to 150 times above the DRI, or 500 to 3,000 milligrams a day. In these doses, niacin can have major side effects, including liver inflammation, headaches, itching and flushing of the skin, gout, internal bleeding, high blood sugar levels, and sexual dysfunction.

All in all, niacin is a poster boy for the case against unregulated nutritional supplements. It actually is a nutrient, and it does work—two things that many supplements do not have going for them. But preparations vary substantially in potency and purity, so a man cannot be sure what he is getting when he swallows a niacin tablet. And in the doses that work, niacin can have major side effects.

Do not take niacin on your own. But if you have a high LDL and a low HDL that does not respond to diet and exercise, ask your doctor to consider niacin among your medicinal options. If your doctor recommends niacin, use it carefully: Pick one preparation and stick with it; increase the dose gradually, listen to your body to detect problems, and have regular medical tests to detect side effects.

Although it is sold as a nonprescription supplement, in therapeutic doses niacin is actually a powerful drug. Treat it as such, using it only under your doctor's supervision.

Selenium

Selenium is a trace element that is essential for health. Only small amounts are required; the DRI for men is just 55 micrograms. Selenium is provided by many foods, including tomatoes, shellfish, poultry, garlic, meat, and whole grains and vegetables grown in selenium-rich soils.

Scientists have been interested in selenium because it functions as an antioxidant. As a result, doctors have wondered if selenium might help prevent heart attacks or cancer. To date, the evidence is mixed.

In 1982, a Finnish study reported that people with low blood selenium levels had an increased risk for developing coronary artery disease, and a 1991 study of Finnish men linked low selenium levels to atherosclerosis of the carotid artery. In 1995, however, the Physicians' Health Study cast considerable doubt on the hypothesis that selenium protects the heart. In fact, in American men, high selenium levels were associated with a slight increase in heart attack risk.

To learn if selenium supplements might reduce the risk of recurrent skin cancer, a team of scientists headquartered in Arizona administered either 200 micrograms of selenium or a placebo to 1,312 volunteers with an average age of sixty-three; the participants took their tablets daily for an average of four-and-a-half years. When the study ended in 1996, the researchers were disappointed to learn that there was no difference in the occurrence of skin cancer between the two groups, but they were startled to find that there were about 50 percent fewer cancer deaths in the selenium group. Selenium was linked to a significant reduction in deaths from lung, colon, esophageal, and prostate cancer; protections appeared strongest for prostate cancer, with 63 percent fewer deaths in the men who took selenium. These results were greeted with great interest but also with caution; some doctors felt they were too good to be true, and most stressed the need for further research.

In 1998, the Health Professionals Study provided some of that additional research. Instead of administering supplements, the researchers evaluated the mineral intake by analyzing the selenium content of toenail clippings submitted by 33,737 men. The men who had the highest selenium levels were only about one-third as likely to develop advanced prostate cancer as the men with the lowest levels. The Harvard team calculated that a daily intake of 159 micrograms of selenium would achieve the protective levels.

Despite these two encouraging studies, it is too early to make a blanket recommendation for selenium. Still, until more data are available, a supplement of 200 micrograms a day would be a reasonable choice for men, particularly those with an increased prostrate cancer risk (see Chapters Three and Twelve). Remember, though, that excessive amounts of selenium can be toxic; hair loss and skin disorders begin to appear at levels above 400 micrograms a day.

Chromium

Chromium is another trace metal that is important for carbohydrate metabolism; the precise daily requirement is not known, but the Food and Nutrition Board of the National Academy of Sciences suggests a daily intake of 35 micrograms a day. Dietary sources of chromium include brewer's yeast, peanuts, legumes, and whole grains as well as meat and cheese.

Do not believe most of what you hear about chromium. A compound called chromium picolinate is heavily promoted for weight loss, increased energy, and other "benefits." Unfortunately, there is no evidence to support any of these claims, and in test-tube experiments, large amounts of chromium picolinate may cause cell damage.

Although chromium does not live up to its hype, it may have one benefit that can help some men. Between 1968 and 1982, six independent trials suggested that chromium might raise HDL cholesterol levels, but these studies were small and flawed. In 1991, however, doctors in North Carolina tested an organic form of chromium against a placebo in sixty-three men with low HDL levels. Over a two-month period, the mineral produced a 16 percent rise in the average HDL levels without any apparent side effects. It is only one trial and only lasted two months. More research is needed to see if chromium can produce a sustained rise in HDLs. Until new information is available, men with low HDLs can consider trying the North Carolina regimen of a form of chromium called *glucose tolerance factor* (GTF) in a dose of 200 micrograms three times a day. Needless to say, though, no one should turn to GTF without first trying to raise his HDL through quitting smoking (Chapter Eight), exercise (Chapter Five), weight loss and diet (Chapter Four), and possibly low-dose alcohol (Chapter Seven).

Other Supplements

If you do not believe that supplements are a big business, just stroll down the aisles of a few drug stores, supermarkets, or health food shops. The array of products is bewildering, the claims made for them no less overwhelming.

Aside from the supplements we have discussed here and possibly calcium (see Chapter Four), there is no reason for healthy men to consider any of these products. A few may be useful for men with specific health problems, but because these products are unregulated, there is no assurance about efficacy or safety, potency or purity. Here is a quick run-down on some of the most popular supplements.

Saw Palmetto

It is an herbal extract sold under many names for the treatment of prostate disorders. Studies in Europe suggest that it may alleviate symptoms of *benign prostatic hyperplasia* (BPH), but there is no evidence that it will prevent BPH, much less prostate cancer. Saw palmetto has no effect on sexual function. Despite scientific uncertainties, men with BPH who do not respond well to prescription medications might consider a trial of saw palmetto—after checking with their doctors, of course (see Chapter Eleven).

Fish Oil

Doctors first became aware of the potential benefits of fish oil in 1971, when Danish scientists reported that the Eskimos of Greenland had a very low rate of heart attacks despite eating large amounts of fat. They postulated that protection depended on *eicosapentaenoic* acid (EPA) and *docosahexaenoic* acid (DHA), two omega-3 fatty acids found in fish oil.

Over the past thirty years, researchers have accumulated a substantial body of evidence that eating fish is beneficial. In one study, people who consumed at least 8.75 ounces of fish a week enjoyed a 38 percent reduction in fatal heart attacks, and in another, heart attack survivors who ate fish twice a week were 29 percent less likely to suffer recurrent attacks than comparable patients who did not eat fish. Although not all studies agree that eating fish protects against heart attacks, fish consumption has been linked with a reduced risk of sudden death, hypertension, and stroke (see Chapter Four).

If eating fish is helpful, perhaps men should skip the shopping and cooking and take their fish oil straight up. Indeed, fish oil was a popular supplement in the 1980s, but it began to fade when studies reported little sustained benefit.

Two 1999 studies are reviving interest in fish oil supplements. Doctors in Germany administered capsules containing fish oil or vegetable oil to 223 heart patients. After two years, the people who took fish oil (6 grams a day for 3 months, then 3 grams a day) had fewer cardiac events and better angiograms than their peers, but the protection was modest. A much larger Italian study of 11,324 heart attack survivors was more positive, reporting that just 882 milligrams of EPA and DHA a day appeared to reduce the risk of cardiac events by 10 percent.

It is far too early to recommend fish oil supplements for everyone, or even for all cardiac patients. For now, eat your fish and stay tuned for the results of additional research.

GARLIC

Garlic (*Allium satirum*) traces its origins to central Asia. Although the plant grew wild for centuries, it now exists only as a cultivated crop. About 2 million tons are harvested annually. Most garlic is processed into a dry powder, but some medicinal preparations use oil that is extracted from the cloves. Garlic can also be aged and fermented to remove its odor. Garlic powder is considered the most medically active preparation, deodorized garlic, the least.

Of the nearly 100 chemicals in garlic, the most important appears to be *allicin,* a sulfur-containing amino acid. Allicin is not present in fresh garlic, but it is formed instantly from its parent chemical when cloves are crushed or cut. Scientists believe that allicin is responsible for the biologic activity of garlic; cooks know it is responsible for the characteristic odor that has earned the name "stinking rose." Most garlic powder preparations are standardized to contain a specified amount of allicin. Laboratory experiments have studied either whole garlic or purified extracts, but most clinical trials have used garlic powder.

Garlic is widely promoted to fight heart disease. Experiments in animals and test tubes suggest that garlic may help in several ways, by lowering cholesterol, reducing blood pressure, keeping arteries supple, and fighting clot formation. Experiments in test tubes and rats do not necessarily translate into benefits for humans. In the past ten years, however, there have been credible human studies of garlic and health, but the results are mixed.

The possibility that garlic could lower cholesterol in humans got a big boost in the early 1990s. First, studies in Germany found that a popular garlic powder (Kwai) could lower cholesterol levels by 12 percent. In 1993 researchers in New Orleans reported that tablets providing 900 milligrams of garlic powder a day could reduce LDL ("bad") cholesterol levels by 11 percent; garlic was particularly effective in people with high cholesterol levels. A 1994 British meta-analysis of sixteen trials also reached a favorable conclusion, predicting a 12 percent reduction in cholesterol.

Unfortunately, subsequent research has been less encouraging. Two groups of Australian researchers broke the bad news. A 1995 study of twenty-eight subjects and a 1996 investigation of 115 people with high cholesterol levels found no benefit from garlic, even though both used the same tablets that appeared effective in Germany. A 1996 American study that used a different preparation, aged garlic extract, was more optimistic, but it demonstrated a cholesterol reduction of just 6 percent. Even those results, though, look good in comparison to more recent research: A German study of garlic oil extract and Canadian and American studies of garlic powder have all reported no benefit.

Garlic is nearly as popular as a remedy for high blood pressure as it is for high cholesterol. As with cholesterol, there is a whiff of evidence that it may help. A British meta-analysis of eight trials of garlic powder reported a 7 millimeter drop in *systolic blood pressure* (the higher blood pressure number, measured while the heart is pumping blood into the arteries) and a 5 millimeter drop in *diastolic blood pressure* (the lower number, measured when the heart is refilling with blood between beats).

Investigations of garlic's effects on arteries themselves have received less publicity but may be more significant in the long run. A 1997 study from Germany evaluated the *elasticity* (flexibility) of the body's main artery, the *aorta*. Researchers compared 101 adults who had been using garlic powder for at least two years with an equal number who had not taken garlic. All the subjects were between fifty and eighty years of age and none were taking cardiovascular medications. Although blood vessels grew stiffer with age in both groups, ultrasound testing showed that the garlic users in all age groups had more flexible arteries.

Although the 1997 investigation of elasticity is interesting, it is not a randomized clinical trial. But in a 1999 study that evaluated the *carotid* (neck) and *femoral* (leg) *arteries* in 152 patients with atherosclerosis who were randomly assigned to receive garlic powder or a placebo over a two-year period, garlic appeared to slow the progression of cholesterol-laden plaques, which even regressed in some subjects.

The major side effect of garlic is obvious. In Shakespeare's *A Midsummer Night's Dream*, Bottom advised his fellow actors to "eat no onions nor garlic, for we are to utter sweet breath." In addition to bad breath, garlic can induce *gastroesophageal reflux disease* (GERD) and heartburn. Less common problems include flatulence and rashes. Because garlic may reduce blood clotting, people taking aspirin, *warfarin* (Coumadin), or other *anticoagulants* (blood thinners), should use garlic with care.

Is garlic right for you? That depends on your goals. If your aim is to make a great pasta sauce, the answer is yes. But if you are interested in garlic for health, the only realistic answer is maybe.

Garlic may help reduce cholesterol levels, lower blood pressure, and protect blood vessels, but the evidence of benefit is mixed, even contradictory. Preliminary studies hint that garlic may have a role in reducing the risk of gastrointestinal cancer, but this potential benefit is even more speculative. If you decide to give garlic a try, remember that tablets containing garlic powder have the best shot at helping. A reasonable dose is 300 milligrams of garlic powder three times a day. But, like all dietary supplements, garlic pills are not subject to FDA standards for purity or contents. You should pick a brand that promises to deliver 1 to 1.5 percent allicin, but there are no assurances that it will live up to that goal. Unfortunately, deodorized preparations are less likely to deliver the active chemical.

Above all, do not count on garlic. If you are attracted to the herb, and if you and your companions don't mind the odor, use garlic to supplement things of proven benefit. For cholesterol and blood pressure, regular exercise, weight control, tobacco avoidance, and a diet low in saturated fat, cholesterol, and salt but high in fruits, vegetables, and fiber is the way to start.

GLUCOSAMINE-CHONDROITIN SULFATE

Glucosamine is a natural compound present in most human tissue, including joints, where it has an important role in the metabolism of various proteins in cartilage. Chondroitin is a larger substance composed of many glucosamine molecules linked to sugar molecules.

Best-selling books to the contrary, glucosamine-chondroitin sulfate is not an "arthritis cure." Several randomized clinical trials, though, do suggest that it may be mildly effective in relieving the pain of osteoarthritis, and a 2001 study suggested that it may actually slow the progression of joint damage. A recent meta-analysis of all the trials concluded that although these studies demonstrate benefits, most have technical flaws that prevent firm conclusions.

Glucosamine-chondroitin sulfate may be worth a try for men with arthritis pain that does not respond satisfactorily to standard therapies, including weight loss, exercise, joint protection, heat and cold applications, and pain relievers or anti-inflammatory medications. Patients with diabetes should be cautious, since glucosamine may increase blood-sugar levels. The supplement may interact with anticoagulants; the long-term safety and efficacy of glucosamine-chondroitin sulfate is not known.

ST. JOHN'S WORT

Botanists know it as *Hypericum perforathum,* but it got its common name centuries ago because it is a plant ("wort" in old English) that produces its bright yellow flowers in June, around the time of John the Baptist's birthday. By any name, it has become a best-selling herbal remedy for depression, outselling Prozac by four to one in the United States.

St. John's wort is available in the United States without prescription. It is licensed for the treatment of depression, anxiety, and insomnia in Germany, and it has been widely used throughout Europe. A meta-analysis of twenty-three trials involving 1,757 patients with mild to moderate depression concluded that St. John's wort is as effective as *tricyclic antidepressants.* In most of these studies, however, the diagnosis of depression was not well established, the dosage of prescription antidepressants was low, and the observation periods were brief.

St. John's wort is less expensive than prescription antidepressants and it has fewer side effects, though a few patients have reported dry mouth, dizziness, constipation, and other mild disturbances. However, additional studies will be required to confirm its efficacy and to compare it with the newer prescription antidepressants.

The active ingredient in St. John's wort appears to be *hypericin,* a chemical that inhibits the uptake of *serotonin* and other *neurotransmitters.* As a result, it may not be safe to take St. John's wort along with prescription antidepressants. The dose of hypericin varies from brand to brand. The contents, potency, and purity of the preparations sold in America have not been evaluated by the FDA or any other reliable source.

Like many herbal medications, St. John's wort is heavily promoted. It may have some benefit, but it is not a cure-all for depression, and it should never be used as a substitute for standard therapy. More studies will be needed to evaluate its role.

GINGKO

Dating back 200 million years, *gingko biloba,* the maidenhair tree, is the oldest species of tree alive today. Extracts of gingko leaves have been used in Asia for centuries, and it is currently one of the most widely used medications in Germany. Gingko extract contains numerous chemicals; various *flavonoids* are among the most active ingredients. In animal and laboratory experiments, gingko extracts appear to increase blood flow, inhibit *platelet-activating factor,* and neutralize oxygen free radicals.

Gingko is principally promoted to improve memory and enhance the circulation. A highly-publicized 1997 American study of 203 individuals reported that a particular gingko extract, EGb761, was able to stabilize or improve cognitive performance and social function in patients with Alzheimer's disease or *multi-infarct dementia,* another common cause of mental deterioration in the elderly. However, the improvement occurred in only 27 percent of patients and was modest at that. Unfortunately, a 2000 study in 123 patients with dementia found no benefit from gingko, and there is no good evidence to support claims that gingko prevents mental deterioration or enhances cognitive function in healthy people (see Chapter Eight). European studies suggest that gingko may improve pain-free walking in patients with *intermittent claudication* caused by peripheral vascular disease (see Chapter Fourteen). Few side effects have been recorded.

Given the limited alternatives, it may be reasonable for caregivers to administer gingko to patients with cognitive impairment. It is also possible that people with intermittent claudication might experience improvement. The EGb761 formulation has been best studied; a common dose is 40 milligrams three times a day or 80 milligrams twice a day.

Despite the paucity of evidence that gingko can help healthy people, it has become the third best-selling herbal supplement in America, to the tune of $270 million a year.

ECHINACEA

Although many herbal medications trace their origins to Asia, echinacea is a native American, the purple cornflower. It is used in Germany to treat infections of the respiratory and urogenital tracts and to enhance wound healing. In the United States, where echinacea is the best-selling herbal medication, it is heavily promoted to prevent and treat colds. Studies of echinacea have recorded mixed results; most are methodically flawed. The most optimistic studies suggest that echinacea may shorten the duration of cold symptoms by about a third. Few side effects have been reported; despite this apparent safety, there seems little reason to recommend echinacea.

Ginseng

Extracts from the ginseng root have been used in Asia for more than 2,000 years. Today it is one of the most popular herbal products in the world. It is also one of the most expensive. Perhaps because this slow-growing perennial has a shape that reminds some observers of the human form, it is popularly known as the "man root" and is touted to enhance all parts of the body. In the United States, ginseng is touted as a general tonic to enhance energy, relieve stress, slow the aging process, improve sexual performance, and promote vitality.

Despite the popularity of ginseng, its chemical ingredients are poorly understood. Most products contain only 2 to 3 percent of the presumed active components know as *ginsenosides*. Human studies are scant, contradictory, and methodologically flawed. Few side effects have been reported; disappointment may be the most common.

Zinc

Claims that zinc helps the prostate are unfounded, and claims that zinc lozenges can ease the symptoms of colds are based on contradictory data. Zinc is often recommended for macular degeneration, and a recent study shows that it appears to help, at least when it is combined with antioxidant vitamins.

Melatonin

Anecdotal evidence is cited to support occasional use of melatonin for jet lag or insomnia. Extravagant claims that melatonin helps fight aging, cancer, and other problems are unfounded. The long-term safety of melatonin is not known.

Creatine

One of the twenty natural amino acids that the body uses to make proteins, creatine is present in many of the body's tissues. Creatine is particularly concentrated in muscle, where it has an important role in generating energy. But the body can produce 1 to 2 grams of creatine a day on its own, and the average diet will provide another gram or two, mostly from meat, fish, and milk.

Very high doses of creatine, 20 grams a day, about the amount contained in ten pounds of steak, can increase muscle performance, but only for very brief, high intensity, repetitive tasks such as weight lifting, and only to a modest degree, perhaps 4 percent. Away from the lab, field trials of creatine have found little or no benefit on actual athletic performance. Preliminary studies suggest that creatine may help certain patients with severe neuromuscular diseases. The long-term safety of creatine is not known. Sammy Sosa notwithstanding, creatine cannot be recommended as a supplement.

ANDROSTENEDIONE (ANDRO)

Since Mark McGwire revealed that he took andro during his epic seventy home run season, andro has become wildly popular as a performance-enhancing supplement. It is sold as a nutritional supplement, but it has no role in human nutrition. Instead it is an *androgen,* a male hormone (see Chapters One and Ten). Recent studies suggest that it does not enhance performance but may have serious side effects. Do not take it.

DEHYDROEPIANDROSTERONE (DHEA)

Like andro, dehydroepiandrosterone (DHEA) is not a nutrient but a steroid hormone. DHEA is produced in the adrenal gland; its function is a mystery, but it is converted into androgens and estrogens, male and female hormones.

Because DHEA levels are high in young adulthood but low in old age, it has been hyped relentlessly as an antiaging supplement that will burn away body fat, build muscle, enhance sexual performance, slow memory loss, boost the immune system, and fight heart disease and cancer, among other things. There is no evidence that it works, and some reasons to worry that long-term use could have serious side effects, including benign prostate hyperplasia and prostate cancer. Do not take it.

MORE TO AVOID

Other supplements to avoid include yohimbine, sold for potency; lecithin, sold for cholesterol; coenzyme Q, sold for heart disease; and ephedrine, sold for weight reduction but often used for "herbal high." In fact, it is a good idea to stay away from any product that has not been evaluated by competent, unbiased medical scientists.

Perspectives

When it comes to supplements, the stakes are high, both in money and in health. It may be entirely reasonable for you to use a supplement, but before you do, consider these facts:

- The 1994 Dietary Supplement Health and Education Act removed supplements from the jurisdiction of the Food and Drug Administration (FDA). That's because they are classified as dietary aids even when they are actually sold to improve health. Since they are not subject to the strict FDA standards that govern prescription and nonprescription drugs, supplements can be manufactured, distributed, and promoted without proof that they are safe and effective. In fact, there are no assurances that a product will provide the active ingredients that it purports to contain, or that it is free of impurities.
- Anecdotes and testimonials should never be accepted as substitutes for scientific evidence of efficacy—even if the testimonial is offered by someone with no financial interest in the product. Only controlled trials in which a medication, herbal or conventional, is compared to an inert placebo can establish that a product is effective and safe.
- Most studies of herbal products have been performed in Europe, particularly Germany and France, where herbs are enormously popular. Many of the trials lack controls and methods that meet current American scientific standards.
- Supplements are often very expensive, and they are rarely covered by health insurance.
- Even if a product is "all-natural," it is not necessarily safe. The *eosinophilia-myalgia syndrome* is a cautionary tale; caused by "all-natural" supplements of the amino acid *tryptophan,* it cost thirty-six Americans their lives and made more than 1,500 seriously ill before the problem was recognized in 1990.
- Supplements can interact with standard medications. If you use herbal remedies, be sure to let your doctors and pharmacists know what you are taking.
- Vitamins, minerals, and herbs should never be used in place of good nutrition and standard medical care. If you choose to take herbal medications, you should use them as supplements, rather than substitutes, for traditional treatments.

Medical science is finally starting to give supplements the study they need so badly. Along with other research, the Harvard men's health studies suggest that low-dose aspirin may have an important preventive role, at least for men over fifty and for everyone with atherosclerosis who can take aspirin. Because they provide folate and vitamins B_6, B_{12}, and D, multivitamins make sense for nearly everyone. However, vitamin E has been disappointing, vitamin C has not been proven helpful, and beta-carotene may do more harm than good. In contrast, selenium may prove beneficial. Men with low HDL cholesterol levels may benefit from chromium or niacin, but they should only be used as part of a comprehensive, medically supervised program. A few herbal products may merit consideration in special circumstances, but men should not rely on them as panaceas, and they must remember that there is no proof that unregulated products are safe or effective.

Caveat emptor, buyer beware!

CHAPTER SEVEN

An Answer for Some, a Peril for Others: Alcohol

IS IT A NUTRIENT that can favorably affect the body's metabolism or a source of empty calories that can contribute to both obesity and malnutrition? Is it a substance that reduces the risk of heart disease or one that raises the blood pressure and damages the heart muscle? Is it a relaxing social lubricant or a highly addictive drug that can destroy individuals and rip families apart? Is it principally a hazard for men or does it pose greater dangers for women? Is it a supplement that can prolong life or a toxin that produces illness, robs years of life, and drains the economy of $185 billion a year?

Although these questions are very important, you do not have to spend long hours searching for the answers. In fact, the answer to each of these queries is yes. That's because the subject is alcohol, the Jekyll and Hyde of preventive medicine.

In terms of health, alcohol is neither good nor evil; instead, it is both. It sounds like a paradox, but it is not. In fact, alcohol can be salutary or destructive, depending on who is raising the glass, when he is drinking, and, above all, on how much he is drinking. In the past twenty years, medical research has demonstrated that alcohol is a double-edged sword; it's important information, but it confirms what John Seldon wrote more than 300 years ago: " 'Tis not the drinking that is to be blamed, but the excess."

It all started about 10,000 years ago, when men learned to cultivate crops. Barley may not have been the first crop, but it probably was not too far behind; man learned to brew beer almost as soon as he learned how to farm. It took another 5,000 years or so for men (or, quite possibly, women) to learn how to ferment fruits, but they have been drinking wine ever since. And if the pleasure of wine dates to antiquity, so too does the realization that alcohol can be destructive. In 850 B.C., Homer warned, "Inflaming wine, pernicious to mankind/[it] unnerves the limbs and dulls the noble mind."

Like many modern health problems, the hazards of alcohol escalated when a technological breakthrough made distilled liquor widely available at a low price. The "gin epidemic" struck England in the early eighteenth century, prompting the College of Physicians of London to warn of drinking spirits as "a great and growing evil."

Alcohol has been a part of American life ever since colonial times. The Eighteenth Amendment to the Constitution tried to prohibit the sale of alcohol, but it failed miserably and was rescinded in 1933 after only thirteen years. Alcohol has been perfectly legal ever since, though nearly all states raised the legal drinking age from eighteen to twenty-one during the 1980s.

At the start of the twenty-first century, 61 percent of all adult Americans, and 72 percent of all American men, use alcohol. That makes it the most widely used drug, and the most widely distributed toxin, in the country. According to a 1997 analysis of tax receipts, the average American adult consumes 116 beers, twenty-three glasses of wine, and fifty-one shots of liquor a year. That is a lot, about six pints of pure alcohol, but averages are misleading. If everyone consumed the average amount, alcohol would be an asset to the nation's health; since many people drink much more while others consume much less, alcohol trails only smoking among the leading preventable causes of death in the United States.

Men drink for many reasons. Some drink for personal pleasure, others to facilitate social interactions or to be one of the boys, still others to calm their nerves or lift their spirits. Because alcohol is a big business, many people are swayed by corporate persuasion; each year, the alcohol industry spends more than $1.5 billion to promote its products to Americans. And because alcohol is addictive, up to 19 million Americans drink because they have become alcohol-dependent; the majority of them are men.

Men drink for many reasons, but few drink to improve their health. Properly used, however, alcohol can do just that. But before you decide if drinking is right for you, consider the pros and cons of alcohol. It is an important decision and a personal choice each man must make for himself.

Potential Benefits

Alcohol *can* improve health if it is used by the right people, at the right time, in the right amount. Along with other research, the Harvard men's health studies report that most of the benefit depends on a reduced risk of heart disease. But the Health Professionals and Physicians' Health Studies have also identified other ways that alcohol may help.

Alcohol and Atherosclerosis

More than 2,400 years ago, Socrates said that "good men eat and drink that they may live." Physicians have been recommending a healthful diet ever since, but it was not until 1786 that Dr. William Heberden, the great English physician, prescribed alcohol for patients with angina. Still, it took about 200 years more for researchers to begin unraveling the complex relationship between alcohol and the heart.

In 1991, the Health Professionals Study conducted a careful evaluation of drinking and the risk of coronary artery disease. It found drinking was protective. Compared to abstainers, light drinkers (one-third to two drinks a day) enjoyed a 28 percent reduction in heart attacks, bypass operations and angioplasties, and cardiac deaths; moderate drinkers (two to three drinks a day) experienced a 48 percent reduction in risk. Because so few of the 51,529 men in the study consumed more than three drinks per day, the researchers were unable to evaluate the effects of heavier drinking.

Starting with the 1980 Honolulu Heart Study, other research on men had also reported that light to moderate drinking reduces the risk of coronary artery disease. But skeptics argued that these studies were flawed because they may have counted former drinkers who were forced to quit because of illness as nondrinkers, and because they failed to consider the impact of diet. The Health Professionals Study answered both of those arguments. Alcohol was just as protective even if former drinkers were excluded from the analysis. Moreover, since the drinkers actually consumed more fat and less fiber than the nondrinkers, diet was not responsible for the apparent protective effect of alcohol. Finally, the benefit of alcohol was confirmed even after other cardiac risk factors such as smoking, blood pressure, and cholesterol were taken into account.

The Health Professionals Study has provided additional information about alcohol and cardiac risk. It found that men who drink on three or four days each week are 34 percent less likely to develop heart disease than men who drink just once a week or less. It also found that beer, wine, and distilled liquor are all protective; if anything, liquor had a slight edge over the other beverages. Finally, the study reported that drinking was associated with higher levels of HDL ("good") cholesterol.

In 1997, the Physicians' Health Study confirmed that drinking reduces the risk of heart attacks, and it added the information that alcohol reduces a man's risk of developing angina. As compared with abstainers, men who averaged one drink a day enjoyed a 31 percent lower risk of angina and a 35 percent lower risk of heart attack; men who averaged two or more drinks a day experienced even greater benefit, reducing their risk of angina by 56 percent and of heart attacks by 47 percent. As in the Health Professionals Study, the apparent benefit of alcohol held up even after obesity, diabetes, exercise, family history, and other cardiac risk factors were considered. The scientists also found that aspirin use did not influence the results.

In 1998, the Physicians' Health Study answered another question about alcohol and the heart when it reported that alcohol protects men who already have had heart attacks as well as men with healthy hearts. In cardiac patients, low doses of alcohol were best; two to four drinks a week reduced the risk of a recurrent heart attack by 28 percent. In 1999, the study determined that low doses of alcohol also reduce the risk of sudden cardiac death, which is often caused by arrhythmias, abnormalities of the heart's pumping rhythm. And a 2001 report from another group of Harvard scientists linked low-dose alcohol to a reduced risk of congestive heart failure.

More recently, the study added the information that men who metabolize alcohol slowly derive more benefit from low-dose alcohol than rapid metabolizers, probably because they get a little extra boost from a small amount. But since you cannot tell your rate of alcohol metabolism without sophisticated testing, men who choose to drink should simply keep to the safe range of one to two drinks a day. Of greater practical importance, the study reported that men who consume little or no alcohol early in adult life derive cardiac protection if they begin modest drinking later on.

Both the Physicians' Health Study and the Health Professionals Study have also provided insights into the relationship between drinking and diabetes. Although heavy drinking increases the risk of developing diabetes, light to moderate drinking is actually associated with a decreased incidence of the disease. Finally, men who already have diabetes derive the same cardiac benefits from light drinking as nondiabetics do.

Peripheral artery disease is another manifestation of atherosclerosis. In this case, cholesterol-laden plaques produce blockages in the arteries that carry blood to the legs. The Physicians' Health Study found that drinking protects the legs nearly as much as the heart; men who averaged one or more drinks a day were 26 percent less likely to develop peripheral artery disease than nondrinkers, even after taking other atherosclerosis risk factors into account.

A third major manifestation of atherosclerosis is *ischemic stroke* (see Chapter Three). For years, doctors have considered heavy drinking as a stroke risk factor because it raises blood pressure and increases the risk of *hemorrhagic strokes,* which develop when small arteries in the head burst, releasing blood into the brain (see Chapter Three, Figure 3.2). But ischemic strokes are four times more common than hemorrhagic strokes, and because they result from blockages in the arteries that carry blood to the brain, they are manifestations of atherosclerosis. Two 1999 studies suggest that low-dose alcohol may help. The Physicians' Health Study found that men who consume one to seven drinks a week are about 20 percent less likely to have strokes than teetotalers. Similarly, researchers from New York reported that an alcohol intake of up to two drinks a day was associated with a 50 percent reduction in the risk of ischemic strokes in men and women, even after taking heart disease, hypertension, diabetes, smoking, and obesity into account. Indeed, the Stroke Prevention Guidelines of the National Stroke Association cite light to moderate drinking as a way to reduce the risk of stroke. But the New York study provides an important note of caution; whereas light drinking appeared protective, heavy drinking (four or more a day) increased the risk of ischemic stroke.

Alcohol and Mortality

Even committed teetotalers who review the data will have to agree that light to moderate drinking appears to reduce a man's risk of angina, heart attack, sudden cardiac death, and ischemic stroke. Since heart attacks and strokes account for 40 percent of the deaths in the United States, it seems possible that light drinking will also reduce a man's overall risk of death. It is a hopeful possibility, but is it a reality?

To find out, researchers in Australia reviewed more than 2,700 studies of alcohol and health. From this huge pool, they identified sixteen scientifically sound studies that investigated the relationship between the level of alcohol consumption and the risk of death. All in all, they found that men who averaged 10–19 grams of alcohol per day (roughly one drink a day) had a 16 percent lower death rate than teetotalers. But even slightly larger amounts diminished the returns, and moderate to heavy drinking was clearly harmful. Men who consumed 40 grams of alcohol a day (roughly three drinks) had the same mortality rate as nondrinkers, but by 60 grams (about five drinks a day), the death rate was one and one-third times higher than in abstainers. For women, incidentally, the maximum benefit was observed at about 9 grams of alcohol a day (about three-quarters of a drink), and mortality began to rise above 20 grams a day (about one and a half drinks).

Epidemiologists describe these results as a J-shaped mortality curve: Death rates fall with light drinking, then rise sharply with increasing alcohol consumption. Several studies completed after the 1996 Australian meta-analysis add weight to the observation. In 1997, the Physicians' Health Study confirmed a J-shaped relationship between alcohol consumption and mortality, but it reported a lower optimal dose than the meta-analysis. Among 22,071 men, those who averaged two to four drinks a week enjoyed a 28 percent lower risk of dying than nondrinkers; men who consumed more than two drinks a day had a one-and-one-half times higher mortality rate than abstainers. A 1997 study of 18,244 Chinese men found that men who drank up to two drinks a day had a 19 percent lower death rate than nondrinkers. A 1997 study of 490,000 American men and women also found that death rates were lowest among people who averaged about one drink a day.

HOW DOES ALCOHOL HELP?

The most important benefit of alcohol is its ability to boost HDL ("good") cholesterol levels. It does not take much alcohol to do the job—just one to two drinks a day will elevate HDL by 5 to 10 percent. A ten-point rise in HDL whether achieved by exercise, weight loss, smoking cessation, diet, or alcohol, is associated with a 40 percent reduction in cardiac risk. It is no coincidence that most studies of low-dose alcohol report reduction in cardiac risk of about 40 percent.

Alcohol may help in other ways, too. Most heart attacks are triggered by blood clots that form on cholesterol-laden arterial plaques. Even in low doses, alcohol appears to inhibit the activity of platelets, the fragmentary blood cells that trigger the clotting process. In addition, alcohol may help dissolve clots after they form; in 1994, the Physicians' Health Study found that drinking appears to boost levels of *tissue-type plasminogen activator* (t-PA), the same "clot buster" that doctors now use to treat heart attack victims. Three recent European studies report that drinkers have lower levels of clotting protein *fibrinogen* and two other newly identified cardiac risk factors, *C-reactive protein* and *homocysteine* (see Chapter Three). Finally, insulin resistance and high insulin levels are cardiac risk factors in diabetics and nondiabetics alike. Low-dose alcohol appears to improve tissue insulin sensitivity, reducing insulin levels.

OTHER POSSIBLE BENEFITS

From a personal perspective, men may find a drink or two relaxing and pleasurable. From a medical perspective, the major benefit of low-dose alcohol is a reduced risk of heart disease that results in a lower all-over mortality rate. It is an important benefit, indeed, but it is not alone. In fact, the Harvard men's health studies have identified other potential benefits of light-to-moderate drinking.

The most important additional benefit of low-dose alcohol is a reduced risk of diabetes. Like the Physicians' Health Study, the Health Professionals Study found that men who drink moderately, consuming two to three drinks a day, are 39 percent less likely to develop diabetes than nondrinkers. Doctors are not sure why alcohol is linked to improved blood sugar control, but increased tissue sensitivity to insulin is a likely explanation.

The Health Professionals Study has identified two other possible benefits, a lower likelihood of painful gallstones and a reduced risk of bothersome symptoms of *benign prostatic hyperplasia* (BPH). Scientists do not know why alcohol reduces the risk of gallstones, but in the study, men who consumed one to two drinks on most days were 15 to 30 percent less likely to develop gallbladder attacks than nondrinkers. The news about BPH is particularly interesting, since many doctors advise men with the disorder to avoid alcohol, especially late in the day. That's because of alcohol's well-documented diuretic properties. It reduces the brain's production of *ADH*, a hormone that regulates urine volume, so even a drink or two can increase the flow of urine—hardly a welcome event for a man with an enlarged prostate. Surprisingly, perhaps, the Harvard study found that men who average two to three drinks a day are 41 percent less likely to develop BPH symptoms than teetotalers. The protective mechanism is unknown, but may involve lower testosterone activity in drinkers. In any case, the Health Professionals Study found that low-dose drinking is associated with another benefit, a reduced risk of erectile dysfunction. Men who consume one to two drinks a day are 33 percent less likely to be impotent than either nondrinkers or heavy drinkers—but the study also reported that men who drink heavily face an increased risk of impotence.

IS RED WINE REALLY BETTER?

In theory, it is. That is because red wine contains substances from grape skins that are absent in white wine, beer, and liquor. These potentially protective ingredients include *flavonoids* and other *phenols* that have antioxidant properties and *resveratrol,* a chemical that may help lower cholesterol levels.

Theory is one thing, practice another: Are red-wine drinkers really better off? In 1991, the Health Professionals Study found no significant difference between wine, beer, and liquor. In 1999, the Physicians' Health Study agreed, adding that all three beverages produced similar protective elevations in HDL cholesterol levels. To settle the issue, researchers from those two Harvard studies joined with scientists from California and the Netherlands to analyze twenty-five studies from around the world that allowed direct comparisons between the various alcoholic beverages. The result of this meta-analysis was a dead heat or, more properly, a live heat, since all forms of alcohol were equally beneficial as long as the dose was right.

The Best Dose

Will alcohol improve your health or will it harm you? The answer depends on how much you consume, when you drink, and whether or not you have problems that increase your personal risk.

Dose is the most important factor. Most studies suggest that the optimal dose for men is 15 to 30 grams of alcohol a day; for women, the best dose is just half as much. There are two reasons for the gender difference. Women metabolize alcohol at a slower rate than men, and even small amounts of alcohol increase a woman's risk of breast cancer, probably by boosting estrogen levels.

You never would walk into a restaurant and order 15 grams of alcohol with dinner. How does that amount translate into common beverages? In a sense, the answer depends on where you are. In Austria, for example, one drink is defined as containing 6.3 grams of alcohol. In Britain it is 8 grams, but in Japan it is as high as 19.75 grams. Standards vary in the United States, but most authorities count 13 to 15 grams of alcohol as a standard drink. That is the amount you will get in twelve ounces of beer, five ounces of wine, or one and a half ounces of 80 proof liquor.

A man who averages seven to fourteen drinks a week can expect to benefit from alcohol, but, as in so many things, only if his timing is right. If your seven to fourteen drinks are consumed on just one or two days of the week, you are asking for trouble. Binge drinking increases the risk of death, even if the total weekly dose is modest. And just a drink or two can be lethal for a man who drinks before he drives or operates heavy machinery. Even small amounts of alcohol can slow reflexes and impair judgement.

Properly timed, one to two drinks a day will help protect men from atherosclerosis, but that does not mean every man should drink. Even small amounts of alcohol can interact adversely with medications, particularly sedatives and tranquilizers; if you are taking medications, check with your doctor or pharmacist before you decide to drink. Similarly, even light drinking can be very dangerous for people with certain alcohol-sensitive health problems; liver disease and uncontrolled high blood pressure head the list. The calories in alcohol can contribute to obesity; at seven calories a gram, alcohol is a caloric-dense food, so a standard drink will give you about 100 extra calories, without counting the mixers.

Age is another factor in the alcohol equation; most of the benefits of alcohol show up in men older than forty-five, but many of the risks occur in younger men. It is also true that surprisingly small amounts of alcohol can trigger important behavioral problems in vulnerable individuals. Last but not least, low doses of alcohol can lead to higher doses; problem drinking starts with one drink at a time. That's why it is important to consider the adverse effects of excessive drinking before you decide if alcohol is right for you.

Potential Risks

A little alcohol will fight atherosclerosis and promote longevity, at least for healthy men who drink responsibly. But if a little alcohol is good, more is not. In fact, excessive drinking kills 100,000 Americans each year; the majority are men.

In excessive amounts, alcohol can damage virtually every organ in the body. Although alcohol tolerance varies, the risks of alcohol rise steeply in people who consume more than three drinks a day.

Although small amounts of alcohol can protect the heart, larger amounts are toxic for the cardiovascular system. The Health Professionals Study found that two drinks a day will not raise a man's blood pressure, but a large body of research shows that heavier drinking increases the risk of hypertension, and with it, stroke. In sensitive individuals, even modest amounts of alcohol can trigger rapid or erratic heart beats, the so-called holiday heart syndrome. Large amounts of alcohol can directly damage the heart muscle, leading to *alcoholic cardiomyopathy* and congestive heart failure. When alcohol abuse is accompanied by malnutrition, as is often the case, it can produce another type of congestive heart failure, *beriberi*.

Although small amounts of alcohol reduce the risk of the nation's leading cause of death, heart disease, larger amounts increase the risk of the second leading killer, cancer. In women, even light drinking increases the risk of breast cancer; in men, heavy drinking may increase the risk of prostate cancer. In both genders, excessive drinking increases the risk of cancers of the mouth and throat, esophagus, stomach, liver, and pancreas. In addition, the Health Professionals Study found that men who eat poorly and drink excessively have an increased risk of colon cancer.

Liver disease is one of the major complications of excessive drinking. Alcohol can cause enlargement of the liver, abnormal deposits of fat in the liver, and inflammation of the liver (*alcoholic hepatitis*). Even worse is *cirrhosis*, irreversible scarring of the organ that can lead to fatigue, yellow eyes and skin, massive accumulation of fluid in the abdomen and legs, breast enlargement, life-threatening bleeding, and infections, confusion, coma, and death. Alcohol explains why the combination of chronic liver disease and cirrhosis is the tenth most common cause of death in the United States, and cirrhosis is 2.3 times more common in men than women.

Alcohol can also be very toxic to the organ system it hits first, the intestinal tract. Drinking can cause inflammation and bleeding from the esophagus or stomach and it can aggravate ulcers and prevent them from healing. Alcohol is a major cause of *pancreatitis*, a highly painful inflammation that can be lethal in its acute phase or can cause lifelong pain and malnutrition, often accompanied by diabetes.

Alcohol can also take its toll on the body's metabolism. In 1991, the Health Professionals Study reported that men who drink add the calories from alcohol without reducing their calories from other sources. Similarly, a recent study from the Netherlands found that aperitifs really do stimulate the appetite; people who drink consume more calories from food than people who do not. And a new study from France demonstrates that alcohol's calories do count: Drinkers had larger waists and higher waist-to-hip ratios than abstainers. But if alcohol contributes to obesity, it can also produce malnutrition. That is because people who abuse alcohol for long periods of time often eat poorly. As a result, they can experience muscle wasting and weakness, as well as low blood levels of vitamins, proteins, sugar, magnesium, calcium, and phosphorous.

Excessive drinking can also damage the musculoskeletal system, causing muscle damage and osteoporosis. Nor is the skin immune; alcohol is a cause of *rosacea*. If that is not enough, the Physicians' Health Study found that drinking appears to increase the risk of cataracts. Blood disorders are even more serious, including anemia, low-white-blood-cell counts, low-platelet counts, abnormal bleeding, and depressed immune function. People who drink heavily are susceptible to many infections, including pneumonia.

Some men drink in the belief that alcohol will give them a sexual lift. It is a mistake, a big mistake. In fact, alcohol reduces libido and heavy drinking can cause impotence. As usual, Shakespeare got it right; in Act II of *Macbeth* he reminds us that excess alcohol "provokes the desire but takes away the performance." Alcohol also lowers sperm counts, contributing to infertility. Men can also develop large breasts from drinking. It's bad news for the reproductive tract, and it is even worse for women, who face an increase of breast cancer as well as abnormal pregnancies and fetal damage.

Alcohol is a major cause of injuries and traumatic deaths, both from accidents and violence. Of the 100,000 deaths attributed to alcohol annually, nearly half are due to trauma, including 44 percent of all traffic fatalities and a substantial proportion of deaths from drownings, fires, homicides, and suicides. It is no wonder that accidents are the fifth leading cause of death in the United States, or that men are much more likely to die from accidents, homicides, and suicides than women.

The nervous system is particularly vulnerable to the effects of alcohol. In the long run, excessive drinking can cause many types of neurologic damage. It can injure peripheral nerves, interfering with sensation, and it can damage the brain permanently, causing incoordination, memory loss, confusion, and dementia. In the short term, alcohol can cause acute intoxication. In legal terms, intoxication occurs at blood levels of 80 to 100 milligrams per deciliter but judgment, coordination, and cognitive function can be impaired at levels of just 20 to 30 milligrams per deciliter—and in the average man, it takes just two drinks to reach those levels within thirty minutes. At 200 milligrams per deciliter, alcohol will produce unconsciousness, and at 300 to 400 milligrams per deciliter, death. In large doses, alcohol is a poison.

Last but not least, drinking can lead to a vast array of psychosocial and economic problems. That is why every man who uses alcohol, or is considering it, should pause to ask himself if he may be at risk for problem drinking.

Problem Drinking

In 1633, George Herbert advised, "Drink not the third glass, which thou canst not tame/when once it is within thee!" It's good advice, but it is hard to follow; that's why surveys report that drinking has caused problems in one of three American families.

Problem drinking is distressingly common in the United States. Various community surveys have disclosed that the prevalence of alcohol abuse and dependence during the course of a year vary by age and gender.

Alcohol abuse takes a tremendous toll on the nation's health. It is responsible for about 20 percent of all hospitalizations and nearly 5 percent of all deaths. Drinking also drains the country's wealth, accounting for about 12 to 15 percent of all health care expenditures for adults, or approximately $185 billion

Table 7.1: PREVALENCE OF ALCOHOL ABUSE

AGE	MEN	WOMEN
18–29	17–24%	4–10%
30–44	11–14%	2–4%
45–64	6–8%	1–2%
65 and over	1–3%	Less than 1%

a year. Alcohol is also responsible for innumerable social and psychological difficulties; an estimated 27 million American children are at risk for emotional trauma as a result of a parent's alcohol abuse.

HOW MUCH IS TOO MUCH?

The World Health Organization (WHO) has a simple but accurate answer. Any man who averages more than two drinks a day or who consumes more than four drinks on a single day is an at-risk drinker. It is a broad definition, but it brings home the fact that a narrow line separates healthful drinking from hazardous drinking.

The American Psychiatric Association (APA) has devised a classification system based on the behavioral and biological effects of excessive alcoholic consumption:

Alcohol Abuse is defined as a maladaptive pattern of alcohol use leading to significant impairment or distress that is manifested by one or more of the following within a twelve-month period: (1) failure to fulfill obligations at work, school, or home; (2) recurrent use of alcohol in hazardous situations; (3) legal problems related to alcohol; and (4) continued drinking despite alcohol-related social problems.

Alcohol Dependence is defined as a maladaptive pattern of drinking that includes three or more of the following over a twelve-month period: (1) tolerance to alcohol, characterized by either an increase in the amount of alcohol consumed or a decrease in the effects of a given dose of alcohol; (2) physical or emotional distress provoked by alcohol withdrawal; (3) use of greater amounts of alcohol over a longer period than intended; (4) a persistent desire to control alcohol use or an inability to gain control; (5) a great deal of time spent on obtaining alcohol, drinking, or recovering from drinking; (6) reducing important social, occupational, or recreational activities; and (7) continued drinking despite physical or psychological problems.

Alcoholism is defined by the National Council on Alcoholism and Drug Dependence and the American Society of Addiction Medicine as "a primary chronic disease with genetic, psychosocial, and environmental factors . . . often progressive and fatal . . . characterized by impaired control over drinking, preoccupation with the drug alcohol, use of alcohol despite adverse consequences, and distortions in thinking, most notably denial."

ARE YOU AT RISK?

Defining alcohol abuse is difficult, recognizing it harder still. Over 700,000 Americans are currently being treated for alcoholism, but they are just the tip of the iceberg. According to current estimates, 15 million people in the United States abuse alcohol—that is 11 percent of adult men and 4 percent of women.

Doctors have devised a variety of tests to identify alcoholism. The CAGE questionnaire is simple but accurate. To see if you may be at risk, ask yourself these four questions:

1. Have you ever tried to cut down on your drinking?
2. Have you ever been annoyed by criticism of your drinking?
3. Have you ever felt guilty about your drinking?
4. Have you ever had a morning "eye opener"?

Answering yes to one or more of these questions does not mean you are an alcoholic, but it does suggest you may be at risk—and that even low-dose alcohol may not be good for you, despite its potential cardiac benefits.

Serious as it is, alcohol dependence occupies just one pole of the broad spectrum of hazardous and harmful drinking. To see if you may be at risk for alcohol-related problems, ask yourself the ten questions of the Alcohol Use Disorders Identification Test (AUDIT):

1. How often do you have a drink containing alcohol?
    - (0) Never
    - (1) Monthly or less
    - (2) 2 to 4 times/month
    - (3) 2 to 3 times/week
    - (4) 4 or more times/week

2. How many drinks do you have on a typical day when you are drinking?
   - (0) None
   - (1) 1 or 2
   - (2) 3 or 4
   - (3) 5 or 6
   - (4) 7 to 9

3. How often do you have 6 or more drinks on one occasion?
   - (0) Never
   - (1) Less than monthly
   - (2) Monthly
   - (3) Weekly
   - (4) Daily or almost daily

4. How often during the last year have you found that you were not able to stop drinking once you had started?
   - (0) Never
   - (1) Less than monthly
   - (2) Monthly
   - (3) Weekly
   - (4) Daily or almost daily

5. How often during the last year have you failed to do what was normally expected from you because of drinking?
   - (0) Never
   - (1) Less than monthly
   - (2) Monthly
   - (3) Weekly
   - (4) Daily or almost daily

6. How often during the last year have you needed a first drink in the morning to get yourself going after a heavy drinking session?
   - (0) Never
   - (1) Less than monthly
   - (2) Monthly
   - (3) Weekly
   - (4) Daily or almost daily

7. How often during the last year have you had a feeling of guilt or remorse after drinking?
   - (0) Never
   - (1) Less than monthly
   - (2) Monthly
   - (3) Weekly
   - (4) Daily or almost daily

8. How often during the last year have you been unable to remember what happened the night before because you had been drinking?
   - (0) Never
   - (1) Less than monthly
   - (2) Monthly
   - (3) Weekly
   - (4) Daily or almost daily

9. Have you or someone else been injured as a result of your drinking?
    (0) Never
    (1) Yes, but not in the last year
    (2) Yes, during the last year

10. Has a relative or friend or a doctor or other health worker been concerned about your drinking or suggested you cut down?
    (0) Never
    (1) Yes, but not in the last year
    (2) Yes, during the last year

An AUDIT score of eight or higher is considered positive; it does not mean you are a problem drinker, but it does indicate risk, and that you should consider getting help before you experience the dark side of alcohol.

GETTING HELP

Doctors do not fully understand the causes of alcohol dependency; in most cases, genetic factors, biochemical differences, and psychological influences contribute to the problem, though to varying degrees. Without understanding what causes the problem, it has not been possible to devise a completely effective treatment plan. Still, help is available. The first stage is to withdraw from alcohol, often with the help of sedatives and sometimes with a brief in-patient stay. The next, harder step is to stay away from alcohol. For many men, self-help groups such as Alcoholics Anonymous are most effective. For others, counseling or psychotherapy is best, either in individual sessions or in groups. Family therapy, workplace interventions, and various psychosocial and religious supports are also available. Researchers are working hard to develop medication to treat alcohol dependency; *disulfiram* and *naltrexone* have helped many people recover from alcohol dependency, but more research is needed to develop better treatment methods, both medicinal and behavioral.

Alcohol dependency is a life-long problem—but even if a "cure" is not possible, treatment can be effective. Most problem drinkers bear little overt resemblance to the stereotypical down-and-out drinker. A man can be at the peak of professional success and still be at risk. He can appear healthy and have a peaceful family life while drinking more than he should. Before you hoist a toast to the health benefits of low-dose alcohol, ask yourself if you are vulnerable to alcohol-related problems—and if you are, take action before those problems develop.

Alcohol and Health: Good or Evil

The French say "*A votre santé,*" the Italians say, "*Salute,*" and the Germans say, "*Prost.*" In Russian it is "*Na Zdorovya,*" in Yiddish "*L'Chaim.*" All around the world, it seems, people use alcohol to toast health. But is it really possible? Can alcohol really improve a man's health?

It hardly seems possible, but it is true. Alcohol is good for health *if* the dose is right, the timing is right, and the drinker is right. By now, a massive amount of medical evidence supports this news, but even as the data came in during the eighties and nineties, most doctors were reluctant to recommend alcohol for health. Since many physicians spend considerable portions of their professional lives wrestling with problem drinkers and alcohol-related illnesses, they can hardly be blamed.

The American Heart Association notes that 100,000 deaths in the United States can be attributed to alcohol-related diseases each year. But if all current drinkers were to abstain, about 80,000 extra deaths from heart disease would occur annually. If you drink a little, you can reduce your risk of dying from heart disease, but if you drink too much, you will increase your risk of dying from many causes, including cancer, liver disease, trauma, and even heart disease.

Is drinking right for you? It is a personal decision. Men are better candidates for low-dose alcohol than women. Older men are better candidates than younger men, and men with heart disease risk factors, particularly low HDL cholesterol levels, are the best candidates of all, as long as they have no specific reason for abstaining.

If you choose to drink, limit yourself to one to two drinks a day, counting twelve ounces of beer, five ounces of wine, or one and a half ounces of distilled liquor as one drink. But do not drink at all before you drive or operate dangerous machinery.

Do not drink at all if you have liver disease or other alcohol-related problems, such as uncontrolled hypertension or congestive heart failure, pancreatitis, or very high triglyceride levels. Do not drink if you take medications that interact adversely with alcohol. Check with your doctor to see if alcohol is safe for you.

Drink with extra care, or not at all, if you have a family history of alcohol abuse. Do not force yourself to drink if alcohol causes unpleasant symptoms such as heartburn, palpitations, headaches, or untimely drowsiness.

Despite all these precautions, do not shun all thoughts of alcohol. Most men can drink safely and responsibly, and men who do so will benefit from up to two drinks a day. If you are one of these men and you enjoy a drink or two, drink up.

To your health!

CHAPTER EIGHT

The Answers: Behavior Modification and Stress Control

MOST MEN DO NOT THINK ABOUT HEALTH often enough or carefully enough; it's one reason they do not live as long as women. And when men get around to thinking about their health, they tend to focus more on "physical" ailments than psychosocial issues. It is a typical concrete, action-oriented, hard-edged male response, and it is another reason that men have more health problems than the "weaker sex."

A look at the ten leading causes of death in America will convince you that men really should pay heed to the psychological and behavioral aspects of health. For men, accidents, suicides, and homicides rank as the third, eighth, and tenth leading causes of death, but only one of these psychosocial issues, accidents, makes the top ten for women—and although it is in sixth place for women, accidental deaths are still 2.4 times more common in men.

Accidents and violence are the most dramatic examples of the way behavior affects health, but psychological influences are also important for even the most careful and peaceful of men. Heart disease is the leading killer of American men, and heartfelt emotions rank among its important risk factors. In addition, two behavioral issues, smoking and drinking, are among the reasons that cancer, chronic lung disease, and liver disease rank as the second, fourth, and tenth leading causes of death in America, and each is about one and a half times more common in men than women.

To a greater or lesser degree, psychosocial factors directly contribute to six of the ten leading causes of death in men. It is an impressive illustration of the mind's importance, but it is just the tip of the iceberg. Emotions play a role in many other "bodily" ailments. The list includes headaches, thyroid disorders, asthma, palpitations, gastritis, diarrhea, back pain, chronic fatigue, itching, and skin rashes. Psychological factors can also play a role in sexual dysfunction. In addition, strong emotions can affect the immune system, perhaps impairing its ability to ward off cancer and infections.

Psychological illnesses are no less important in their own right. According to the U.S. Surgeon General, one of every five Americans will experience a significant mental disorder this year, but only a fraction will recognize the problem for what it is and seek help. In all, psychological woes will strike half of all Americans during the course of their lives. Anxiety heads the list, affecting about 15 percent of all adults; with a prevalence of more than 7 percent, depression is in second place. The distress and suffering are enormous, both for patients and their families, and the economic costs are also staggering. In 1996, the last year for which complete figures are available, treatment of mental disorders drained $69 billion from the American economy. Add the $17.7 billion dollars spent on Alzheimer's disease and the $12.6 billion spent for the treatment of drug and alcohol abuse, and you will see why mental illness consumes more than 7 percent of our health-care dollars, not counting indirect costs like lost work days.

In the final analysis, mind and body are not separate entities; instead, they are but two aspects of a single human being. Nearly 2,400 years ago, the great Greek physician Hippocrates recognized that a sound mind and a sound body are equally important determinants of human health and well-being. It's an important message, but it is lost on many of today's men. T. S. Eliot noted: "Men tighten knots of confusion/Into perfect misunderstandings." It is time to untie the knots: By addressing both emotional and physical health, men can follow Plato's injunction to "tune the strings of the body and mind to perfect spiritual harmony."

Risky Behavior

Is nature to blame or is it nurture, is it testosterone and the Y chromosome or role models and cultural norms? Nobody knows, but as for most complex questions, the likely answer is not one or the other, but both. Whatever the explanation, the facts are clear: Men are risk takers, and risky or aggressive male behavior has a negative impact on the health of both men and women. It is part of the reason men have a much higher risk of death from injury, homicide, suicide, and AIDS, while women have a much higher risk of injury from domestic violence.

ACCIDENTS AND VIOLENCE

Accidents are the third leading cause of death in American men, and the leading cause in men younger than forty-four. Motor vehicle accidents account for almost 42,000 of the nearly 94,000 accidental deaths each year; falls are in second place, accounting for about 17 percent, followed by poisoning (10 percent), drowning (4 percent), fire (4 percent), and firearm accidents (1 percent). As bad as they are, accidental deaths are just the tip of the injury iceberg. Sixty-eight million accidents severe enough to restrict activity or require medical care occur in the United States each year. In all, the medical care and lost productivity attributed to accidents consumes about 1 percent of the nation's gross domestic product.

Accidents will happen, but only if we let them. Some accidents are truly chance events, random and unpredictable. But most begin with risky or careless behavior, which is why the *British Medical Journal* banned the word "accident" from its pages in 2001, except presumably for "acts of God" and other truly random events. By any name, most accidents are caused by human misbehavior, just the thing at which young men excel. When the Centers for Disease Control and Prevention surveyed the nation's youth in 1999, they found that males were far more likely than females to engage in risky behaviors, such as not wearing seatbelts, riding motorcycles (and not wearing helmets), drinking when driving and drinking to excess, abusing drugs, carrying weapons, fighting, and having unsafe sex. Less dramatically, but just as injuriously, a broken stair-rail, loose rug, or ill-placed electrical cord can lead to injury or death from falling; older people are at particular risk.

Like accidents, violence is predominantly a male problem. Men are the principal perpetrators and victims of homicide and suicide and are responsible for most domestic violence.

Traumatic injuries and deaths can be prevented. Measures such as wearing seat belts; avoiding dangerous or excessive alcohol use; wearing helmets when biking; using flotation devices while boating; placing fences around swimming pools; installing smoke alarms, fire extinguishers, and carbon monoxide detectors; restricting access to firearms; and performing household safety checks would help enormously. Though human behavior (or misbehavior) is at the root of many injuries, and is much harder to change, men should still do the simple things that can protect themselves and their families.

Smoking

Until recently, smoking was mostly an issue for men, but that started to change with the U. S. Surgeon General's Report on Smoking and Health in 1964. In the mid-twentieth century, nearly 55 percent of American men were smoking, a rate more than two times higher than for women. At present, only a quarter of American adults smoke, and the rate is only slightly higher for men (25.7 percent) than women (21.5 percent). It is great progress, but it should not breed complacency. In fact, the quitting rate has leveled off, and men are threatened by the resurgent popularity of cigars. Even worse, about 3,000 of our children, both boys and girls, take up the habit every day.

Taking about 430,000 lives each year, smoking is the leading preventable cause of death in the United States. Table 8.1 summarizes smoking-related illnesses in men. It is long list, and getting longer all the time. In 2000, for example, the Physicians' Health Study added colon cancer and Type 2 diabetes to the tobacco hit list, and the Health Professionals' Study added community-acquired pneumonia. In all, smoking is responsible for one of every five American deaths.

The Harvard Alumni Study found that smoking is the most dangerous lifestyle risk factor, increasing a man's risk of dying during the study by 76 percent. That's the bad news. But the study also found some good news: Quitting reduced the death rate by 41 percent.

Quitting is difficult, but it is possible; since 1964, in fact, more than 46 million Americans have kicked the habit, and more types of help are available now than ever before. The time honored "cold-turkey" approach to quitting is still the place to start. Support groups, counseling, and hypnosis can also help many men who smoke. A wide range of pharmacological assists are also available. They include the prescription drug *buproprion* (Wellbutrin, Zyban) as well as nicotine replacement patches, gums, nasal sprays, and inhalers.

Men who smoke should quit. Men who do not smoke should never start. And all men should avoid exposure to all other forms of tobacco, including second-hand smoke and smokeless tobacco.

Alcohol and Drug Abuse

Smoking is no longer a predominately male concern, but alcohol and drugs are still. Alcohol, the most widely abused drug in the world, is discussed in Chapter Seven. It is a complex story, since low doses of alcohol can actually help protect some men from disease while larger amounts (and ill-timed drinking of

Table 8.1: HEALTH CONSEQUENCES OF SMOKING IN MEN

Heart	Coronary artery disease Angina Heart attacks Sudden cardiac deaths Arrhythmias (irregular heart beats)
Circulation	Hypertension Blockages of arteries Aneurysms of the aorta
Central Nervous System	Strokes Brain hemorrhages
Lungs	Lung cancer Mesotheliomas (cancer of the lung lining) in conjunction with asbestos exposure Bronchitis Emphysema Pneumonia Asthma
Head and Neck	Cancer of the mouth, tongue, and larynx (voice box) Allergies Sinusitis Periodontal disease Tooth loss Macular degeneration Cataracts Hearing loss
Digestive Tract	Cancers of the esophagus, stomach, colon, and pancreas Gastritis Ulcers
Urinary Tract	Cancers of the kidneys and bladder
Male Reproductive System	Impotence
Skeletal System	Osteoporosis Fractures
Skin	Premature wrinkling
Psychiatric	Addiction Depression
Trauma	Burns and smoke inhalation
Blood	Decreased oxygen-carrying capacity Increased white and red blood cell counts Leukemia Multiple myeloma
Metabolism	Decreased HDL cholesterol Increased waist-to-hip ratio (truncal obesity) Altered metabolism of various medications Type 2 diabetes

even modest amounts) harm all men. But for drugs, the bottom line is simple: The only safe dose is zero. Even if the goal is simple, getting there can be very difficult.

Substance abuse does not respect gender, and the sex differences in the prevalence of drug use and the dependence vary according to age, ethnicity, and the particular agent. In every category, however, men outnumber women by ratios that range from as low as two to one all the way up to seven to one.

Like tobacco and alcohol abuse, drug abuse causes a huge range of medical problems ranging from infections (HIV and AIDS, hepatitis B and C, pneumonia) to heart attacks and respiratory failure to drug overdoses and withdrawal syndromes. In addition to innumerable cases of illness, drug abuse takes 5,000 to 10,000 lives each year and drains the economy of about $3.2 billion in health care costs alone.

The medical, personal, and social consequences of drug abuse are vast. Solutions to the problems are complex, and progress has been slight at best. Like men who abuse alcohol, those who abuse drugs, both illicit street drugs and prescription medications, need professional help. Society needs help, too, both in the drug-producing underdeveloped world and in the drug-consuming industrialized countries.

Men are driven to abuse tobacco, alcohol, and drugs by complex social pressures, biological factors, and psychological problems ranging from the anxiety disorders to depression to isolation. In turn, alcohol and drugs can exacerbate mental problems. Whether or not they engage in risky or abusive behavior, all men should know how to recognize, prevent, and treat these common, important psychosocial problems.

Stress and Anxiety

Stress is a fundamental, and normal, human response to threat. In the early years of the twentieth century, Dr. Walter B. Cannon of Harvard Medical School pioneered medical study of the "fight or flight" reaction. Stress produces a state of arousal. The mind becomes more vigilant and the pupils widen to admit more light. Breathing speeds up, and the bronchial tubes widen to admit more oxygen. The heart beats faster and pumps more blood, raising the blood pressure. Blood is directed away from the intestinal tract and the skin, which feels cold and clammy. More blood is delivered to the muscles, which become tense and ready to spring into action.

Stress also affects the body's metabolism. *Adrenaline* and *cortisone* are pumped into the blood. In contrast, insulin levels fall and blood sugar rises to provide instant energy to the brain, heart, and muscles. And the blood itself changes, as the clotting system is activated to staunch any wounds.

STRESS AND HEALTH

Stress is a basic human response that served men well when it was triggered by a physical threat such as a saber-toothed tiger. Even today, it helps men mobilize their maximum physical resources to put out a fire or catch a fourth-quarter-touchdown pass. But stress can trigger a similar reaction in boardrooms and highways, where it can get in the way of a smooth response to a raging chief executive officer or a sticky traffic jam.

Stress can be good or bad for health. If it helps a man get pumped up to meet a challenge, it is a plus, but if it is triggered inappropriately, is unduly severe, or is excessively prolonged, it is harmful. Excessive stress produces exhaustion and illness. *Acute stress reactions* triggered by traumatic events, such as accidents, and *adjustment reactions,* caused by more protracted life events, such as financial setbacks or marital woes, are examples of harmful stress. Fortunately, many stress reactions respond to simple measures, such as deep breathing exercises, counseling, temporary tranquilizing medications, and, above all, the passage of time.

ANXIETY

Anxiety is different. Stress is the body's response to an external threat, but anxiety is the response to an internal stimulus. Stress may be helpful or harmful, but anxiety is always unpleasant and unwelcome.

About 8 percent of adult men are troubled by persistent and disruptive anxiety at some time in their lives. In most cases, it lasts for six months or longer. The most common variety is *generalized anxiety disorder,* which usually begins gradually in early adulthood or mid-life. It is characterized by excessive worry that lasts at least six months and is accompanied by physical symptoms, such as muscle tension and aches, hypervigilance, irritability, shakiness, dry mouth, light headedness, excessive sweating, and intestinal complaints. The other anxiety disorders include *post-traumatic stress disorder, panic attacks, social anxiety disorder,* various *phobias,* and *obsessive-compulsive disorder.*

Anxiety can disrupt a man's work and his family. It can bring on alcohol, tobacco, and substance abuse. And it can lead to physical illness; in particular, many studies suggest that anxiety increases a man's risk of heart disease.

RECOGNIZING ANXIETY

Like other illnesses, anxiety disorders can be treated. The first step is to recognize the problem for what it is. To find out if you may be suffering from anxiety, answer the simple questions in table 8.2. Add up your score; totals above 61 suggest severe anxiety; scores between 46 and 60, moderate anxiety; numbers between 31 and 45, mild anxiety; scores below 30 do not suggest a problem with anxiety.

TREATMENT

The first step in treating anxiety is to check for correctable medical or lifestyle issues that can mimic or exacerbate anxiety. Thyroid disease is an example of the former, excessive caffeine use an example of the latter. Next, try to simplify life by removing or minimizing stress whenever possible. Remember that exercise is an excellent way to dissipate tension (see Chapter Five). Consider learning autoregulatory techniques, such as deep breathing, progressive muscular relaxation, and meditation. Above all, get expert help. Talking therapy is effective for anxiety. Many varieties are available, ranging from counseling to traditional psychotherapy to cognitive-behavioral therapy. Finally, medication can be extremely beneficial. A rapidly expanding roster of antianxiety and antidepression drugs are available by a doctor's prescription.

Anger and Hostility

Do real men express their feelings and emotions? In our culture, as in most others, a large number of pressures, overt and subtle, are arrayed against male expressiveness. But there is an exception: outbursts of anger are tolerated, even encouraged. It is an unfortunate exception. Although people benefit from expressing most emotions, men who unbottle their anger too freely can be left with a shattered bottle.

Anger and hostility can damage relationships and disrupt work. Road rage and domestic abuse are but two examples of the way anger can lead to violence. Anger can also cause internal damage; in particular, two recent studies from Harvard demonstrate that it can be heartbreaking.

THE HOSTILE HEART

Ever since 1961, scientists at Harvard Medical School and the Harvard School of Public Health have been observing 2,280 men as part of the Normative

Table 8.2: A TEST FOR ANXIETY

	Almost never	Sometimes	Often	Almost Always
1. I am "calm, cool, and collected."	4	3	2	1
2. I feel that problems are piling up so that I cannot overcome them.	1	2	3	4
3. I feel my heart racing or pounding without exercising.	1	2	3	4
4. Some unimportant thought runs through my mind and bothers me.	1	2	3	4
5. I feel secure and at ease.	4	3	2	1
6. I feel I am dizzy, lightheaded, or faint.	1	2	3	4
7. I wish I could be as happy as others seem to be.	1	2	3	4
8. I feel joyful and confident.	4	3	2	1
9. I feel worried and tense.	1	2	3	4
10. I am afraid of people and things.	1	2	3	4
11. I have stomach pains or indigestion.	1	2	3	4
12. I am inclined to take things hard.	1	2	3	4
13. I sleep poorly or have nightmares.	1	2	3	4
14. I enjoy sitting quietly.	4	3	2	1
15. I feel rushed or hurried.	1	2	3	4
16. I get headaches or neck pains.	1	2	3	4
17. I get flushed or sweaty without exercising or I get hives.	1	2	3	4
18. I am eager for new challenges and tasks.	4	3	2	1

Source: Spielberger, C. D., *Manual for the State-Trait Anxiety Inventory.* Palo Alto, California: Consulting Psychologists Press.

Aging Study. In 1986, 1,305 men with an average age of sixty-one completed the Minnesota Multiphasic Personality Inventory, a test that can quantify anger. Each participant received a score that indicated his level of anger and hostility. The men returned for comprehensive medical examinations every three to five years, at which time they were checked for heart disease and cardiac risk factors such as smoking, hypertension, and high cholesterol. All the men were free of coronary artery disease when the study began, but during seven years of observation, 110 of them developed heart disease. The men with the highest anger scores were at the greatest risk for developing heart disease. The risk was substantial; coronary artery disease was diagnosed three times more often in the angriest men than in the men with the least anger. The link between anger and heart disease was not explained by differences in blood pressure, smoking, or other cardiac risk factors; hostility was heartbreaking in its own right.

Another Harvard study examined factors that might modify the effects of anger. Doctors interviewed 1,623 patients about four days after they suffered heart attacks; 69 percent of the patients were men. The participants used a standard test to evaluate the intensity of any episodes of anger they experienced within two hours of their attacks. As reported in an earlier study, anger was clearly dangerous for the heart, more than doubling the incidence of heart attacks. But anger was far less likely to trigger a heart attack in well-educated people. Among individuals who never completed high school, a spell of anger increased the risk of a heart attack 3.3 times, but among people who had at least some college education, anger boosted risk only 1.6 times. The difference was not explained by variations in the intensity of anger or by other behavioral factors. Instead, having an educated head was what seemed to protect the angry hearts. And in a related study, Harvard scientists reported that taking a single aspirin tablet prevents about 40 percent of anger-induced heart attacks, suggesting that hostility harms the heart in part by activating the blood-clotting system (see Chapters Three and Six).

Heartbreaking hostility is not unique to patients seeing Harvard doctors. In fact, studies from around the world have confirmed the link between anger and coronary artery disease. In a study of 3,750 middle-aged Finnish men, for example, a high hostility rating was associated with a high risk of dying from heart disease. In the landmark American Multiple Risk Factor Intervention Trial (MR. FIT), men with a high potential for verbal or physical expressions of anger suffered 50 percent more heart attacks than their more docile peers. The risk was even greater for male physicians who were observed for twenty-five years by researchers at Duke University; angry docs were five times more likely to have heart attacks than were mild-mannered medics.

COOLING DOWN

Like stress and anxiety, excessive hostility can be treated. In fact, it will respond to many of the interventions that are used to manage anxiety. But if you have a short fuse, you can also help yourself. Consider learning how to meditate. Or you can experiment with breathing exercises:

- Breathe in through your nose slowly and deeply, pushing your abdomen out so your diaphragm contracts maximally.
- Hold your breath for a few seconds.
- Exhale slowly through your mouth, thinking "relax."
- Repeat the sequence five to ten times, concentrating on breathing slowly and deeply.

You can also use behavioral techniques to help stay calm. Practice during daily life, so you will be able to keep your cool in times of stress:

- Drive your car in the slow right-hand lane.
- Use your car horn only to prevent car accidents, not to vent frustration.
- When you drive up to a toll plaza, join the longest line, even if you have exact change.
- Eat slowly.
- Talk slowly, trying not to interrupt.
- Do not put in the last word in an argument, even if you think you are right.
- Do not shout or raise your voice in anger.
- Do not use expletives; substitute less hostile phrases like "darn" or "rats."
- Do not permit outbursts of anger. Instead wait for a few moments, take a few deep breaths, and express yourself calmly.
- Try not to grimace or clench your teeth; practice smiling.

It is also very important to structure your life to reduce stress. Identify the things that bother you most and try to change them. Learn to recognize warning signs of building tension, such as a racing pulse, fast breathing, or a jumpy, restless feeling. When you recognize anger signals, take steps to relieve tension before it builds to the boiling point. Often something as simple as a brief walk or a snack can cool things down nicely. Build strong relationships and talk out your feelings instead of bottling them up inside. If it is difficult for you to talk out your anger, try writing a letter that expresses your feelings. Establish priorities; set realistic expectations and pace yourself, building in time to relax. Get enough sleep. Do not try to calm yourself with nicotine, alcohol, or drugs. Think positively and make time for activities that are stimulating and enjoyable.

Depression and Bereavement

Because it is more common in women, depression is often considered a "female disease." It is a widespread misconception that has the unfortunate effect of making it harder for men to correctly identify symptoms of depression, and it even deters doctors from properly diagnosing depression in men. In fact, depression does not respect gender. If you doubt statistics, remember the case of Sir Winston Churchill, who recognized his own recurring depression as a "black dog" that turned up without warning. Similarly, TV newsman Mike Wallace felt his depression as "endless darkness." Or consider the case of Pete Harnisch, who could not finish pitching the opening game of the 1997 season for the New York Mets because of exhaustion: "I felt very withdrawn, I felt very much to myself: the sleeping problem was back . . . there was a lot of anxiety. . . . I wasn't eating anything. I had a lot of things going together." Team doctors placed Harnisch on the disabled list and evaluated him for a variety of medical problems before diagnosing depression. With treatment he was back on the mound four months later.

WHAT IS DEPRESSION?

Everyone feels sad and down from time to time. It is a normal emotional reaction to loss or disappointment. But true depression is more than ordinary sorrow or grief. It is an excessive, maladaptive response to a loss or other setback, and the loss itself may be a matter of personal perception rather than an actual life event.

The most common feature of clinical depression is the loss of self-esteem. People who are depressed feel hopeless, helpless, and worthless. They often feel they are a burden to others. Pessimism is universal and guilt common. Loss of interest in the world around them causes people who are depressed to become isolated and withdrawn from social and professional contacts. They cannot remember, concentrate, or focus normally. Instead of engaging in productive tasks, they are indecisive and preoccupied with themselves, often plagued by recurrent thoughts of illness and death. Despite all this self-preoccupation, depressed people often exhibit self-neglect, especially in matters of appearance, hygiene, nutrition, and exercise. Physical symptoms are nearly universal, often including disturbances of sleep and appetite, loss of sexual interest, aches and pains, and abnormal bowel function. Many depressed people are physically inactive and lethargic, but others are anxious and agitated.

In its full-blown version, depression is easy to recognize. But the symptoms can be subtle, often masquerading as a physical illness. To assist in establishing a correct diagnosis, the American Psychiatric Association has established criteria for the diagnosis of major depression (see Table 8.3).

The American Psychiatric Association criteria apply to one of the most serious types of depression, major depression. But there are other variants: *Dysthymia* is less severe than major depression, but is a low-grade condition that persists for years. Because it is so chronic, many people mistake dysthymia for a pessimistic personality, thus depriving themselves of the opportunity to get effective treatment. *Adjustment disorder with depressed mood,* formerly called reactive depression, is a depressive episode that is clearly triggered by major life stress or loss. *Seasonal affective disorder* (SAD) occurs on a seasonal pattern, usually beginning in the fall and resolving in the spring. As in all forms of depression, sadness and fatigue are two major symptoms, but unlike other types of depression, SAD is usually accompanied by overeating, weight gain, and excessive sleeping. SAD is more common in northern latitudes and has been attributed to lack of daylight. *Bipolar disorder* or *manic depressive illness* is a very serious illness in which periods of depression alternate with episodes of *mania,* periods of inappropriate elation, increased energy and activity and diminished need for sleep, inflated self-esteem, and expansive plans with little concern for consequences. Finally, *psychotic depression* is another severe illness in which deep depression is accompanied by the thought disorders characteristic of psychosis.

Table 8.3: CRITERIA FOR THE DIAGNOSIS OF MAJOR DEPRESSION

To meet these criteria for major depression, patients must exhibit symptoms that are not explained by medical conditions, drugs, or recent bereavement nearly every day for at least two weeks.

At least one of these two symptoms should be present:

- Depressed mood
- Severely diminished interest in or pleasure from activities that are usually pleasurable

In addition, at least four of these seven symptoms should be present:

- Substantial change in appetite or weight loss or (less commonly) gain amounting to about 5 percent of body weight in one month
- Insomnia or (less commonly) excessive sleep
- Fatigue or loss of energy
- Diminished physical activity or (less commonly) agitation
- Impaired ability to think, concentrate, or make decisions
- Diminished self-esteem with feelings of worthlessness or inappropriate guilt
- Recurrent thoughts of death or suicide

Adapted from: *Diagnostic and Statistical Manual of Mental Disorders,* American Psychiatric Association, Fourth Edition, 1994.

Recognizing Depression

Depression has many faces. Shakespeare identified it as "the sad companion, dull-eyed melancholy," but many people have a harder time recognizing their own depression. To find out if you may be depressed, ask yourself the questions in Table 8.4, then add up your answers. A score below 30 is reassuring; scores between 31 and 45 suggest mild depression, those between 46 and 60, moderate depression, and scores above 61, severe depression. Remember that these results provide a guideline, but not a diagnosis. If your results suggest depression, consider following them up with a professional evaluation.

The Mind-Body Connection

Nearly all depressed patients experience physical symptoms and many seek medical evaluations rather than psychological help. It can be hard for a doctor to determine if a complaint is caused by depression or bodily illness. To make things even more confusing, physical illnesses often produce depression. In

Table 8.4: A TEST FOR DEPRESSION

	Almost Never	Sometimes	Often	Almost Always
1. I feel blue or sad.	1	2	3	4
2. I feel confident and hopeful.	4	3	2	1
3. I feel like a failure.	1	2	3	4
4. I do not enjoy things the way I used to.	1	2	3	4
5. I feel guilty.	1	2	3	4
6. I have a feeling that something bad may happen.	1	2	3	4
7. I am pleased with myself.	4	3	2	1
8. I blame myself for everything that goes wrong.	1	2	3	4
9. I have crying spells.	1	2	3	4
10. I get irritated or annoyed.	1	2	3	4
11. I am interested in people and enjoy being with them.	4	3	2	1
12. I am unsure of myself and try to avoid decisions.	1	2	3	4
13. I feel that I look attractive and healthy.	4	3	2	1
14. I sleep poorly and am tired in the morning.	1	2	3	4
15. I am energetic and eager to take on new tasks.	4	3	2	1
16. My appetite is not as good as it used to be.	1	2	3	4
17. I am as interested in sex as I used to be.	4	3	2	1
18. I am concerned about my stomach and my bowels.	1	2	3	4
19. I feel healthy.	4	3	2	1
20. I have trouble doing my work.	1	2	3	4

SOURCE: Beck, A. T., et al. "An Inventory for Measuring Depression," *Archives of General Psychiatry* 4. 1961:561–65.

Table 8.5: SOME MEDICAL CAUSES OF DEPRESSION

Medications	Beta-blockers, older antihypertensives, corticosteroids, tranquilizers and sleeping medications, antihistamines, drugs that block stomach acid, digitalis, drugs for abnormal heart rhythms, levodopa, pain relievers
Substance-related problems	Alcohol, cocaine, withdrawal from stimulants (including nicotine and caffeine)
Endocrine and metabolic disorders	Thyroid disease, adrenal disease, diabetes, high blood calcium, low blood sodium, lead toxicity
Neurologic disorders	Alzheimer's disease and other dementias, strokes, head injuries, Parkinson's disease, brain tumors, multiple sclerosis, seizure disorders
Infections	Influenza, mononucleosis, HIV and other viral infections, Lyme disease
Nutritional disorders	Vitamin B_3 or B_{12} deficiencies
Malignancies	Pancreatic cancer and most other malignancies
Cardiovascular disease	Congestive heart failure
Other disorders	Chronic pain from any cause, lupus, polymyalgia, fibromyalgia, chronic fatigue syndrome, sleep apnea, end-stage kidney or lung disease

fact, about 10 percent of all depression stems from a medical illness, and about 25 percent of patients with serious chronic medical problems become depressed as a result of their illnesses. Table 8.5 lists some important medical causes of depression.

The multiplicity of medical difficulties that can cause depression testifies to the close link between body and mind. Even as medical problems can cause mental symptoms, so too can emotional disorders cause physical ills. Suicide is the most obvious and lethal complication of depression, taking some 30,000 American lives each year. Not so obvious is the link between depression and cardiovascular disease. Many studies have established a link between depression and an increased risk of heart attacks, congestive heart failure, and cardiac death, and most indicate that men are much more vulnerable to the heart-breaking effects of depression than women. And a broken heart is not the only potential medical consequence of depression. In fact, it increases the risk of hypertension and predicts a poor functional outcome from most major medical illnesses.

TREATMENT

Like other psychological disorders, depression can respond to "talking therapies," medications, or combinations of the two. Among the many forms of psychotherapy, two—interpersonal psychotherapy and cognitive-behavioral therapy—were specifically developed to treat depression. Studies indicate they can be as effective as medication for mild to moderate depression. People with milder cases of depression may choose to try psychotherapy first, but more severely depressed individuals should usually include medications in their initial treatment program.

Many antidepressant medications are available; they appear equally effective if given in the proper doses for a sufficient period of time. Most doctors favor the newer antidepressant drugs because they act more rapidly and produce fewer side effects. St. John's wort is a nonprescription herbal medication that is widely promoted for depression (see Chapter Six); medical studies suggest that it may help, at least for mild depression, but more research is needed. Self-treatment should never substitute for a comprehensive, medically-supervised program. Depression is a complex problem that requires competent, comprehensive treatment.

Talking therapies and medications are the main treatments for depression, and a combination of the two is even better than either alone. But other things can also help. Exercise has a mood-elevating effect. In fact, the Harvard Alumni Study found that men who exercise regularly are less likely to develop depression than their sedentary peers. Along with sound nutrition, exercise promotes the good general health that is so important for good mental health; healthy bodies and healthy minds go well together.

BEREAVEMENT

Like depression, bereavement is sometimes misclassified as a women's problem. In fact, since women live longer than men, widows outnumber widowers; eleven out of twelve American wives outlive their husbands. And since women express their feelings more freely than men, their grief is more open and visible.

The loss of a spouse is more common for women. By age sixty-five, more than half of all women have lost at least one husband. But bereavement is a man's problem, too. By age sixty-five, 10 percent of all American men have been widowed. And spousal bereavement is actually more serious for men. A 1995 study from California tells just how serious it is. The study did not measure the psychological and socioeconomic burdens of bereavement, though they are obviously enormous. Instead, the researchers focused on another impact of spousal bereavement, the mortality of the surviving spouse.

The study tracked 12,522 married couples from 1964 to 1987. During that time, 1,453 men and 3,294 women lost their spouses. Subsequently, 30 percent of the widowers died, while only 15 percent of the widows succumbed. Healthy men who lost a wife were 2.1 times more likely to die than healthy men who were not bereaved, even after age, education, and other predictors of mortality were taken into account. For men with preexisting medical problems, bereavement boosted the risk of death 1.6 times. The risk was greatest from seven to twelve months after the loss, but an elevated death rate persisted for more than two years. Shakespeare was right when he wrote of "deadly grief."

Why do men who lose their wives face an increased risk of death? Doctors do not know the answer, but they can speculate about several possible explanations. The loss of a caregiver could be part of the answer, but since the impact is substantially greater in healthy men than in ill men who may depend on a spouse for care, that cannot be the whole story. Most likely, intense grief adversely affects the body's stress hormones, nervous system, and immunologic apparatus. It is the same way extreme fright and natural disasters can trigger sudden cardiac death.

Grief is a normal reaction, but it can have many features in common with depression, including extreme sadness, sleep and appetite disturbances, guilt, anxiety, social withdrawal, and loneliness, forgetfulness, and anger. People who are grieving are usually preoccupied with a recent loss and feel an incessant longing for the return of the lost loved one. Grief reactions begin abruptly with an obvious loss. Usually it is the death of a close relative or friend, but it can be the loss of a job or the loss of good health.

Although grief reactions are terribly painful, they are normal. More than that, they actually pave the way to healing and recovery. But the grief reaction also can be abnormally severe and prolonged. Pathological grief needs professional help; normal grief does not, though mourners can benefit from care and support. Here are some ways you can help ease the pain of a bereaved relative or friend:

- Help him anticipate the loss. Often there is plenty of warning before a loss, but the warning signals are often denied or overlooked. Dire predictions or intrusive reminders will not help, but gentle discussions and balanced realism can prepare people for the inevitable.

- Encourage the bereaved individual to express his feelings, even, or especially, if these feelings are accompanied by tears.
- Stay close during the early phase of anger and denial, but stay neutral. Do not try to crash through expressions of denial and do not argue defensively with expressions of anger, even if they are clearly unrealistic. Acknowledge feelings of guilt as valid emotions without reinforcing inaccurate notions of culpability.
- Be empathetic and patient, sympathetic and nonjudgmental. Understand that grief is a powerful emotion that cannot be mitigated by simple advice to "cheer up," much less by well-intentioned reminders that "it could be worse." It may be easy for you to adjust to a loss, but it is hard and slow for a surviving spouse. Shakespeare again: "Everyone can master a grief but he that has it."
- Be available. It is especially important to "be there" when it is the hardest, when the mourner is disorganized and isolated. Do not try to force yourself on anyone or to trick a bereaved person into social contacts before he is ready. But keep in touch and do not let a series of rejections halt your invitations—sooner or later, your companionship will be welcomed.
- As bereavement enters its final phase of reorganization and acceptance, let the mourner know that it's okay to recover, that a return to work and play is not a sign of disloyalty or disrespect. Share his happiness as it returns, even as you shared his pain at its worst.

Social Networks and Isolation

Bereavement is particularly difficult for a man because the loss of a wife often deprives him of his main link to friends and community. It is a prime example of the importance of social networks and the hazards of isolation.

TIES THAT BIND

"No man is an island," wrote John Donne, some four hundred years ago. But in twenty-first century America, many men seem to be very insular indeed. A survey conducted by the New England Research Institute examined the primary social supports for men and women and found a striking gender difference:

Table 8.6: THE SOCIAL SUPPORTS OF MEN AND WOMEN

Primary Support	Men	Women
Spouse	66%	26%
Relatives	10%	40%
Friends	9%	28%
Co-workers	2%	1%
None	10%	4%

Men benefit from intact, supportive marriages. A reduced risk of cardiovascular disease is an important medical gain (see below), but there are others. For example, although research does not generally implicate psychological factors in cancer, a study from the University of Miami demonstrated that an intact marriage improves the outcome of men with prostate cancer. The researchers tracked 143,063 men who were diagnosed with the disease between 1973 and 1990. They found a surprisingly strong protective effect of marriage. The median survival for married men was sixty-nine months, for divorced men fifty-five months, for single men forty-nine months, and for separated and widowed men just thirty-eight months. That means the average married man lived nearly twice as long after diagnosis as the typical widower. The differences were not explained by age, the stage of the disease at the time of diagnosis, or the type of treatment that was administered. All in all, unmarried men were about 30 percent more likely to die from prostate cancer than married men.

Marriage is the most important social support for men, so important that it has a major impact on health. A 1990 study for Princeton University, for example, found that unmarried men have twice the mortality rate as married men. But marital strife has the opposite effect. Recent studies from Toronto and Salt Lake City show that marital cohesion protects against hypertension, while marital conflict sends the blood pressure soaring, particularly in men. Divorce doubles the suicide rate in men but does not change the rate in women, which is much lower to begin with. Divorce also substantially increases the rate of illness during the first year of separation.

Although marriage is the main social support for men, others are available. Studies from California, North Carolina, Connecticut, and elsewhere have linked attendance at religious services to lower blood pressures and longer survival. The benefits may depend on faith, but an investigation from Sweden suggests that it may derive simply from sharing communal activities. Researchers tracked more than 12,000 people over a nine-year period. Even after accounting for previous health, smoking, exercise, education, income, and other factors, attending cultural events was associated with longevity. In all, people who attended concerts and plays rarely or never were 2.8 times more likely to die during the study period than were people who attended frequently; occasional concert-goers were in between, with a death rate 1.6 times lower than frequent attendees.

LONELY HEARTS

People are good medicine, and the converse is also true: isolation is heartbreaking. A landmark study from the 1960s evaluated nearly 7,000 adults in Alameda County, California. After checking numerous risk factors, researchers identified one that more than doubled a man's risk of dying during the nine-year study period. This crucial risk factor was not smoking, drinking, lack of exercise, or poor nutrition. In fact, it was social isolation: Men with the fewest social ties had the highest risk of dying from heart disease, circulatory ailments, and even cancer.

Isolation has its greatest impact on the heart. Many studies have linked low social support to an increased risk of heart attacks and a shortened survival following attacks. And a recent study from the Harvard School of Public Health demonstrates that isolation affects the mind as well as the heart; it linked social disengagement to a two-fold increase in the incidence of cognitive decline.

For health, heart, and mind, men should reach out and establish ties with individuals and community. It does not come easily to many men, and it is particularly hard to build bridges that do not rely on a spouse. Hard or not, it is the smart thing to do, particularly when men confront the transition from work to leisure.

Work and Retirement

According to Freud, a man's mission in life is "to work and to love." Love can cement the social networks that protect a man's health, but in this modern world careless love can be very hazardous indeed (see Sexually Acquired Diseases, Chapter Ten). But what of work? Does it have the same dual capacity to either promote or impair health?

On the Job

Work presents health hazards of the most basic sort. In 1998, for example, private employers in the United States reported 5.5 million work injuries and 390,000 cases of occupational illness. In 1997, the most recent year for which such data are available, 5,255 civilian workers died from their injuries; 93 percent were men. According to the National Safety Council, occupational injuries and illnesses drain the economy of over $125 billion annually.

The combined efforts of the Occupational Safety and Health Administration (OSHA), responsible employers, and concerned workers' groups have greatly improved workplace health. Still, all employees must protect themselves from accidents and injuries. It is a particular problem for men, who constitute 78 to 100 percent of the workforce in the ten most dangerous occupations. Add risk-seeking behavior and alcohol and drug abuse, and you will see why work can be physically hazardous to men.

From a psychological point of view, work can either boost a man's health or hinder it. Men tend to be more competitive than women, often dividing the world into winners and losers, as if there were no middle ground. Striving for success (or struggling to avoid failure) can turn men into workaholics. Men who succeed derive emotional satisfaction from work, particularly if their jobs entail creativity, independent judgment, and challenge without undue stress. But work can also deprive men of the family relationships and social networks that are particularly important when illness or retirement keep men from their work.

Can a man actually work himself to death? The Japanese think so. In fact, *karoshi* or "death from overwork" is a recognized diagnosis that is backed up by compensatory payments to survivors in Japan. But does overwork also affect Western men? In 1997, a British team answered the question by performing a meta-analysis of twenty-one studies of work and health. The researchers confirmed an association between hours of work and ill health; the effect was small but consistent and significant.

Although working hours are important, working conditions have an even greater impact. Studies from Sweden, Denmark, and Italy demonstrate that men who have low control over their jobs, men who have high mental stress but low physical activity at work, and men who have low social support from their coworkers face an increased risk of heart attacks and death. Although OSHA and its friends have improved the physical safety of work, the mental aspects are not getting better. On the contrary, changing gender roles, globalization, rapidly evolving technologies, economic imperatives, and rising productivity standards are adding to the stress men face at work. Worst of all, perhaps, is the erosion of autonomy and control. Just ask any doctor who works for an HMO.

OUT TO PASTURE

Work may be a heartbreaker, but is retirement any better? Yes and no. If retirement is involuntary or unexpected, it will reduce a man's self-esteem and add to his stress. But if retirement is preceded by realistic anticipation and planning, it can mark a happy new chapter in a man's life.

Three major changes accompany retirement: the loss of income, the loss of workplace relationships, and the loss of identity as a worker. The key to a successful retirement is to anticipate all three, and to plan accordingly. The need for financial planning is obvious. Not so obvious, but just as important, is the need to build relationships to replace those at work. Similarly, a man should cultivate interests and activities to make the leisure of retirement as rich and rewarding as the challenges of work.

The key is a gradual transition, ideally extending over a period of years. Men should think of retirement as a career change, not the end of productivity. People who develop hobbies, interests, and relationships in advance should be able to anticipate retirement with eagerness, not dread. Above all, perhaps, men should heed the lifestyle lessons revealed by the Harvard studies of men's health (see Chapters Three through Seven). Men who stay healthy and age successfully will have the physical and mental resources to enjoy retirement. In turn, mental stimulation and physical activity should help keep men alert and happy during their "golden years."

Memory Loss

It is ironic. Over the years, every man accumulates a sizable array of things he would like to forget but cannot, yet over the years, particularly in advancing years, every man forgets things he would like to remember. Forgetting names can be an embarrassment, misplacing eyeglasses a bother, losing the car keys a real nuisance. But when the little lapses seem to mount up, they add another dimension: worry about "losing it," about severe mental impairment, and Alzheimer's disease.

Those worries are understandable. Although severe cognitive impairment, or *dementia* in medical lingo, is uncommon in younger people, it becomes increasingly prevalent with advancing age; only a minority of sixty-five-year-olds meet the medical criteria for dementia, but the prevalence rises steadily thereafter. By age eighty-five, 16 to 35 percent of Americans suffer severe cognitive impairment—and at least half of it is due to Alzheimer's disease.

Worry about memory loss is understandable, but in most cases it is unwarranted. In the past few years, scientists have learned a lot about normal mental aging and how to keep the mind young. Doctors have developed ways to distinguish normal forgetfulness from serious memory loss, and they can use simple tests to identify treatable causes of dementia. And at last researchers are making great strides in understanding the causes of Alzheimer's disease, progress that offers real hope for the future.

Normal Memory

In today's cyberspace culture, the human brain is often likened to a computer. Not yet, anyway. The brain is smarter, faster, much more complex, and infinitely more creative than even the most sophisticated supercomputer. The brain is also more fragile, but the body has good ways to protect it, providing the body stays healthy itself.

According to current estimates, the brain has about 100 billion nerve cells. It is an awesome number, but the vital connections that allow nerve cells to communicate with each other are even more spectacular, amounting to some 100 trillion interconnections or *synapses*. Each nerve cell transmits information in the form of electrical impulses that race through the cell at 200 miles per hour. But to pass information along to other cells, the electrical impulses are converted into chemical signals called *neurotransmitters*. More than twenty chemical messengers have been identified, and each seems suited to a particular neurologic function. *Acetylcholine* is the neurotransmitter most intimately linked to memory, and it is the brain chemical that is depleted in Alzheimer's disease.

Although the brain weighs less than three pounds, it is subdivided into many highly specialized zones, each responsible for a particular function, such as word recognition, speech, vision, sensation, locomotion, coordination, and so forth. New research using the technique of *functional magnetic resonance imaging* (fMRI) suggests that at least two areas of the brain play key roles in memory. The *hippocampus* appears particularly important for long-term memory, while the *frontal lobes* contribute more to short-term memory.

Whether you are concentrating to read this *Guide*, relaxing under a tree, or fast asleep, your brain is always hard at work. Although it accounts for less than 2 percent of body weight, the brain receives 15 percent of the body's blood flow and consumes 25 percent of its oxygen supply. While other organs can burn carbohydrates, fats, or protein for energy, the brain depends entirely on glucose (sugar), which is why it accounts for up to 70 percent of the body's glucose consumption.

A good memory requires many things, including a healthy heart and blood vessels, a good supply of oxygen and glucose, and the right mix of neurotransmitters. Scientists are working hard to develop medications to influence neurotransmitters, and they have already succeeded in manipulating several important chemical messengers including *dopamine* (Parkinson's disease), *serotonin* (depression), and even *acetylcholine* (Alzheimer's disease). But you do not have to depend on doctors and drugs to keep the brain's supply of blood and oxygen up to par. If you remember to take care of your cardiovascular health and metabolism, your memory will benefit enormously.

NORMAL FORGETTING

You do not have to be neuroscientists to understand the importance of memory. Shakespeare called memory "the warden of the brain." But forgetting is as normal as remembering; as Shakespeare tells us: "But men are men; the best sometimes forget."

Just as memory involves different regions of the brain, forgetting involves the loss of different types of memory. *Long-term memory* retains information learned in the past, while *short-term memory* stores information from the present. Long-term memory is designed to be highly durable, while short-term memory can be temporary, like forgetting a phone number as soon as you have written it down.

If you did not forget information stored in short-term memory, your mind would soon be cluttered with all sorts of useless information. More than simply normal, that type of forgetting is adaptive and helpful. Forgetting items in your long-term memory bank is different, but even here there are important distinctions. Long-term memory can be *episodic* (remembering when you last rode your bicycle, for example), *semantic* (remembering facts and principles, such as knowing what a bicycle is), or *procedural* (remembering how to ride a bike or how to perform arithmetic). It is perfectly normal to forget episodic memories, but semantic and procedural memories should be much more deeply entrenched.

TIME MARCHES ON

Every part of the body changes over time, and the brain is no exception. The changes occur at different rates for different people, but the average brain shrinks by about 10 percent during maturity, with a corresponding increase in the volume of the *cerebrospinal fluid* that bathes the brain. Brain cells do die as people age, but the standard estimate of 100,000 cells a day is now considered high, even if it amounts to just a hundred thousandth of the brain's total cell population. Also changing is the conventional wisdom that brain cells cannot regenerate or repair themselves. Exciting new research shows that new cells can be added to the aging brain.

Even if the brain does not shrink as much as scientists originally believed, it does change with age, and its functional abilities also change. But here, too, new research is clarifying the impact of aging. Healthy elders experience little decline in abstract reasoning, visual-spatial ability, and language skills, though there is often some slowing in these processes. Long-term memory is also well preserved, but short-term memory does weaken; new learning occurs at a slower pace, new information is processed more superficially, and details tend to slip.

Normal age-related changes in memory can be annoying, but you can learn to cope with them (see the list on page 238 for tips). But do you need to worry about further deterioration? In most cases, you do not. In fact, people who are sharp enough to worry about misplacing their keys or forgetting a name, probably have little real cause to worry. But there are exceptions; Table 8.7 presents some simple guidelines to help you determine if memory lapses are normal or worrisome.

Memory *lapses* are normal, even inevitable. True memory *losses,* on the other hand, are legitimately worrisome, even frightening. But here, too, there are degrees. *Mild cognitive impairment* (MCI) is an abnormal condition, but memory and judgment are preserved well enough to allow independent function. In most patients, MCI remains relatively stable, but in some it progresses to full-blown *dementia*.

EVALUATING DEMENTIA

Call it dementia or use the old term senility, by any name, severe memory loss is a terrible, terrible disability. It is becoming progressively more common as people live longer, but it was well known in 1864 when the poet Swinburne wrote that "the world shall end when I forget."

Table 8.7: EVALUATING FORGETFULNESS

NORMAL AGING	ABNORMAL FORGETTING
Independence in daily activities preserved.	Person becomes critically dependent on others for key independent living activities.
Complains of memory loss but able to provide considerable detail regarding incidents of forgetfulness.	May complain of memory problems only if specifically asked; unable to recall instances where memory loss was noticed.
Patient is more concerned about alleged forgetfulness than are close family members.	Close family members much more concerned about incidents of memory loss than patient.
Recent memory for important events, affairs, conversations not impaired.	Notable decline in memory for recent events and ability to converse.
Occasional word finding difficulties.	Frequent word finding pauses and substitutions.
Does not get lost in familiar territory; may have to pause momentarily to remember way.	Gets lost in familiar territory while walking or driving; may take hours to eventually return home.
Able to operate common appliances even if unwilling to learn how to operate new devices.	Becomes unable to operate common appliances; unable to learn to operate even simple new appliances.
Maintains prior level of interpersonal social skills.	Exhibits loss of interest in social activities; exhibits socially inappropriate behaviors.
Normal performance on mental status examinations, taking education and culture into account.	Abnormal performance on mental status examination not accounted for by education or cultural factors.

SOURCE: Modified from *Diagnosis, Management, and Treatment of Dementia*. American Medical Association: 1999.

In most cases, true dementia is irreversible, but even in these situations there are important ways to help. However, some causes of dementia can be corrected. Here are some things that doctors look for:

- *Drug Toxicity.* We live in a medicated society. Drugs can be life-saving, but they can also have serious side effects. Older folks are particularly sensitive, and a wide variety of medications, ranging from antihistamine to sedatives, pain relievers, and antihypertensives can produce mental changes that resemble dementia.

- *Substance Abuse.* It is high on the list when young people have mental status changes, but it can affect older adults, too. Alcohol ranks first (see Chapter Seven).
- *Depression.* When typical symptoms are present, depression is easy to recognize, but masked depression can produce mental slowing that resembles dementia (see pages 220 to 225).
- *Thyroid Disease.* An overproduction of thyroid hormone can produce confusion and delirium, but in most cases many other symptoms differentiate it from dementia. But an underactive thyroid can be tricky, sometimes mimicking dementia. A simple blood test can tell the tale.
- *Vitamin B_{12} Deficiency.* Also known as *pernicious anemia,* it too can be tricky, producing dementia before other problems surface. A simple blood test can make the diagnosis.
- *Other Metabolic Derangements.* These can also be detected with simple blood tests; examples include abnormalities of sodium, calcium, or glucose metabolism and advanced cases of liver failure or kidney disease. In most cases, the primary medical problem is quite apparent, even without blood tests.
- *Anatomic Abnormalities.* Structural changes in the brain may produce irreversible dementia, but some others can be corrected. Examples include *hydrocephalus* (excessive "water on the brain"), *subdural hematomas* (blood clots around the brain), and some brain tumors. A careful neurologic exam will usually provide clues to those problems, but to be safe many doctors obtain CT or MRI scans of the brain as part of a thorough dementia evaluation.

Preserving Memory: The Body's Role

It is much easier to prevent dementia than to correct it. Although dozens of neurologic diseases can cause dementia, two stand out: Alzheimer's disease and *vascular* or *multi-infarct dementia.* Vascular dementia occurs when small vessels in the brain become diseased or blocked, depriving brain cells of the oxygen and glucose they depend on. If enough brain cells are killed off by this process, memory cannot be restored. But vascular dementia can be prevented, and measures that protect the brain's blood supply can also lessen the impact of other dementing illnesses, even Alzheimer's disease. The key is to reduce cardiovascular risk factors. Here is a quick review of the main precepts from Chapters Three through Eight:

- Do not smoke.
- Maintain a normal blood pressure; medications may be needed.
- Maintain optimal levels of LDL ("bad") and HDL ("good") cholesterol; medications may be needed.
- Maintain a normal or near-normal blood-sugar level; medications may be needed for diabetics.
- Follow a good diet: reduce your intake of saturated fat, trans fatty acids, and cholesterol. Favor monounsaturated and omega-3 fats from olive oil, fish, nuts, and possibly canola oil. Eat lots of high fiber foods, including whole grains, fruits, and vegetables. Reduce your intake of processed foods and sodium (salt). Maintain a good intake of low- or nonfat dairy products.
- Exercise regularly. Two 2001 studies linked regular physical activity to a reduced risk of cognitive decline.
- Avoid obesity.
- Reduce stress.
- Take a multivitamin that provides 100 percent of the recommended daily allowance of folic acid and vitamins B_6 and B_{12}.These three Bs lower blood levels of homocysteine, and a major 2002 study linked higher levels of the amino acid to an increased risk of dementia.
- Limit your alcohol consumption to two drinks a day.
- Consider low-dose aspirin (81 to 325 milligrams a day).

PRESERVING MEMORY: THE MIND'S ROLE

Mind and body are inseparable aspects of the human organism. A healthy body will help keep your mind alert, and an active mind will also help itself stay young and sharp. The guys in the locker room were right after all; for the mind, as for the body, the watchword is use it or lose it. As Samuel Johnson said in 1754: "It is a man's own fault, it is from want of use if his mind grows torpid in old age." Here are some tips:

- Keep learning. Read, take courses, explore new hobbies, do anything that is stimulating, interesting, and, above all, new.
- Try mental gymnastics. Do word puzzles, jigsaw puzzles, or math problems. Play computer games or chess.
- Try things that take manual dexterity as well as mental concentration. Drawing, ceramics, sculpture, and square dancing are examples.
- Reduce stress in your life.
- Get enough sleep.
- Be sure your hearing and vision are good.
- Establish a social network. Spend as much time as possible with other people. Meet new people and expand your contacts.

Scientists do not have proof that exercising the mind will keep it sharp, but all the clues point in that direction. If you do not believe the neurobiologists, consider the case of Oliver Wendell Holmes. When the great jurist was asked why he was reading Plato at age ninety-two, he replied, "To improve my mind." Or consider the advice of Cicero some 2,000 years earlier: "Old men retain their mental faculties, provided their interest and application continue." If computer games are not your thing, you could do worse than reading Plato or Cicero or, for that matter, one of the Harvard Medical School books or newsletters.

Managing That Senior Moment

Memory lapses are normal, even universal. But they do increase with age, even in people with healthy bodies and brains. Here are a few ways to compensate:

- *Write it down.* Make lists, jot memos to yourself, and use a calendar to note your appointments and obligations.
- *Rehearse.* If you have a complex task or trip ahead, review all the steps in your mind until they become second nature.

- *Concentrate.* Work at learning new information by focusing your mind and repeating the information until it is yours. Do one thing at a time.
- *Simplify.* Eliminate distractions. Put routine things on automatic pilot so you will not waste mental energy on them. For example, always put your keys and eyeglasses down in the same place.
- *Stay alert.* Get enough sleep. Minimize your use of alcohol, sedatives, even antihistamines.
- *Reduce stress.* The last thing you need is to be distracted by worry or anxiety.
- Be sure your hearing and vision are up to par. It can be hard enough to recognize a face, let alone identify one that is blurred.
- Be honest and ask for help when you need it: "I'm having a senior moment, please remind me of your name."

ALZHEIMER'S DISEASE

Although many neurologic illnesses can cause dementia, two dominate. Evidence is emerging that vascular dementia can be prevented by a comprehensive program to ensure cardiovascular health. But *Alzheimer's disease* is quite another matter; while lifestyle measures may help, the real hope here lies with basic research that is just now uncovering the causes of the problem, thus laying the groundwork for better methods of diagnosis, treatment, and even prevention.

The characteristic findings of Alzheimer's include the presence of *neurofibrillary tangles* and *neuritic plaques* in the brain. Initially scant and scattered, the tangles and plaques progressively increase in number and size until they destroy nerve cells. But not all parts of the brain are equally vulnerable. Instead, the *hippocampus,* which is principally responsible for memory, is hit the hardest.

It took the better part of 100 years, but scientists have finally figured out how the plaques and tangles come into being. Normal nerve cells produce *amyloid precursor protein* (APP), which protrudes from the surface of the nerve cell. Unlike the quills of a porcupine, however, APP is harmless until it is snipped by two enzymes (*gamma-* and *beta-secretase*), releasing a small, sticky fragment called *beta-amyloid.* Another series of proteins called *presenilins* regulates the activity of the all-important snipping enzymes, while still other proteins determine whether the beta-amyloid is cleared away or simply accumulates in the brain. If the beta-amyloid builds up, it is toxic to nerve cells. First, it interferes with nerve function, blocking production and release of the neurotransmitter *acetylcholine,* which is essential for nerve cells to communicate with each other. Eventually, beta-amyloid destroys the nerve cells themselves. There is some evidence that vascular damage and inflammation triggered by oxygen free radicals contribute to the damage.

WHO GETS ALZHEIMER'S DISEASE?

Although Alzheimer's disease usually becomes apparent in old age, it is actually a genetic disorder. In fact, genetic abnormalities on at least six different chromosomes have been identified in patients, and more are sure to be discovered as research accelerates. These genes determine when the disease begins and how quickly it progresses, as well as the overall risk of developing Alzheimer's. For example, mutations in the *presenilin-1* and *-2* genes govern early-onset Alzheimer's, while the better-studied mutations of the gene for *apolipoprotein E* (ApoE, a cholesterol-carrying protein that helps repair nerve-cell membranes) determine the much more common late-onset familial and sporadic forms of the disease.

Even if it is "all in the genes," additional factors contribute to Alzheimer's. As noted, inflammation and oxidative damage may add insult to the injury produced by beta-amyloid itself. Impaired blood flow to the brain and serious head injury have also been implicated as risk factors. For example, recent studies tell us that high systolic blood pressure, high cholesterol levels, and low levels of vitamin B_{12} and folic acid increase risk. In contrast, exercise, the cholesterol-lowering statin drugs, and *non-steroidal anti-inflammatory* drugs (NSAIDs, such as aspirin) may reduce risk. More research will be needed to establish the true importance of these potential risk factors and protective influences; recent studies have ruled out previous risk candidates, including exposure to aluminum and dental amalgam.

SYMPTOMS

Although the range of Alzheimer's is variable, the typical patient progresses steadily through three stages, each lasting about three years. Memory, reasoning and judgment, and personality and behavior are all affected, usually in that order. It is a grim scenario, but brighter days lie ahead. New insights into the causes of this dread disease may soon lead to improved methods of diagnosis, treatment, and prevention. Even now, medications may be able to slow the disease or blunt its complications, and social networks can provide enormous support and comfort to patients and their caregivers alike.

DIAGNOSIS

Alzheimer's disease cannot be diagnosed by a single test. Instead, physicians use mental status tests to establish the presence of dementia, then order blood tests and neuroimaging studies such as *computed tomography* (CT scans) or *magnetic resonance imaging* (MRI) of the brain to rule out other causes of dementia. Genetic testing cannot establish a diagnosis of Alzheimer's disease, but in some cases it may identify people at increased risk. Routine testing is not advisable, and some experts caution against any genetic testing until better methods of prevention and treatment become available. People with a strong family history of early-onset Alzheimer's may wish to discuss the issue with their physicians.

TREATMENT

Several drugs are available to treat Alzheimer's disease; the *cholinesterase inhibitors,* which increase brain levels of the neurotransmitter acetylcholine, are the most helpful, but they produce only modest benefits.

Since medications produce only modest gains, many people are turning to supplements. Can they help? The leading candidate is *gingko biloba*. Hope is based principally on a 1997 study of 203 individuals with vascular dementia or Alzheimer's disease. The herb appeared to stabilize or improve cognitive function and social performance, but the improvement was modest and only 27 percent of the patients achieved those slight benefits. Unfortunately, a 2000 study in 123 older individuals with vascular dementia, Alzheimer's disease and age-related memory loss found no benefit from gingko. Because the options are limited, gingko may still be a reasonable choice for people struggling with dementia, but there is no evidence that it can prevent dementia or help with age-related memory lapses.

It is the same story for vitamin E. Although a single 1997 trial showed that very high doses of the supplement appeared to slow the progression of Alzheimer's disease, there is no evidence that it will stave off dementia or improve working memory. In fact, a study of more than 1,000 elderly Pennsylvanians found no benefit from vitamin E or other antioxidants such as vitamins C and A, beta-carotene, and selenium.

At this point, your best bet is a simple multivitamin. That is because high levels of the amino acid *homocysteine* have been linked to an increased risk of dementia as well as heart disease and stroke. The folic acid, vitamin B_6, and vitamin B_{12} in multivitamins will lower homocysteine levels with minimal cost and few, if any, side effects. It is a logical step, though there is still no proof that it will actually protect your head or your heart. Still, try to remember your daily multivitamin.

Prevention

Although there is no proven way to prevent Alzheimer's disease, several strategies may help. The most important involve measures to preserve vascular health. Smoking, high fat diets, low levels of B vitamins, the lack of regular exercise, and head trauma have all been linked to an increased risk of Alzheimer's. Clearly, it is important to avoid these risks. In contrast, long-term use of aspirin or other nonsteroidal antiinflammatory drugs has been associated with a decreased risk of Alzheimer's. The National Institute on Aging has begun a trial of NSAIDs in 2,600 people over the age of seventy to evaluate the benefits and risks of preventive treatment. Until the results are in, it is still too early to recommend routine use of these mediations, but low-dose aspirin makes sense for men at risk of atherosclerosis (see Chapter Six). The same is true for the cholesterol-lowering statin drugs. Four recent observational studies suggest that people who take these medications enjoy a substantially reduced risk of Alzheimer's disease, but clinical trials will be required to prove the point.

New Horizons

Although Alzheimer's disease remains a terrible problem, there is hope that recent research breakthroughs will be translated into new methods for prevention and treatment. Not this year, to be sure, but perhaps soon enough to help still healthy people at risk, and possibly in time to help some patients who already have early disease.

One approach is to develop drugs that will prevent nerve cells in the hippocampus from over-producing beta-amyloid, the toxic protein that causes brain damage. Now that scientists have identified the enzymes that convert the harmless amyloid precursor protein into beta-amyloid, they have likely targets for new drugs.

Another approach is to develop a vaccine. Experiments in mice have already demonstrated the feasibility of this technique. Since mice do not get Alzheimer's, the first step was to create genetically altered mice that would develop Alzheimer's. Next, biotech scientists injected the mice with a vaccine made from synthetic beta-amyloid. The antibodies appeared to protect the mice, even reversing some of the damage in older animals with the disease, but human trials in France were halted in 2002 due to serious side effects. Harvard scientists have had success with another vaccine administered into the nasal passages of mice. They have also been able to dissolve plaques by applying anti-amyloid antibodies directly to mouse brains through tiny holes in their skulls. It will take years for doctors to learn if either approach will be useful for humans. Still, it is wonderful to see a glimmer of light at the end of the dark Alzheimer's disease tunnel. But it is long tunnel, and it will take time to bring new possibilities to fruition. Even so, basic research is at last promising to advance what Milan Kundera called "the struggle of memory against forgetting."

Staying Mentally Well

Just as moderation is the key to physical health, balance is the key to psychological health. Balance work with play, exercise with rest, discipline with indulgence. Balance stimulation and challenge with relaxation and recovery, excitement with calm. Balance independence with interdependence, solitude with companionship. Balance practical realities with hopes and expectations, effort with relaxation, routine with spontaneity. Balance your needs with those of your family and community.

Balance your mind and body to keep both active, healthy, and happy.

PART III

The Maladies of Men

CHAPTER NINE

Disorders of the Penis, Scrotum, and Testicles

In the Beginning: Boyhood

The child is father of the man.

When William Wordsworth wrote those words in 1807, he could not have known much about developmental biology, but the poet certainly understood the human heart. He knew that childhood experiences have effects that last throughout life, playing an important role in establishing the personality structures and behavioral patterns that determine a man's psychological health (see Chapter Eight). Nearly two centuries later, scientists have learned that Wordsworth's observation is as valid biologically as psychologically. For several decades, doctors have been accumulating evidence that atherosclerosis, the leading killer of American men, gets its start in childhood. And new research suggests that a man's risk of disease in adulthood may even start taking shape before birth; fetal nutrition and other prenatal influences appear to have a lifelong effect on the risk of cardiovascular disease, diabetes, and possibly even prostate cancer.

Fetal development is extremely complex, and a lot can go wrong. Fortunately, serious problems are really very uncommon. You will need expert medical help to care for major problems in your sons, but you should understand the approach to some basic issues that can have ramifications in adulthood.

Normal Development

Humble beginnings indeed. After a sperm and egg unite, the future human being is but a tiny single-cell embryo, which goes through thousands of cell divisions and intricate differentiations to form all the organs and tissues of the human body, including uniquely male components such as hormones and genital tract organs.

From the moment of conception, males are different from females because they have a Y chromosome (see Chapter One). But until about seven weeks of pregnancy, males and females are otherwise exactly alike. At about seven to eight weeks of fetal life, hormones from the mother's placenta trigger the production of *testosterone* by cells that will ultimately become the *Leydig cells* of the testicles. Testosterone makes the boy as well as the man; without it, precursor cells would not develop into the male genital tract. But if testosterone is necessary, it's not sufficient. *MIS*, another hormone that is introduced by the future *Sertoli cells* of the testicle, is required to prevent the fetus from also developing a set of female reproductive organs.

Testosterone levels remain high throughout fetal life, dropping sharply just before birth. Except for a brief blip at about six months of age and another at about six years, testosterone levels stay low until puberty, when they rise rapidly, reaching maximum adult levels in the mid-teen years.

The testicles begin to mature midway through the first trimester of pregnancy. At that time, even though hormone production is underway, the testicles are still very rudimentary. In fact, they are located high in the rear of the abdomen, near the kidneys. At about seventeen weeks of pregnancy, the testicles begin their descent through the abdomen. They arrive at the groin five to ten weeks later, then cross through the *inguinal canal* into the newly formed scrotum by the thirtieth week of pregnancy (see Figure 9.1).

What is the purpose of this unique fetal migration? To produce sperm, the testicles need to be relatively cool, which is why they move from the body's warm interior to the cooler scrotum (see Chapter Ten). But like all trips, things can go wrong. In some cases, the testicles do not complete the whole trip (see The Undescended Testicle, page 251) and in others, the inguinal canal does not close properly, setting the stage for groin hernias (see Chapter Ten).

The tissues of the penis begin to develop during the second month of fetal life. The *urethra* develops first, but is soon surrounded by the tissue that becomes the shaft of the penis. The shaft of the penis ends in a rounded structure called the *glans*. The skin of the penis gradually grows forward, until the glans is covered by a thin layer of skin, called the *prepuce* or foreskin. Later in embryonic development the foreskin separates from the glans beneath it. Circumcision is the now-controversial operation that removes the foreskin, usually shortly after birth (see page 252).

The penis and testicles remain small until puberty, which occurs between the ages of nine-and-a-half and thirteen-and-a-half in 95 percent of American

FIGURE 9.1. THE DESCENT OF THE TESTICLES

3 Month Fetus

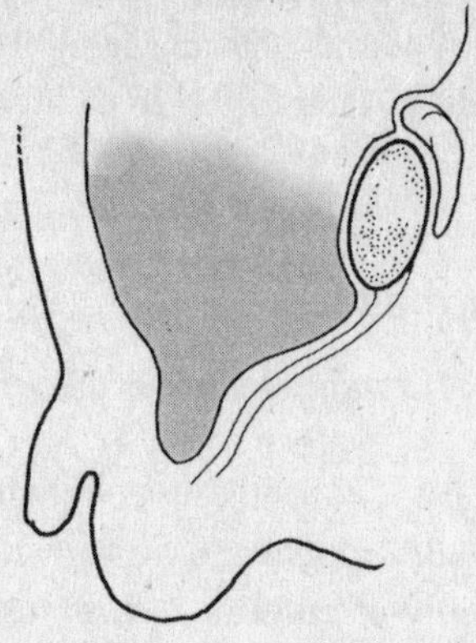

6 Month Fetus

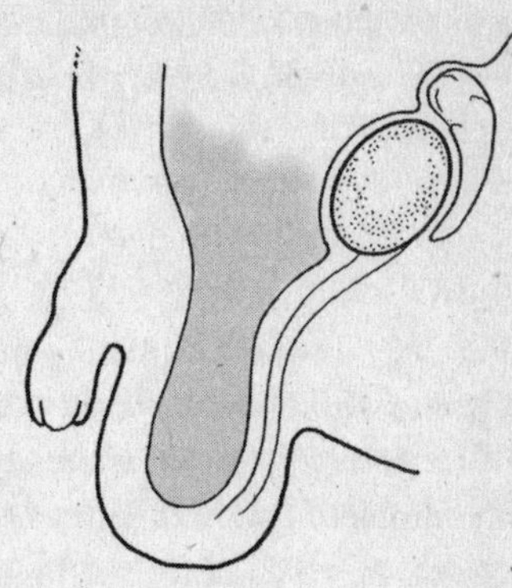

At Birth

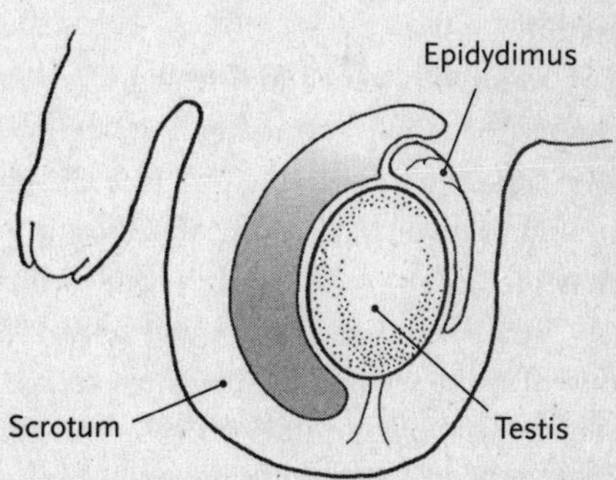

The testicles begin to mature midway through the first trimester of pregnancy. At that time, even though hormone production is underway, the testicles are still very rudimentary. In fact, they are located high in the rear of the abdomen, near the kidneys. At about 17 weeks of pregnancy, the testicles begin their descent through the abdomen. They arrive at the groin 5–10 weeks later, then cross through the inguinal canal into the newly formed scrotum by the 30th week of pregnancy.

boys. When testosterone levels rise, the genitals begin to enlarge and become fully functional. The average boy produces sperm and is able to ejaculate by age fourteen. Hormonal changes produce temporary breast enlargement in about 60 percent of adolescent boys (and in nearly all newborns).

Testosterone also accounts for the growth spurt of adolescence and for the secondary sex characteristics that mark the beginning of manhood: large muscles, strong bones, a deep voice, oily skin, and the growth of facial and body hair (the loss of scalp hair comes much later). Puberty also marks the beginning of sexual urges or libido. Gender identity, which actually begins to form in early childhood, is usually established firmly during adolescence. And as any parent will testify, the combination of hormones, libido, and cultural pressures continue to produce the behavioral roller coaster that is so common in young teens.

Uncommon Abnormalities

It's a long way from conception to manhood. For most, the trip is uneventful, but for some it's a bumpy, even tortured, road.

In rare cases, the testicles are absent or fail to function properly. A more common problem that occurs in as many as one of every 500 males is *Kleinefelter syndrome,* which is caused by the presence of an extra X chromosome. Since these boys have a normal Y chromosome as well as the two X's, they look normal at birth. But behavioral abnormality may appear in childhood; puberty is delayed, and sexual and reproductive abnormalities become evident in maturity. Testosterone replacement therapy is very helpful, but will not restore fertility.

Even with genes and testicles, abnormalities of the *pituitary gland* hormones that should stimulate testosterone production can produce delayed puberty and reproductive failure (see Chapter One and Ten). On the other hand, premature overproduction of testosterone by the testicles or adrenal glands may produce *precocious puberty* and *virilization.*

The penis and urethra may also develop abnormally; occurring in about one of every 250 births, the most common problem is *hypospadias,* in which the urethral opening develops on the shaft of the penis instead of at the tip. Less often, the penis can be small or *inconspicuous,* and the external genitals can be *indeterminate* or *ambiguous.*

Structural abnormalities of the genital tract require the expert attention of pediatric urologists, who also care for various abnormalities of the kidneys, bladder, and urinary tract that can afflict both boys and girls. Functional abnormalities, such as bedwetting (*enuresis*) are usually treated by pediatricians and psychologists. Pediatric endocrinologists can help sort out and treat hormonal abnormalities, and the overall care of a pediatrician is always essential. Family counseling also helps people cope with urogenital abnormalities. But parents themselves will have to decide about circumcision, and they should be knowledgeable about undescended testicles and other abnormalities of the scrotum.

The Undescended Testicle

Scrotal abnormalities are common in childhood. Hernias, hydroceles, varicoceles, and related problems can appear at any time from birth to adulthood. Occurring most often between ages twelve and eighteen, testicular torsion (twisting) is a true medical emergency that parents must be able to recognize in order to get prompt surgical help. This chapter will discuss all these issues in detail.

An undescended testicle is the most common inborn disorder of the genital tract. In about 4 percent of boys, one or both testicles have not completed their descent into the scrotum by the time of birth; because the migration occurs late in fetal life, the abnormality is up to five times more common in preemies.

When a pediatrician examines a newborn boy, he will always feel the testicles to be sure both are in the scrotum. If he cannot feel the testicles in their proper place, he will diagnose the condition as *cryptorchism* and will carefully examine the baby's groins to see if he can feel a testicle in the inguinal canal.

There are two reasons why it is important for doctors to diagnose cryptorchidism. The first is an increased risk of malignancy; undescended testicles are about eleven times more likely to develop testicular cancer than those that are normally positioned (see page 262). The second reason is infertility; testicles that are exposed to the warmth of the body's interior are damaged and lose their ability to produce sperm (see Chapter Ten).

Since the consequences of an undescended testicle are so important, the next step may seem surprising: it is simply doing nothing. That's because as many as two-thirds of all undescended testicles will enter the scrotum on their own during the first year of life.

Even if the testicle has not descended by the boy's first birthday, there is still time to act, since irreversible damage to the testicle will not occur until age two. But sometime between ages twelve months and two years, doctors will reposition the testicle surgically, using an operation called *orchidopexy.* If a hernia is also present, doctors will repair it during the operation. Orchidopexy succeeds in salvaging nearly all undescended testicles, but if doctors cannot feel the testicle in the groin, they will first have to find it by *ultrasound, computed tomography* (CT), or *laparoscopy.* But although orchidopexy can improve fertility if it is done early enough, it does not reduce the risk of testicular cancer, so these boys need careful surveillance until they reach early middle age (see page 263).

What if doctors are unable to feel one or both testicles in an older child or adolescent? The first step is to try again. The scrotum has a muscle (the *cremasteric*) that can pull the testicles up toward the abdomen. It is a protective reflex that is stronger in youth, but it can make a normal testicle difficult or impossible to feel. A warm bath followed by a repeat exam when the boy is relaxed will usually reveal that the *retractile testicle* is back where it belongs. Retractile testicles do not have an increased risk of malignancy.

Doctors are divided about how to best manage a truly undescended testicle in older children and adults. Most would perform an orchidopexy if the problem is discovered before puberty, but remove an undescended testicle in teenagers and young adults. No action is necessary beyond the age of thirty-five, since the risk of testicular cancer declines with age. It is important to keep an eye on all boys who have had undescended testicles to be sure they produce enough testosterone at the time of puberty and beyond.

Circumcision

Circumcision is one of the oldest surgical procedures, dating back more than 4,000 years to the ancient Egyptians and the biblical Hebrews. It's one of the most common operations in the United States, where it is performed more than 1.2 million times each year, and it is one of the fastest, taking just three to five minutes from start to finish. But circumcision has also become one of the most controversial procedures, stimulating debate among physicians and sparking emotional arguments between nonmedical advocacy groups on both sides of the question. All parents should understand the operation before deciding if it is right for their sons.

The foreskin is the skin that covers the tip of the penis or glans. In most newborns, the foreskin still adheres tightly to the glans. During the first years of life, however, these tissues continue to separate; by age five, the foreskin can be retracted away from the glans in more than 90 percent of boys. In adolescents and adults, the foreskin covers the glans when the penis is flaccid, but retracts when the penis becomes erect, leaving the glans exposed.

SURGICAL CONSIDERATIONS

Circumcision is the surgical removal of the foreskin; after circumcision, the glans is exposed when the penis is flaccid as well as when it is erect. Modern surgical technique uses a clamp to protect the glans during the operation; doctors generally prefer the *Gomco clamp*, but many practitioners of ritual

Jewish circumcisions use the *Mogen clamp*. In either case, a scalpel is used to remove the foreskin after the protective clamp is in place. Although newborn circumcision has been performed without anesthesia for centuries, there is no reason to continue that practice today. In fact, effective pain control can be accomplished by injecting a local anesthetic into the penis; an anesthetic cream, EMLA, is also helpful but it appears somewhat less effective than the injected medication. A sugar-coated pacifier can also reduce discomfort, as can acetaminophen (Tylenol and other brands). However, these techniques should be used only to supplement anesthetic injections or creams. In older boys and adults, circumcision often requires general anesthesia and somewhat more complex surgical techniques that include stitching the skin's edges together.

CULTURAL AND RELIGIOUS CONSIDERATIONS

The Egyptians were probably the first people to perform circumcisions. The ancient Jews may have learned the practice from them, but the Old Testament ascribes the ritual to a command from God. "And ye shall circumcise the flesh of your foreskin; and it shall be a token of the covenant betwixt me and you"—Genesis XVII. For more than 4,000 years, traditional Jewish circumcisions have been performed on the eighth day of an infant boy's life by trained practitioners called mohels. Muslims also perform circumcision; although the timing is less strict, their ritual usually occurs early in life. A few groups of Native Americans, Australians, and Africans have also practiced circumcision for cultural or ceremonial purposes, but the operation is uncommon in Asia, Northern Europe, and South America.

Although circumcision began as a religious rite, it became a routine medical practice about 100 years ago, when the operation was advocated to improve hygiene and prevent disease. In some circles, circumcision was even believed to promote sexual morality. By the 1950s, about 90 percent of American males underwent newborn circumcision. Since then, medical research has questioned the value of circumcision, and the operation has become less popular. At present, about 60 percent of American boys are circumcised shortly after birth, but the rate is much lower in Canada and England.

POTENTIAL BENEFITS

Although doctors are still debating the pros and cons of circumcision, the American Academy of Pediatrics (AAP) has recently issued a position paper than summarizes the operation's benefits and risks. The potential benefits fall into several categories:

Urinary Tract Infections. The most important benefit of circumcision is a reduced risk of urinary tract infections during infancy. Early studies reported that uncircumcised male infants were ten to twenty times more likely to get urinary tract infections than were circumcised babies. Although recent studies found less benefit, they still report that uncircumcised male infants are three to nine times more likely to develop urinary tract infections. Critics point to flaws and limitations of various studies, but the AAP Task Force on Circumcision concludes that the protection is real. Still, it is a small advantage at best, since urinary tract infections are uncommon even in uncircumcised male infants and most respond well to antibiotic therapy. All in all, seven to eighteen of every 1,000 uncircumcised male infants will develop a urinary tract infection during the first year of life compared with one to two circumcised male infants.

Cancer of the Penis. In the United States, uncircumcised men are about three times more likely to develop cancer of the penis than are circumcised men. It's a statistical plus for circumcision, but it is less important than it seems. That's because cancer of the penis is so rare in America, developing annually in fewer than ten of every one million men. Good hygiene also appears to reduce the risk of penile cancer.

Disorders of the Penis. Phimosis is the inability to retract the foreskin, usually because of inflammation or infection. The condition is usually mild, but it can produce painful erections and other symptoms. By removing the foreskin, infant circumcision prevents phimosis. But good hygiene is also protective, and when the disorder is treated promptly it usually improves rapidly; some men, though, require circumcision in adulthood to correct unusually severe cases of phimosis. Circumcision also prevents *posthitis,* or inflammation of the foreskin, and it appears to reduce the risk of *balanitis,* or inflammation of the glans. Still, these are generally mild conditions that respond well to treatment.

Sexually Transmitted Diseases (STDs). Although circumcision appears to reduce a man's risk of HIV infection, it is incomplete protection at best, and there is no protection against other STDs for a man or his partner. Safe sexual practices are the only ways to protect against STDs (see Chapter Ten).

Potential Risks

If the benefits of circumcision have been overstated by its advocates, its risks have also been exaggerated by its critics. Still, there are potential risks.

Operative Complications. All operations have risks, and circumcision is no exception. In trained hands, however, complications are uncommon, occurring in between two and six of every 1,000 newborn circumcisions. Even when complications occur, they are usually mild, with temporary bleeding and mild infections leading the list. In rare cases, however, complications can be severe or even fatal.

Expense. Although the British National Health Service has stopped covering routine newborn circumcision because it could not document medical benefit, most American insurers pay for the operation. Even so, circumcisions add $150 to $270 million to America's annual medical bill.

Pain. Contrary to some cultural beliefs, infant circumcision is painful. However, effective pain relief is available, and there is no evidence to support concerns about lasting psychological damage from the "trauma" of circumcision.

Sexual Dysfunction. There is no reliable evidence to support the claim that newborn circumcision increases the risk of sexual problems in adulthood or that the operation impairs sexual satisfaction in either partner.

Perspectives

After studying all the scientific data, the AAP Task Force on Circumcision concluded that "Existing scientific evidence demonstrates potential medical benefits of newborn male circumcision; however, these data are not sufficient to recommend routine neonatal (newborn) circumcision." It is a fair statement. Although the statistics favor circumcision, the margin of benefit is so small that parents may reasonably choose to have their infant sons circumcised or to forgo the operation.

It is an individual choice with no wrong answer. Religious convictions, cultural attitudes, and personal beliefs are often the determining factors. If parents are unable to arrive at a decision based on these factors, they may choose to consider the simple advice that a son should look like his father. But if parents choose circumcision, they should be sure that the procedure is performed by an experienced and competent individual, that their son is healthy at the time of the operation, and that modern anesthesia is provided.

Circumcision has been controversial since its earliest days. The controversy is not likely to diminish anytime soon. Doctors will continue to study the pros and cons of infant circumcision, but they have already produced enough information to allow parents to make a calm, rational, individual decision. The best time to make that decision is before birth, when there is quiet time to consider the circumcision choice with circumspection.

The Scrotum and Testicles

The scrotum is one of the most vulnerable parts of the male anatomy. It is a small sack containing vital organs and sensitive tissues that is suspended outside the body with only a thin layer of skin for its protection. But male anatomy is not as perverse as it seems. Vulnerability is the price men pay for procreation. Because the scrotum is outside the rest of the body, the testicles are about six degrees cooler than the body's interior, and that is just the right temperature for sperm production.

The scrotum allows the testicles to perform two jobs: delivering testosterone to the blood, and supplying sperm for ejaculate. But the scrotum contains a variety of structures that participate in these tasks, and any of them can be the source of trouble.

Normal Anatomy

The testicles are at the center of it all, a pair of smooth, oval structures with a slightly spongy texture. An adult's testicle is about two inches long and weighs about one-third of an ounce. Each is covered by a double-layered tissue called the *tunica vaginalis*. The testicle contains two types of cells that are crucial for its function: *Leydig cells* produce testosterone and *germ cells* manufacture sperm. Newly formed sperm enter the many tiny *seminiferous tubules*, and then pass through small ducts that carry them into a single large tube, the *epididymis* (see Figure 9.2). Sperm spend about twelve days in transit through the epididymis, a twenty-foot-long tube that is tightly coiled at the upper rear of the testicle. The epididymis gradually thickens and straightens, continuing on as the *vas deferens*, a muscular tube that travels up from the scrotum into the lower pelvis, where it widens into the *ampulla*. The *seminal vesicles* join the ampulla to

FIGURE 9.2. NORMAL ANATOMY

The scrotum is a small sac that suspends the testicles outside the body, thus providing the cooler environment that is essential for sperm production. The scrotum also contains the epididymis and vas deferens, the tubes that carry sperm to the ejaculate. The testicular artery supplies oxygen-rich blood, and a network of veins removes carbon dioxide and other waste products.

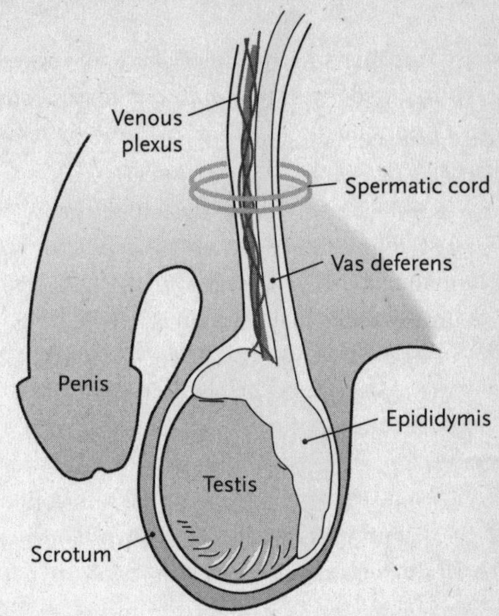

form a common *ejaculatory duct* that travels through the *prostate gland* into the *urethra.*

The scrotum contains several additional structures that are not directly responsible for manufacturing hormones or producing and delivering sperm. The *testicular arteries* bring in oxygen-rich blood, and a network of veins and *lymphatics* drains away fluid and wastes. Along with a network of nerves, these vascular structures are bundled around the vas to form the *spermatic cord.* In turn, the cord is surrounded by the *cremasteric muscle,* which can contract to raise the testicles toward the body when protection is needed.

Any of the tissues in the scrotum can be the source of pain or swelling. If that were not complex enough, swelling can also develop when structures that do not belong in the scrotum force their way in; hernias are the most common. Finally, kidney stones often refer pain to the scrotum, even though all the scrotal structures are perfectly normal (see Chapter Thirteen).

Evaluation

To diagnose a scrotal abnormality, doctors will ask how long the problem has been present, if it developed abruptly or gradually, and if it was preceded by trauma or injuries. Fever is an important indicator, as is the presence or absence of pain. A simple physical exam comes next. The doctor will check for swelling, tenderness, warmth, and discoloration of the scrotum. He may also use a bright light to look for any fluid by *transilluminating* the testicle, and he may also perform a digital rectal exam and urinalysis.

If a history and physical exam do not provide a diagnosis, the next step is often an *ultrasound* of the scrotum. It is a simple, painless, risk-free test. The patient lies on his back with a towel supporting his scrotum. A technician coats the scrotal skin with a coupling gel, then runs the ultrasound transducer across the skin. The transducer beams high-frequency sound waves into the scrotum. The waves that are echoed back from the internal structures are processed by a computer, then projected onto a video screen, and captured in photographic images.

Despite its simplicity, a scrotal ultrasound test allows doctors to diagnose the wide range of ailments that can affect the scrotum. It can help tell doctors which problems are serious and which are not.

Testicular Torsion

Testicular torsion occurs when an abnormally narrow attachment between the testicle and the spermatic cord allows the cord to twist, rotating the testicle (see Figure 9.3). Because the twisting blocks the flow of blood in the testicular artery, testicular torsion is a urologic emergency. Without prompt treatment, the testicle will be irreversibly damaged and will have to be removed.

Testicular torsion is most common in boys and young men but it can occur at any age; 25% of cases develop in men above twenty-one. The key symptom is severe pain in one testicle. It begins abruptly, sometimes after exercise but sometimes at rest or even during sleep. Many patients can recall milder episodes of pain that resolved spontaneously. The pain of torsion is often accompanied by nausea and vomiting. The testicle is swollen, tender, and drawn up high in the scrotum.

Scrotal Doppler ultrasound is the best way to confirm the diagnosis of torsion. Immediate surgery is required to salvage the testicle. If treatment is delayed beyond four hours, the chances of failure increase progressively. Although torsion usually occurs in only one testicle at a time, surgeons should always repair the other side, which may also have an abnormal attachment.

Because torsion is most common between ages twelve and eighteen, doctors may fail to consider the diagnosis in older men with testicular pain. It is a

FIGURE 9.3. TESTICULAR TORSION

An abnormally narrow attachment between the testicle and the spermatic cord may allow the cord to twist. Emergency surgery is required to restore blood flow and prevent permanent damage.

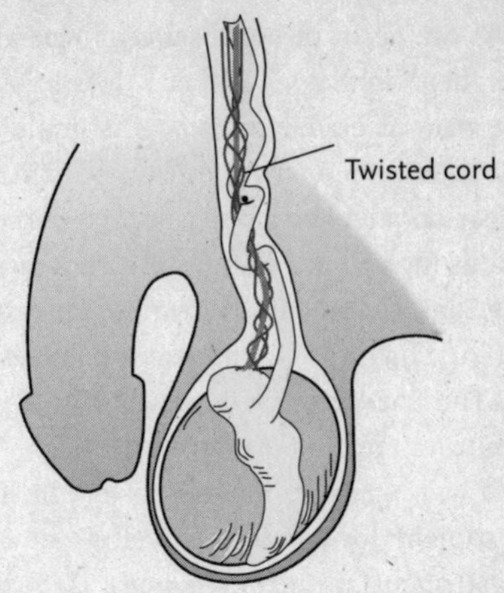

great mistake; although it's uncommon, torsion can even occur beyond age fifty.

Orchitis

Although it is not an emergency like testicular torsion, orchitis is nearly as painful and it is often accompanied by fever. The testicle is swollen and very, very tender to the touch. The skin of the scrotum feels warm and it may be reddened

Orchitis is an infection of the testicle. Mumps is the most common cause, but it is now quite rare in the United States, thanks to childhood vaccinations. This is a very good thing, since there is no specific treatment for mumps' orchitis, which often leaves permanent damage in its wake.

Epididymitis

Despite its unfamiliar name, epididymitis is a common problem that is responsible for more than 60,000 visits to American emergency rooms each year. As the "itis" in its name indicates, it is also an inflammatory disease, in this case involving the epididymis. Bacteria are responsible; the infection starts in the urethra or prostate, then spreads back up into the epididymis. Although sexually active men in their twenties and thirties are most often afflicted, epididymitis can occur in the absence of sexual activity and can strike men right through their eighties.

The pain of epididymitis begins gradually and builds slowly over one to two days; some men also complain of urinary burning and frequency or of a penile discharge. A low-grade fever is common, but the temperature can sometimes be as high as 104 degrees. Doctors can usually feel a swollen, tender epididymis, but if the infection goes untreated, the whole testicle may feel swollen, in which case an ultrasound is needed to be sure epididymitis is the culprit. The patient's urine usually contains white blood cells, but ordinary urine cultures are often negative.

Men with epididymitis can be very ill. They often require bed rest with a scrotal support for comfort as well as nonsteroidal antiinflammatory drugs (NSAIDs), such as aspirin, *ibuprofen* (Motrin and other brands), or *naproxyn* (Aleve). Antibiotics are mandatory; medications in the *fluoroquinolone* family are excellent, and *doxycycline* is a good (and less expensive) alternative. Some men experience low-grade pain and inflammation after the infection is eradicated by antibiotics; in these cases, NSAIDs should help.

Hydrocele

Doctors classify testicular torsion, orchitis, and epididymitis as causes of the "acute scrotum," a broad term for pain and swelling that develop over a matter of hours. A hydrocele is different, producing painless swelling that emerges slowly over a span of weeks or months.

A hydrocele is a collection of fluid between the two membranes that surround the testicles (see Figure 9.4). The testicle itself is normal, but it is hard for doctors to feel the testicle through the large, smooth, soft swelling of a large hydrocele. Because fluid transmits light, a physician can make the diagnosis by simply transilluminating the scrotum with a bright flashlight held up against it. If there is doubt, an ultrasound will confirm the diagnosis.

Hydroceles do not require any treatment unless they are large enough to be embarrassing or uncomfortable. In that case, doctors can draw off the fluid through a needle and syringe, then inject a solution to cause inflammation and scarring of the tunica, obliterating the space. Because the procedure can be painful, men often prefer surgical repair if they need any treatment at all.

FIGURE 9.4. HYDROCELE

A hydrocele is a collection of fluid between the layers of the membranes that surround the testicles. Although the scrotum may be very swollen, the condition is not at all serious.

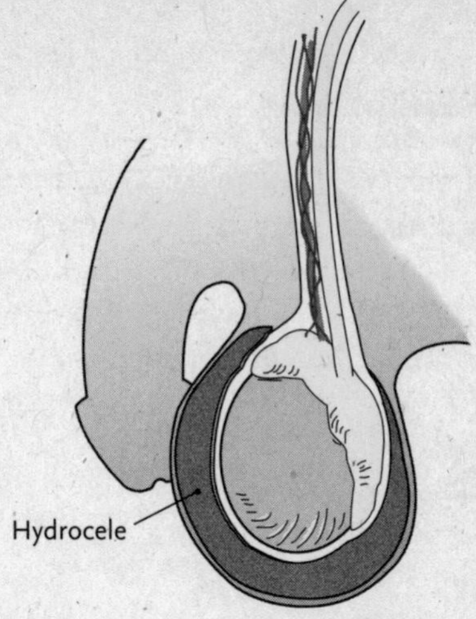

Spermatocele

Spermatoceles are fluid-filled cysts in the epididymis. They usually occur in the upper end and first appear as smooth, painless swellings adjacent to the testicle (see Figure 9.5). Transillumination can usually establish the diagnosis; if necessary, an ultrasound can confirm it. No treatment is needed, but aspiration or surgery can be used for cosmetic reasons.

Varicocele

A varicocele is a swollen, distended network of veins in the spermatic cord. The condition is common, occurring in 15 percent of men. It is painless and is easily recognized by its appearance as a blue-ish "bag of worms" that becomes more prominent when the man is standing (see Figure 9.6); 80 percent are on the left side. Varicoceles are harmless, but they can be associated with infertility; if so, surgical treatment can help (see Chapter Ten).

Massive Edema

In most cases, scrotal swelling originates from a problem in the scrotum itself. But some men with congestive heart failure, liver disease, kidney disease, or other problems retain so much fluid that it accumulates in the scrotum and penis as well as in the legs and abdomen.

FIGURE 9.5. SPERMATOCELE

A spermatocele is a fluid-filled cyst in the epididymis. It is painless and does not require treatment.

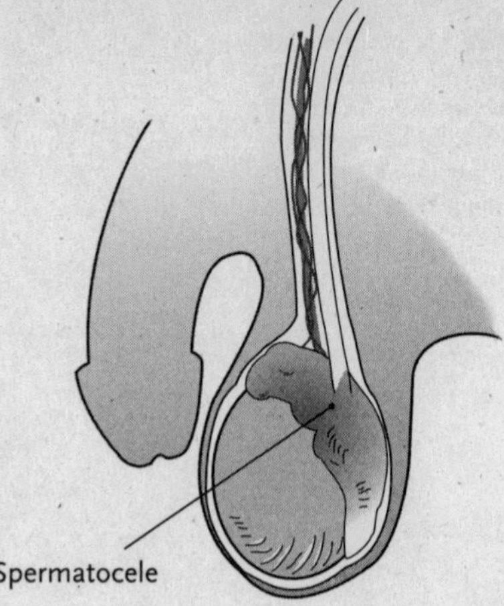

Scrotal swelling that results from blockage of the lymph channels in the groin or scrotum can produce firm swelling that earns the name *elephantiasis* in its extreme form. Fortunately, it is uncommon.

Testicular Trauma

Ouch! A blow to the scrotum is always painful, but the pain usually subsides in a matter of minutes, leaving nothing worse than a bad memory. But if the pain persists, if there is swelling or evidence of bleeding, or if the original trauma is severe, medical attention is mandatory. Ultrasounds can help with diagnosis, and surgery may be necessary to correct problems that can range from bleeding to testicular rupture. That is a big ouch, indeed.

Testicular Cancer

Along with wisdom and experience, testicular cancer is one of the very few good things about growing older. That's because a man's risk of developing the disease declines as he ages. Testicular cancer occurs most often between the ages of twenty and thirty-five. In fact, it is the most common cancer in that age group. But beyond age forty, the disease becomes progressively less common. Still, it is an important disease for all men to understand, particularly since most cases are first recognized by the patient himself, allowing early diagnosis and treatment that can cure this otherwise deadly disease.

FIGURE 9.6. VARICOCELE

A varicocele is a swollen network of veins in the spermatic cord. Surgical treatment may be advisable when the condition is associated with infertility.

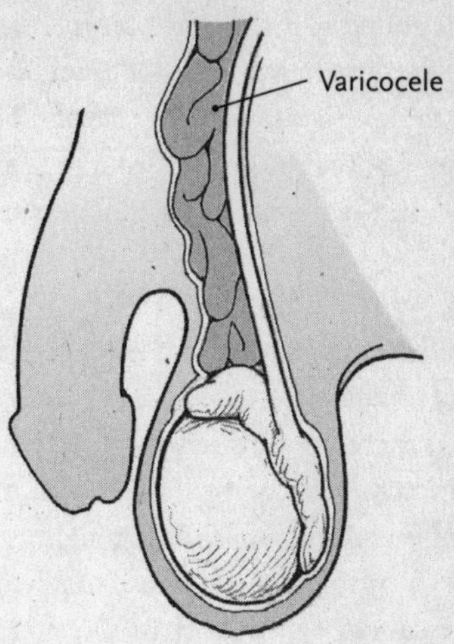

Who Gets Testicular Cancer?

About 7,500 American men will develop the disease this year alone. Except for some very young boys, most patients will be in their twenties and thirties, and most will be white. The disease is seven times more likely to develop in Caucasians than African-Americans; men of Scandinavian descent are at particular risk.

Despite intensive research, doctors do not know what causes testicular cancer. Some, but not all, studies suggest that family history increases risk, raising the possibility of a genetic component. Although neither toxins nor hormones have been firmly implicated, researchers also worry about environmental factors, especially since the incidence of testicular cancer has been rising steadily in the United States and other industrialized countries. In fact, the worldwide incidence has more than doubled over the past forty years. In white Americans, it has increased by 51 percent in just twenty-two years. And as the disease becomes more common, it is also striking younger men. For men born in 1943, the average age of diagnosis was thirty, but for men born in 1968, it is below twenty-five.

Despite these possibilities, the only well established contributor to testicular cancer is cryptorchidism or undescended testicles (see page 251). Testicular cancer is about eleven times more likely to develop in an undescended than a descended testicle. For unknown reasons, risk appears to increase even more if the testicle is biopsied at the time of corrective surgery. Doctors speculate that undescended testicles have an increased risk for cancer because they are exposed to more heat in the abdomen than in the scrotum, which is about six degrees cooler than the body's interior. That theory, however, does not explain the curious fact that the risk of cancer is also increased, though to a much smaller degree, in the normally-positioned partner of an undescended testicle.

GROWING PROBLEMS

In the vast majority of cases, cancer develops in the sperm-producing germ cells of the testicle, and most of these tumors are classified as *seminomas*. Although there are differences between seminomas and the less common types of testicular cancer, most behave in a similar fashion and are diagnosed and treated according to similar guidelines.

A common feature of testicular cancers is their rapid rate of growth. A testicular cancer can double in size in just twenty to thirty days. That is much faster than many other malignancies. Some prostate cancers, for example, may have a doubling time as long as six years or more (see Chapter Twelve). Because of their rapid growth, testicular cancers spread quickly, first to lymph nodes in the abdomen, then to nodes in the chest, and finally to lymph nodes and organs in other parts of the body. Rapid growth accounts for the fact that in about 40 percent of patients, the disease has spread beyond the testicle by the time it is first diagnosed. Fortunately, new treatment programs can cure even men whose cancers have spread. Even so, the rapid growth of testicular cancers underlines the importance of early diagnosis.

DIAGNOSIS

The key feature of testicular cancer is a mass, or nodule, in the testicle. The lump is firm to the touch; although it is classically described as painless, many men complain of aching discomfort, and sharp pain can occur if there is bleeding into the tumor. Symptoms such as weight loss, enlarged lymph nodes, back pain, and swollen breasts suggest widespread disease; fortunately, they are unusual.

Not all scrotal masses are cancerous. In fact, benign disorders are much more common (see pages 259 to 261). Doctors can often recognize benign problems by a simple physical exam. But if a doctor suspects cancer after examining a testicular mass, he will order an ultrasound, which is about 98 percent accurate in distinguishing a true mass in the testicles from other causes of scrotal swelling. If the ultrasound suggests cancer, the patient should have blood tests for *tumor markers*, proteins produced by the cancer cells; *alpha-*

fetoprotein (AFP), *beta-human chorionic gonadotropin* (HCG), and *lactic acid dehydrogenase* (LDH) levels can be used both to diagnose testicular cancer and to monitor its response to treatment.

If clinical findings and ultrasound suggest cancer, a biopsy is mandatory. In nearly all cases, it involves the surgical removal of the abnormal testicle using an incision in the groin rather than the scrotum. Although the operation, called a *radical inguinal orchiectomy,* is surgically straightforward, it is psychologically threatening to many men. It is reassuring, however, to know that sexual function remains intact because the healthy testicle is not disturbed by the operation.

STAGING

A surgical biopsy will permit doctors to diagnose the various types of testicular cancer. To plan the best treatment, though, they will also need to determine if the tumor has spread. Computed tomography (CT) has replaced older tests to identify abnormal lymph nodes in the abdomen and chest. The results of these tests are used to establish a clinical stage. Several systems are in use; in a simplified North American system:

Stage I: Cancer is confined to the testicle and adjoining tissues.

Stage II: Cancer has spread to lymph nodes in the abdomen. Stage II disease can be subdivided according to the size of these nodes:

IIA: Smaller than 2 cm
IIB: 2–5 cm
IIC: Larger than 2 cm

Stage III: Cancer has spread to lymph nodes in the chest and/or other organs.

TREATMENT

Just thirty years ago, 90 percent of men with testicular cancer died from the disease; now, more than 90 percent are cured.

In all patients, the malignant testicle is removed surgically (*radical inguinal orchiectomy*). Most patients with Stage I seminomas receive X-ray therapy to lymph nodes in the pelvis and abdomen. Patients with advanced Stage II or Stage III disease receive chemotherapy. Because nonseminomas are less responsive to radiotherapy, patients with Stage I and even Stage II disease are usually treated surgically by removing the lymph nodes at the rear of the abdomen. Patients with Stage I disease, however, may be cured by orchiectomy alone. Patients with advanced Stage II and Stage III disease receive chemotherapy. Although combinations of drugs are used in chemotherapy, platinum-based medications are the key to success.

Although the results of treatment are excellent, complications can occur. Sexual function remains normal in most men, but infertility is common after chemotherapy. Since the healthy testicle is shielded during treatment, infertility is much less common in men treated with radiotherapy than in men who receive chemotherapy. Because of the risk of infertility, many men choose to store sperm in a sperm bank before treatment begins. Second malignancies develop in a few patients years after successful treatment for testicular cancer.

Do-It-Yourself?

Philosophers proclaim that all men should examine their lives; the American Cancer Society suggests that young men should examine their testicles. It is a logical recommendation, but it has not been validated by scientific data. Since self-examination is quick and painless, however, it's a reasonable approach, particularly for men between the ages of twenty and thirty-five.

Men should establish a regular time for the exam; the first day of each month is easy to remember. The exam is best after a warm shower or bath, when the muscles in the scrotum are relaxed. The procedure is easy to master: Simply roll your testicle gently between your thumb and your first two fingers (see Figure 9.7). Examine one testicle at a time, using both hands for each. Normal testicles are smooth and slightly spongy; you are checking for a firm, pea-sized lump. Learn to recognize the normal rope-like tubular epididymis at the rear of each testicle so you will not confuse it with an abnormal mass. Report to your doctor if you notice an abnormal mass, unusual firmness, or unexpected tenderness of the testicle.

Problems and Progress

Testicular cancer accounts for only 1 percent of all malignancies in men. But its incidence is rising, and it typically strikes young men approaching the prime of life. In most cases, testicular cancer can be cured by various combinations of surgery, radiation, and chemotherapy. Because early diagnosis simplifies treatment and facilitates care, all men should understand the disease, and young men should examine themselves monthly to detect the disease in its earliest stages, when it is easiest to cure.

FIGURE 9.7. TESTICULAR SELF-EXAM

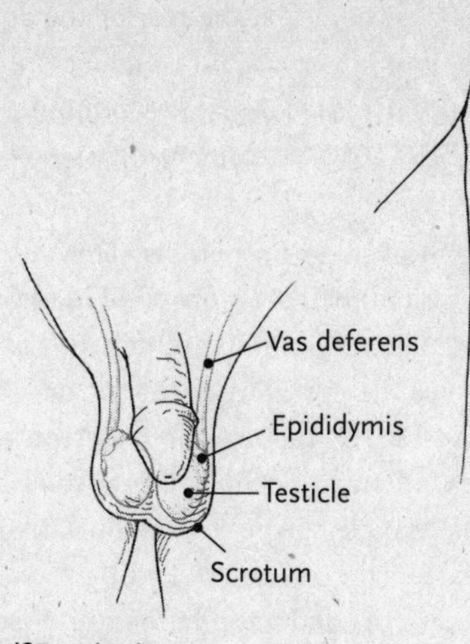

The Scrotal Contents

The largest structures in the scrotum are the testicles, which produce sperm cells and male hormones. The epididymis is at the rear of the testicle; it is a long, coiled tube where sperm mature. The vas deferens or the spermatic duct carries the sperm to the penis during ejaculation. The scrotum also contains veins that can become enlarged.

Self-Examination

Men between the ages of 15 and 40 should examine themselves about once a month, preferably after a warm shower or bath, when the scrotum is relaxed. The technique is easy to master: Simply roll each testicle between the thumb and first two fingers of both hands. Normal testicles feel smooth and slightly spongy. Tell your doctor if you detect swelling, unusual firmness, tenderness, or a lump.

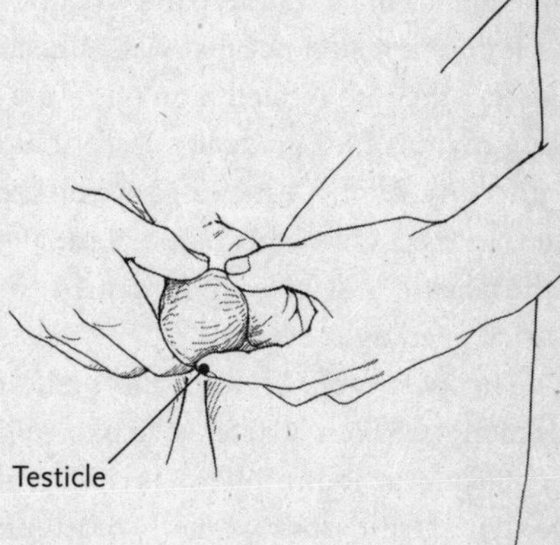

Hernias

As with so much medical terminology, we owe the name hernia to the Greeks, who first used the root word to mean a sprout or the protruding bud of a plant. Although doctors originally used the term to describe any abnormal or unsightly bulge, it is now used to characterize a protrusion through an abnormal opening. As such, hernias can develop in many regions of the body, but for most men, the term is shorthand for a groin hernia. It is understandable, since groin hernias are so common in males; in fact, a man has a 5 to 10 percent chance of developing one at some time in his life. And although hernias are generally considered "minor" problems, they can be serious. They are also expensive; in the United States, hernia operations cost about $3.5 billion a year.

Inguinal Hernias

We can thank the ancients for this term, too. In this case, though, gratitude goes to the Romans who used *inguinis* as a rough synonym for the "private parts."

Inguinal hernias account for 96 percent of all groin hernias. They are a characteristically masculine ailment, occurring nine times more often in males than females. The explanation for this dramatic predominance derives from male anatomy and male behavior. Anatomy is the more important factor. The male generative organs, the testicles, are outside the abdomen in the scrotum, while their female counterparts, the ovaries, are tucked deep within the pelvis. But it does not start out that way. When the testicles begin to develop early in fetal life, they are located high up in the rear of the abdomen. During the ensuing months they gradually descend through the abdomen to the groin (see Figure 9.1). As the testicles pass into the scrotum, they leave an opening behind. In most cases, this inguinal canal will seal over by the time of birth, but if the closure is defective it remains a weak area that may later become an abnormal opening, a hernia.

The most common type of groin hernia, the *indirect inguinal hernia,* develops along the path of fetal testicular migration. Since they develop from congenital defects, indirect hernias can occur at any time of life, from birth to old age, but since tissues weaken with time, indirect inguinal hernias are most common in older men. Advancing age is an even stranger risk factor for the other common variety of groin hernia, the *direct inguinal hernia,* which does not depend on an inborn defect, but is acquired during the course of adult life.

Freud told us that "anatomy is destiny." In the case of indirect inguinal hernias, at least, he was right, since the migration of the testicles explains why males are at such high risk. But behavior is also a male risk factor, since men are more likely to lift heavy objects, increasing abdominal pressure and putting stress on the groin tissues. But if men let it all hang out anatomically and behaviorally, women are equally vulnerable to other factors that can increase abdominal pressure, such as constipation, straining to move the bowels, and obesity.

Femoral Hernias

Accounting for only 4 percent of groin hernias, femoral hernias are actually three times more common in women than men. Femoral hernias typically present as a bulge in the upper thigh, just below the groin. Apart from their location and gender preference, femoral hernias behave very much like inguinal hernias, which will be the focus of the next discussion.

SYMPTOMS

Most men with hernias develop two symptoms: a dull pain or ache, and a bulge in the groin or scrotum. The symptoms usually develop gradually, but they can sometimes begin abruptly, usually as a result of heavy lifting. In some men, an ache or heavy feeling can precede the bulge by weeks or even months. In others, the bulge is entirely painless; sometimes in fact, hernias develop so silently that they are first detected by a physician in the course of a routine physical examination.

Early in the course of a hernia, the bulge is intermittent, noticeable when a man strains or when he stands, but not while he is lying down. The bulge occurs when abdominal contents, a part of the intestine and/or the fatty tissue that surrounds the bowel, protrudes through the opening, pushing on the skin. Hernias that come and go, either spontaneously or as a result of gentle manual pressure on the bulge, are called *reducible hernias.*

Reducible hernias can be uncomfortable or unsightly, but they are not serious. But hernias that cannot be reduced are another matter. Such *incarcerated hernias* are more likely to be painful, and they can develop a second complication, *strangulation,* when pressure interferes with the blood supply of the bowel. All strangulated hernias are painful and tender. In short order, the pain becomes severe and the patients develop nausea, vomiting, abdominal distention, and fever; prompt surgery is mandatory. About 10 percent of indirect inguinal hernias become incarcerated, but a much smaller number go on to strangulate. These complications are much less common in direct inguinal hernias, but are two times more likely to develop in femoral hernias.

DIAGNOSIS

Even in this age of high-tech medicine, the diagnosis of a groin hernia depends principally on a careful physical examination. Most doctors will ask the patient to stand for the exam. The physician will first look at the groin and scrotum, then feel for a bulge in these areas. A direct hernia usually produces an oval bulge near the pubic bone, while a indirect hernia may produce an elliptical swelling lower down toward or within the scrotum (see figure 9.8). If gravity does not bring out the bulge, the doctor places his finger at the base of the scrotum, then asks his patient to cough or strain. As abdominal pressure increases,

FIGURE 9.8. INGUINAL HERNIAS

An inguinal hernia is the protrusion of the intestine or fatty tissue into the groin through a weakness in the abdominal wall. Men are more vulnerable to this type of hernia than women because they are sometimes born with a defect in the inguinal canal, the passage through which the testis descends into the scrotum during fetal life.

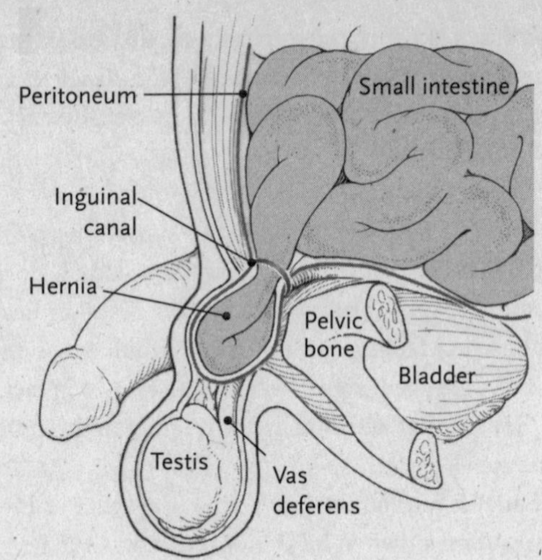

the abdominal contents will bulge through the opening, tapping on the doctor's finger.

Although a simple physical exam will detect most hernias, modern technology can also help. In particular, an ultrasound exam may sometimes detect a very early hernia that produces discomfort but no bulge. The combination of a physical examination and an ultrasound will also detect other conditions that can masquerade as hernias, including enlarged groin lymph nodes, hydroceles, epididymitis, or even testicular cancer.

Treatment

Surgery is the only effective treatment for groin hernias. But that does not mean an operation for every man with a hernia. Most healthy men will choose to have their hernias repaired, but older men with painless, easily reducible hernias may elect to temporize. It is reasonable strategy, particularly in the case of direct hernias, which are less likely to incarcerate and strangulate. In contrast, because femoral hernias are more prone to complications, nearly all should be repaired. Men who choose to live with inguinal hernias must stay alert for the irreducibility, swelling, pain, and tenderness that signal the complications of incarceration or strangulation. They should also make lifestyle changes to reduce abdominal pressure. Men who are obese should reduce, those who strain at moving their bowels should increase their dietary fiber and fluids, and all should avoid heavy lifting and straining (see Chapters Four and

Five). It is also good advice for men who have had surgery, since hernias can sometimes recur, and they can develop on the other side in 10–20 percent of hernia patients. But although lifestyle changes can help, the old-fashioned truss will not prevent hernias from enlarging or incarcerating; they should be used only for comfort, if at all.

Strangulated hernias must be repaired immediately, and incarcerated hernias should be repaired promptly. But reducible hernias can be treated electively, with surgery scheduled at a time of convenience. In nearly all cases, hernia repairs are performed on an outpatient basis, with patients returning home the evening of the operation.

The first hernia repair or *herniorrhaphy* took place in 1887. Since then, surgeons have devised innumerable ways to close the defect. At present, there are three major variations on the theme:

Conventional open repairs use sutures to bring the separated tissues together. It is the way hernias have been repaired for decades, and it still works today. But since the tissues must be pulled together, they are under tension after they are sewn in place. As a result, many patients experience rather prolonged discomfort, and up to 5 to 7 percent develop recurrent hernias because the tissues pull apart.

Tension-free open repairs were pioneered by Dr. Irving Lichtenstein, who introduced the technique in California in 1984. Like conventional surgery, the tension-free repair can be performed as day surgery under local or spinal anesthesia. The difference is that the Lichtenstein repair uses a sheet of mesh to close the defect, avoiding tension on the tissues. Proponents of the tension-free repair report less post-operative pain and fewer recurrences.

Laparoscopic repairs burst on the scene in the early 1990s. Whereas both types of open repairs require a four- to six-inch incision in the groin, the laparoscopic repair requires only three one-half-inch incisions in the abdomen. First, the surgeon inflates the abdomen with carbon dioxide. Next, he inserts a thin fiber optic tube, the laparoscope, through an incision. While watching through a video camera, he then inserts instruments, which he uses to pull the intestinal contents back into place and staple a patch over the defect. Laparoscopic surgery produces less post-operative pain and allows a faster return to work (two to three days versus one to two weeks). But because inflating the abdomen is painful, laparoscopic surgery requires general anesthesia, and because it requires specialized equipment and extra training, it is more expensive than open surgery.

Which type of operation is best? It is a hotly debated question these days, but there is no clear answer. Until studies declare a winner, the best advice is to pick an experienced surgeon who is skilled at hernia operations and allow him to do the operation he does best.

Hernias have plagued men from the very origins of humanity. But with good operations, by whatever technique, surgeons can make a man's hernia part of history.

CHAPTER TEN

Sexuality and Reproduction

EVEN THE MOST STRAIGHT-LACED OBSERVER has to agree that sex is essential for the survival of the species. But for most men, sex is more than procreation; it is also an important element in interpersonal relationships, a means of self-expression, and a source of gratification. When all goes well, sex is a source of a pleasure and affection for a man and his partner, but if problems arise with either sex or reproduction, they can trigger anger and frustration, shame and estrangement. Even worse, perhaps, sex can be the agent of disease; in the worst case, this life-giving activity can actually kill.

Until recently, although most men were thinking about sex and were sexually active, only a few were talking about it. Much has changed. Just as the pill revolutionized sex for women, another pill—Viagra—has transformed it for men. It is a healthy development. Men should know how their bodies function sexually and what can go wrong, and now that many new treatments are available, they should understand how to correct sexual and reproductive dysfunction.

Men at Play: Normal Sexual Function

Although the sex act is a continuous process, researchers have divided it into six stages:

The first necessity is sexual desire or *libido*. The normal sex drive is a prime example of the unity of mind and body; it requires both an appropriate psychological set and sufficient amounts of the male hormone testosterone. Sexual desires begin to develop in puberty, when testosterone levels rise (see Chapter Nine). Although ardor tends to wane with age, most men produce enough testosterone to maintain libido throughout life (see page 314). At any stage of life, however, worry, stress, or depression can reduce or abolish sexual interest, even if a man's physical apparatus remains intact.

Sexual activity itself begins with a state of arousal that leads to an erection. Both elements are complex. Arousal results from various combinations of erotic thoughts and sensory stimulation that may involve the senses of touch,

FIGURE 10.1. NERVOUS SYSTEM AND SEXUAL AROUSAL

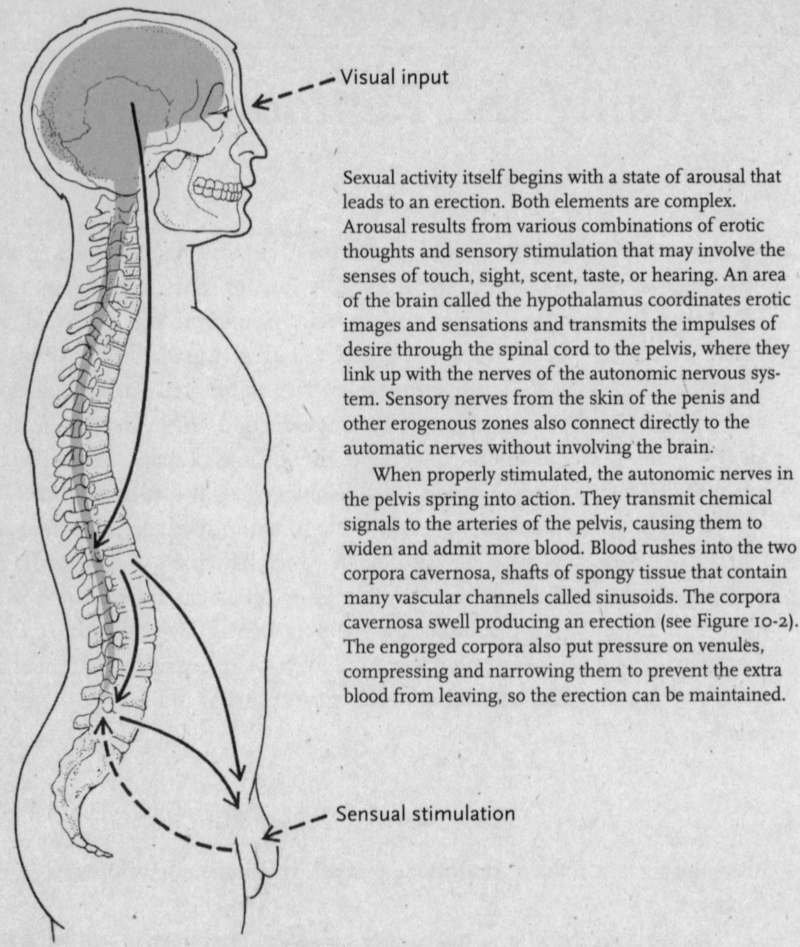

sight, scent, taste, or hearing. An area of the brain called the *hypothalamus* coordinates erotic images and sensations and transmits the impulses of desire through the *spinal cord* to the pelvis, where they link up with the nerves of the *autonomic nervous system*. Sensory nerves from the skin of the penis and other erogenous zones also connect directly to the automatic nerves without involving the brain (see Figure 10.1).

When properly stimulated, the autonomic nerves in the pelvis spring into action. They transmit chemical signals to the arteries of the pelvis, causing

FIGURE 10.2. NORMAL ERECTION

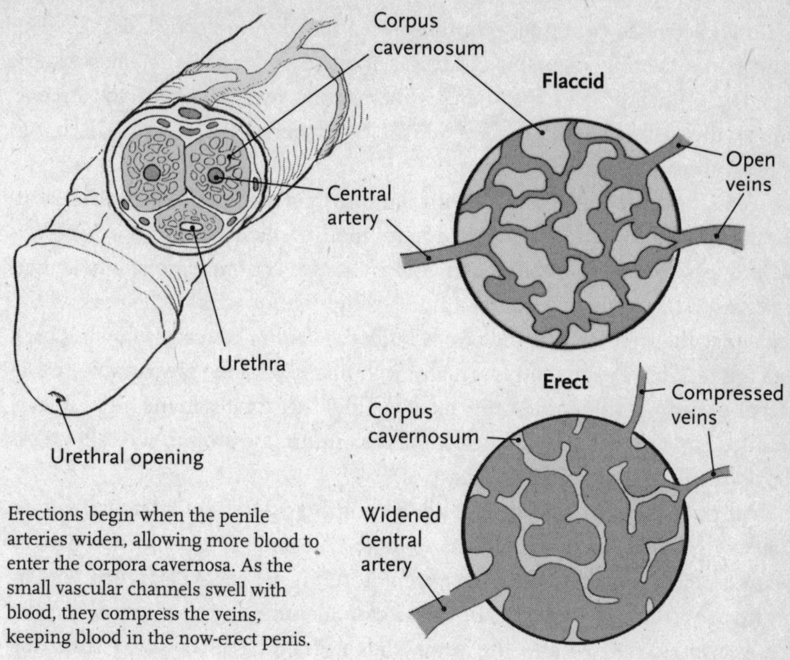

Erections begin when the penile arteries widen, allowing more blood to enter the corpora cavernosa. As the small vascular channels swell with blood, they compress the veins, keeping blood in the now-erect penis.

them to widen and admit more blood. Blood rushes into the two *corpora cavernosa,* shafts of spongy tissue that contain many vascular channels called *sinusoids.* The corpora cavernosa swell producing an erection (see Figure 10.2). The engorged corpora also put pressure on *venules,* compressing and narrowing them to prevent the extra blood from leaving, so the erection can be maintained.

For years, doctors have known that an erection is a hydraulic event that depends on a sixfold increase in the amount of blood in the penis. But new research has revealed that an erection is also a chemical event. A tiny chemical called *nitric oxide* allows nerves to communicate with each other and with the arteries of the penis. Nitric oxide acts on the arteries through an intermediary called *cyclic guanosine monophosphate* (cGMP). It is an exciting discovery for scientists, and it led to important progress for men with erectile dysfunction, since Viagra acts by boosting cGMP levels in the penis (see page 304).

The third stage of sexual activity is aptly called the plateau, which usually lasts from thirty seconds to two minutes. The heart rate and blood pressure rise as sexual activities continue, pumping more blood to the body's tissues. The penis is not the only recipient of increased blood flow; most men also experience facial flushing and the testicles themselves swell by about 50 percent. During the plateau phase, the *prostate* and *seminal vessicles* begin to discharge fluid in preparation for ejaculation.

Sexual excitement climaxes with the fourth stage, ejaculation. The autonomic nervous system is in charge here, too. It tells the muscles in the *epididymis, vas deferens, seminal vesicles,* and *prostate* to contract, propelling semen forward. At the same time, nerve impulses tighten muscles in the neck of the bladder so that semen is forced out through the *urethra* instead of flowing back into the bladder. Ejaculation is usually accompanied by the pleasurable sensation of orgasm. At the same time, most get their heart rates to the highest level produced by sex, which is still below the maximum rate produced by all-out exercise (see Sex and the Heart, page 310).

All good things come to an end. The fifth stage of sexual activity is *detumescence,* when the penis returns to its flaccid state. Detumescence usually follows ejaculation, but it can occur prematurely if the sex act is interrupted by an intrusive thought or event. In either case, detumescence occurs when the penile arteries narrow and the veins widen, draining blood away from the organ.

The final stage in the sex act is the quietest. It is the *refractory period,* a span of thirty minutes (in younger men) to three hours (in older men) during which the penis cannot respond to sexual stimulation.

From a biologic point of view, the point of all this intricate interplay of thoughts, hormones, nerves, and vessels is not sex itself but procreation. Although erection and ejaculation are essential for unassisted reproductive success, they are not sufficient. An additional set of factors is required to produce healthy sperm and deliver them to the ejaculate.

Men at Work: Normal Reproductive Function

Reproduction requires sex (at least until modern technology got into the act), but it also requires a lot more. In fact, a man's reproductive biology is at least as complex as his sexual function. To understand how it works, compare it to the division of labor stages in modern industry (see Figure 10.3).

Management. As in industry, the brain is in charge. In this case, the CEO is the *hypothalamus,* which produces *gonadotropin-releasing hormone* (GnRH). In the

FIGURE 10.3. THE PRODUCTION AND DELIVERY OF SPERM

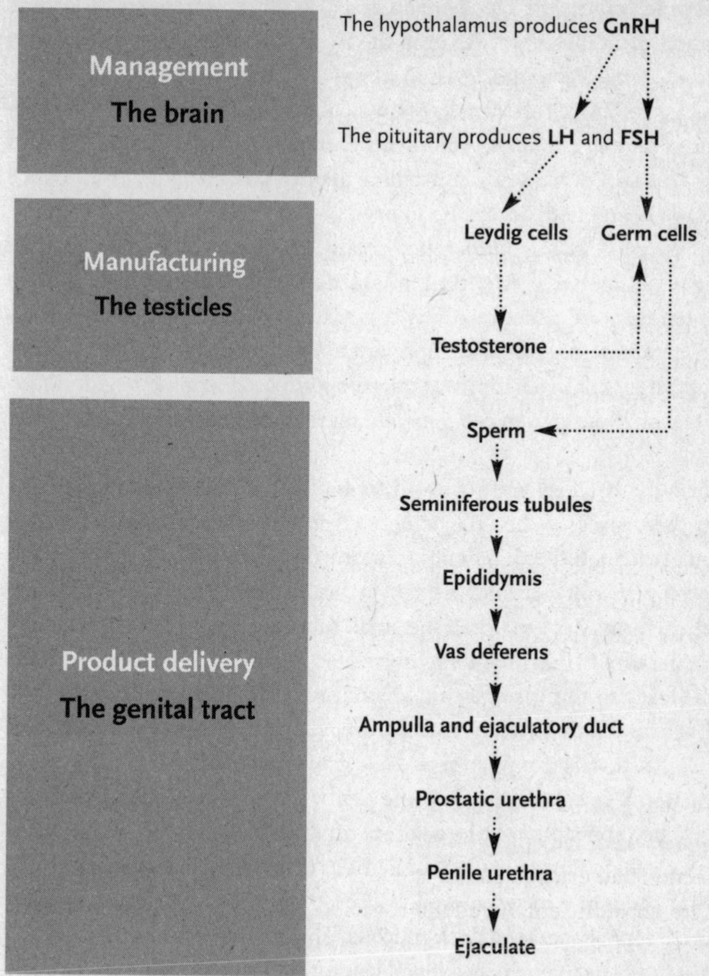

best executive fashion, however, GnRH does not get involved in daily chores. Instead it delegates authority to the *pituitary gland,* which secretes two key hormones, *leutinizing hormone* (LH) and *follicle stimulating hormone* (FSH). LH and FSH travel in the blood to the testicles, where sperm production actually occurs.

Manufacturing. The testicles are factories with two main products, testosterone and the sperm cells themselves. LH stimulates *Leydig cells* to produce the male hormone, which enters the bloodstream and also remains in the testicles in a concentration 100 times higher than in the blood. Testosterone teams up with the second executive hormone, FSH, to stimulate germ cells to produce sperm. Also in the assembly line are *Sertoli cells,* which nurture the germ cells and produce a hormone called *inhibin.* Among other things, testosterone and inhibin join forces in a sort of worker's committee that tells management to produce more or less LH and FSH according to need.

For sperm production to proceed normally, conditions in the factory must be just right. Temperature is critical; production will slow or even grind to a halt if the temperature is not relatively cool, usually about 6 degrees below internal body temperature. It is also important to keep toxic chemicals away from the assembly line. But in a happy workplace, sperm production is astoundingly efficient. Healthy young men can generate more than 1,000 sperm a second.

Product Delivery. It takes seventy-two days for sperm cells to develop in the tubules of the testicles. When they emerge from the assembly line, they look mature but lack motility, the ability to swim that is crucial for fertility. But sperm develop motility during the ten to twelve days they spend traveling through the delivery system. First, the small tubules join together to form the *epididymis,* the thin twenty-foot-long tube coiled behind each testicle. Next, the epididymis leads to the *vas deferens,* which travels up from the scrotum into the lower pelvis, where it widens into the *ampulla,* then forms a common *ejaculatory duct* that travels through the *prostate gland* into the *urethra.*

Ejaculation propels semen from the penis, but product delivery does not end there. When conception is the goal, sperm must be deposited in the vagina within a day or two before ovulation. Semen, which contains fluid from the prostate and seminal vesicles as well as sperm from the vas, coagulates after ejaculation, trapping sperm in thick mucous. That is when *prostate specific antigen,* the protein better known as a blood test for prostate cancer, goes to work. It liquefies semen, freeing sperm to swim through the female reproductive tract to meet their target. All this so just one sperm can penetrate one egg and extend the chain of human life.

Quality Control. Fertility depends on many factors. Sperm must be produced in sufficient numbers, they must have a normal structure, and they have to be able to swim upstream and penetrate the egg. The semen itself must be able to nurture sperm and promote normal function.

The World Health Organization (WHO) has established criteria for normal semen:

CHARACTERISTIC	NORMAL VALUES
Semen volume	1.5–5.0 ml
Sperm count	Above 20 million per ml
Sperm appearance	At least 35 percent normal
Sperm motility	At least 60 percent motile
Forward progression	At least 2+ (on a scale of 1 to 4)
White blood cells	Fewer than 1 million/ml
Sperm clumping	None

Although the WHO values remain the "gold standard" for semen analyses, a 2001 American study has proposed additional criteria that may be helpful. The scientists found that sperm shape was an important determinant of fertility. They also reported that men with sperm counts above 48 million per milliliter, with motility rates of at least 63 percent and a normal shape in at least 12 percent of sperm, were likely to be fertile. In contrast, men with counts below 13.5 million per milliliter, with motility rates below 32 percent and a normal appearance in less than nine percent, were likely to be infertile. Men with intermediate results had variable fertility.

Male reproductive function is as complex as most modern industries, and when all goes well, it is at least as efficient. But like any industry, reproduction functions can go awry with results that are every bit upsetting as sexual dysfunction.

Male Infertility

Few things are more stressful to a couple than the inability to have children. It is heartbreaking and it is common; in the United States about 10 percent of married couples are unable to have even one child, and another 10 percent cannot have a second. In all, Americans spend more than $1 billion a year to treat infertility.

Throughout most of human history, "barren" women have borne the blame for infertility. Not any more. In about 40 percent of infertile couples, a female factor is solely responsible, but in 30 percent male infertility is the only culprit, and both partners have reproductive problems in another 30 percent. Simple arithmetic reveals that a male factor is involved in six of ten cases of infertility.

Doctors at Work: The "Audit"

In most cases, doctors will begin a fertility work-up after six to twelve months of unprotected intercourse has failed to produce a pregnancy. The first step is to be sure the frequency and timing of intercourse is right. To evaluate the male, doctors will perform a simple examination of the genitals and a digital rectal exam to check the prostate. In many cases, the next step is a semen analysis, which is best performed on two separate specimens collected after two to three days of abstinence by masturbating into a specimen jar (not ejaculating into a condom). If the semen is normal, attention turns to the female, but if the semen is abnormal, doctors may order blood tests to check hormones such as LH, FSH, testosterone and *prolactin*. In addition, fertility specialists may request *ultrasound* tests to image the scrotum and prostate. If the sperm delivery system appears blocked, an additional imaging test called *vasography* may be performed. Finally, in a few cases testicular biopsies may also be indicated.

Repair Service: Treatment to Restore Fertility

As with all medical problems, the treatment of male infertility depends on its cause. Men who are exposed to toxins or chemicals that may impair sperm production should end the exposure. Examples include substances of abuse (alcohol, nicotine, marijuana, cocaine), certain over-the-counter and prescription drugs (*cimetidine* [Tagamet], *nitrofurantoin* [Furadantin], *sulfasalazine* [Azulfidine]) and pesticides. Herbs such as *St. John's Wort, echinacea,* and *gingko biloba* may also have an adverse effect on sperm function. Surprisingly, perhaps, taking testosterone and other male hormones also produces infertility. This is because as blood testosterone levels rise, they inhibit LH production so that the testicles make less testosterone and levels in the testicles themselves fall.

Elevated scrotal temperatures will also impair sperm production. Even fevers caused by the flu or other infections can have a deleterious effect, but sperm production recovers to normal within days to weeks. Contrary to a common belief, however, jockey shorts do not raise scrotal temperature enough to reduce sperm counts.

One of the most common treatable causes of infertility is a *varicocele,* a swollen network of veins in the scrotum (see Chapter Nine). Varicoceles do not require any treatment unless they are associated with low sperm counts, in which case blocking off the abnormal veins can improve fertility about half the time.

Infections of the genitourinary tract may also be linked with male infertility. That is why doctors will prescribe antibiotics if they detect abnormal white blood cells in the semen or other evidence of infections such as *prostatitis* (see Chapter Eleven).

A recent study found that men with low sperm counts also tend to have low levels of folic acid in their semen. It is far too early to know if supplements will improve fertility, but the same daily multivitamin that may promote cardiovascular health certainly can't hurt.

The newest and most promising approaches to male infertility involved *assisted reproductive techniques.* The simplest is *artificial insemination,* which involves processing a semen sample and placing purified sperm into the uterus at the time of ovulation. But men with blockages of the sperm delivery system and very low sperm counts require more advanced techniques, such as *in-vitro fertilization* (IVF) and *intracytoplasmic sperm injections* (ICSI). To perform ICSI, doctors harvest sperm from the epididymis and eggs from the ovary. Next they use a micropipette, an eye dropper about 1/10 the thickness of a human hair, to inject a single sperm into an egg. Finally, the fertilized egg is placed in the uterus. ICSI offers the best hope to men with very low sperm counts, but it is emotionally draining, time-consuming, expensive, and even in the best of circumstances it often fails to achieve pregnancy.

ICSI represents exciting progress in the management of male infertility. In time, new research will undoubtedly make further strides in dealing with this difficult problem.

Male Birth Control

Some men have to work hard to promote their fertility, but many have to exercise care to control theirs. Just as infertility was once blamed on women, the responsibility for birth control has been traditionally delegated to females. In fact, men should be equal partners in both areas.

When it comes to birth control, women have many options but men have just two. New research may change that, but for now effective male birth control depends on either condoms or vasectomy.

CONDOMS

This simple device, first used in the sixteenth century to protect against syphilis, has changed dramatically over the years. At first, condoms were made of cloth, then animal intestines. Next came vulcanized rubber, which gave way to latex. Latex remains the preferred condom material, but in today's world condom manufacturers are offering this venerable device in a bewildering variety of textures, colors, and flavors. They are also developing new copolymers such as polyurethane that may be thinner yet more durable than latex. For now, though, unless either partner is allergic to latex, it remains the best choice.

Condoms are at least 95 percent effective if used properly. Here are some guidelines: Use latex condoms labeled "to prevent disease." Store condoms in a cool, dry place out of direct sunlight. Never use condoms that are torn, brittle, sticky, or discolored. Never reuse a condom. If a condom breaks during intercourse, interrupt sexual activity and replace the condom immediately.

Pick a condom that fits properly; fortunately, manufacturers no longer assert that one size fits all. Put on the condom before any sexual contact occurs. The condom should be unrolled completely on an erect penis, covering it entirely but leaving a small space at the tip to collect semen. Some varieties have reservoir tips to accomplish this. Expel air pockets by using pressure directed down toward the base. After ejaculation, the penis should be withdrawn while still erect. To prevent spillage, the condom should be held at its base during withdrawal.

Spermicides that contain nonoxyl-9 confer extra protection against pregnancies but not STDs. Some condoms are manufactured with spermicidal lubricants; water-based lubricants such as surgical jellies are safe for condoms, but oil-based lubricants such as petroleum jelly, mineral oil, hand lotion, and vegetable oil can damage condoms, destroying their effectiveness.

Until recently, condoms were never discussed in polite society. All that has changed. It is a good thing, since changing sexual practices and the spread of HIV and other sexually transmitted microbes have made explicit discussions mandatory (see page 286).

VASECTOMY

Throughout history, men and women have wanted to control their fertility. Until recently, however, the only available methods were abstinence, abstinence during the most fertile days of the menstrual cycle ("the rhythm method"), or interruption of intercourse before ejaculation ("withdrawal" or *coitus interruptus*). Things improved when barrier methods became available, and the male condom and the female diaphragm rapidly became the most widely used methods of birth control. Beginning in the 1960s, things changed again, as birth control pills came into use. Since then, most new birth control methods have focused on the female reproductive system; in the past three decades, doctors have developed safer and more effective birth control pills, implants, injections, intrauterine contraceptive devices, spermicidal jellies, female condoms, and improved tubal ligation techniques, all for women. In contrast, the only addition to a man's contraceptive options has been the vasectomy. It is an old operation with new refinements, and it has been the choice of more than 45 million men worldwide.

The Operation. Vasectomy is a simple operation that divides the *vas deferens* (see Figure 10.4), interrupting the flow of sperm. Because 70 percent of semen derives from the seminal vesicles and 20 percent is produced by the prostate, men who have the operation will not notice the absence of the 10 percent contributed by the vas. And since vasectomy has no effect on hormone production or the nervous system, the operation will not influence masculinity, libido, sexual performance, or erotic sensations. Vasectomy will not even reduce sperm production. After the operation, the testicles continue to generate 50,000 sperm an hour. But since vasectomy stops sperm from entering semen, it does prevent conception. With nowhere to go, the sperm locked in the vas and epididymis die quietly, to be absorbed harmlessly by the body.

Vasectomy is a thirty-minute procedure that is performed in doctor's office under local anesthesia. In the *standard vasectomy,* the urologist makes a small incision in the scrotum just above the testicle (see Figure 10.4). The surgeon pulls the vas up into the incision and clamps it in two places. Next, he divides the vas and removes the short segment between the clamps. Finally, the doctor seals the vas with stitches, clips, or cauterization, then places it back in the scrotum and closes the incision. The procedure is repeated on the other side of the scrotum.

A newer technique, the *no-scalpel vasectomy,* was developed by Chinese doctors in 1974, but was not introduced in the United States until 1985. Instead of making an incision, the surgeon uses a special instrument to make a tiny puncture hole in the anesthetized scrotum. By gently stretching the opening, the doctor can gain access to the vas, which is then clipped and divided in the usual way. The no-scalpel vasectomy requires special training, but it is 40 percent faster than the standard operation and is just as effective. Because the

FIGURE 10.4. VASECTOMY

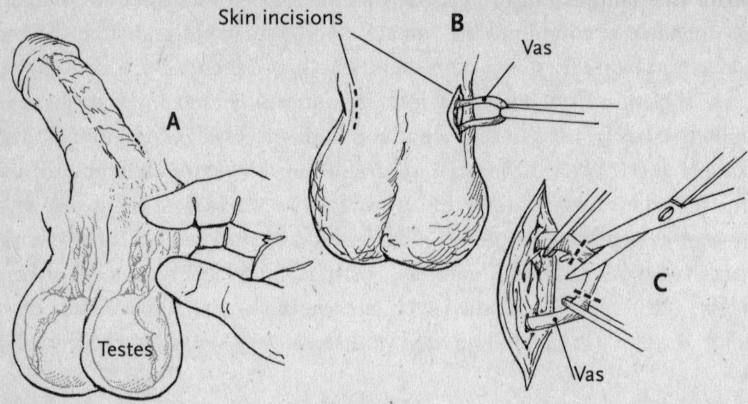

The standard vasectomy is a quick, safe operation that can be performed in a urologist's office. First, the doctor identifies the vas deferens in the scrotum (A). After cleansing the skin and injecting a local anesthetic, he makes a small incision and gently pulls the vas out of the scrotum (B). He then clamps the vas, removes the short segment between the clamps (C), seals the ends of the vas, returns it to the scrotum, and closes the incision with sutures. In the newer, no-scalpel vasectomy, the doctor makes a tiny puncture hole to reach the vas, so skin stitches are not required.

no-scalpel operation does not require an incision or stitches, pain is reduced, healing is faster, and there is a lower risk of complications. Many American urologists now prefer the no-scalpel technique.

Most men recover quickly from a vasectomy. After resting in the doctor's office for about thirty minutes, the patient can drive home for a quiet day of limited activity. Men should avoid strenuous physical exertion and sexual activity for five to seven days before resuming an unrestricted schedule. In fact, sexual activity is essential to the success of a vasectomy. After the operation, the ejaculatory ducts contain live sperm, and it takes twenty to fifty ejaculations to expel them. As a result, men must continue to use other birth control methods until two sperm counts, usually performed twelve and sixteen weeks postoperatively, confirm the absence of sperm.

Efficacy and Safety. Whether performed in a high-tech American urologist's office or in a developing country's birth control clinic, vasectomies are highly effective, with failure rates below 2 percent. Early failures can result from surgical errors, but are more often caused by the patient's unwillingness to use other birth control methods until two semen analyses confirm the absence of sperm. Late failures can result from spontaneous recanalization of the surgically interrupted vas, but these events are rare, occurring in just one of every 40,000 vasectomies.

Although every patient experiences some pain after a vasectomy, the discomfort is usually mild and is easily controlled with mild pain relievers such as *acetaminophen* (Tylenol). A few men develop persistent pain, but it rarely interferes with their quality of life. Local bleeding is fairly common but it usually amounts to nothing more than a small *hematoma* or "black and blue" beneath the skin of the scrotum. Minor infections complicate about 3 percent of vasectomies, and *sperm granulomas,* small pockets of inflammation caused by the body's immune reaction to sperm that leak into scrotal tissues, occur in about 2 percent.

Although the local complications of vasectomies are minimal, concerns have been raised about possible long-term side effects. Up to 60 percent of men develop immune reactions to their own sperm (*antisperm antibodies*), but clinically significant disturbances of the immune system have not been recognized. Similarly, initial concerns about an increased risk of heart attack, stroke, and hypertension have proved groundless. The same is true for kidney stones; although an early study linked vasectomy to an increased risk, subsequent research has refuted these claims. Worries about testicular cancer have also been laid to rest.

The possibility that vasectomy increases the risk of prostate cancer is more complex. Researchers first raised the alarm in 1990, shortly after the worries about cardiac disease had been resolved. Concern flared in 1993 when the Health Professionals Study reported that men who had undergone vasectomies were about one-and-a-half times more likely to develop prostate cancer than men who had not had the operation. The study was careful and large, involving 10,055 men who had vasectomies and 37,800 who had not. Still, many experts were skeptical, pointing out that there were only 300 newly diagnosed cases of prostate cancer in the entire group, and that men who had undergone vasectomy were likely to be under the care of a urologist and might be more likely to undergo tests leading to the diagnosis of early, clinically silent prostate cancer. Indeed, many studies since 1993 have failed to find a link between vasectomy and prostate cancer, and scientists have been unable to identify a biologically plausible reason for vasectomy to increase a man's cancer risk. At present, most authorities, including the National Cancer Institute and the American Urological Association, agree that vasectomy does not increase the risk of prostate cancer. The ongoing Prostate, Lung, Colorectal, and Ovarian

(PLCO) Cancer Trial is taking yet another look at the question, but the results will not be available for several years.

Permanence. As compared to most other birth control methods, a great advantage of vasectomy is that it is permanent. As compared to most other methods, the disadvantage of vasectomy is that it is permanent.

Before a man decides to undergo vasectomy, he should be sure that he does not want to father children in the future. It's an important decision, and most urologists offer counseling to couples to be sure the decision is wise. But life can take unpredictable twists, and even well-reasoned choices may prove regrettable. About 2 percent of men who have had vasectomies later decide to have the operation reversed, usually because of remarriage or a child's death. In about 60 percent of the cases, fertility can be restored, but it is not easy. In fact, delicate microsurgical techniques are required to sew the severed ends of the vas together, allowing sperm to once again transverse its pin-hole sized channel. The operation, called a *vasovasostomy,* requires general anesthesia and relatively lengthy recovery period. A vasovasostomy can cost $7,000 or more, and it is not covered by most insurance plans.

Although it's nice to have a potential way to restore fertility, men who undergo the operation should always assume that a vasectomy is forever.

The Decision. About 500,000 men decide to have vasectomies each year, and the vast majority are satisfied with their decisions. Still, it is important for every man to make his decision carefully and to include his wife in the decision-making process. While the pros and cons of vasectomy usually dominate the discussion, couples should also consider the other birth control options that are available to them. Most involve women, but condoms are a good alternative for many men, and researchers are working to develop new methods of male contraception. But until that research produces results, condoms and vasectomies will remain the only way for men to control their own fertility.

Sexually Transmitted Diseases

A vasectomy will prevent a man from fathering children, but it will not protect him from sexually transmitted diseases (STDs). A condom can do both—if it is used properly.

STDs have plagued men from the earliest days of recorded history. With the discovery of penicillin in the 1940s, many experts thought STDs had been conquered, since a shot of the "wonder drug" was able to cure the two classic STDs, syphilis and gonorrhea. But the experts underestimated both bacterial genetics and human behavior. Penicillin-resistant strains of gonorrhea began to appear early in the antibiotic era and they continue to increase even today. New, drug-resistant STDs have appeared, with AIDS being the most important example. And the sexual revolution of the 1970s increased the spread of STDs through conventional and unconventional sex. All in all, about 15 million Americans acquire STDs each year.

Scientists are developing new ways to diagnose and treat STDs. It is vital work, but it should not have become the top priority that it is today. Researchers are struggling with microbial behavior because people have not been able to control human behavior. In fact, STDs are easily preventable. The best way is to have monogamous sex with an uninfected partner. The next best is to use a condom 100 percent of the time. But since many people neglect to use the "seat belts of sex" men should know what to do about the major STDs.

Gonorrhea

Dating back to the days of the Old Testament, this bacterial infection is the oldest known STD. It was given the name that means "flow of seed" because the penile discharge that characterizes male gonorrhea was erroneously assumed to be semen. In fact, it is pus. The discharge begins three to four days after exposure and is accompanied by burning discomfort in the penis and painful urination. Without treatment, the infection can sometimes spread to the blood, skin, and joints. Doctors report more than 350,000 cases to public health authorities each year, and many other cases are never reported.

Doctors can diagnose gonorrhea by looking at a specimen from the urethra under a microscope and by sending it to the lab to be cultured. A newer test uses DNA technology to identify the bacterium in a urine specimen. A single injection of *ceftriaxone* is the best way to treat gonorrhea, but a variety of oral antibiotics are also effective.

Syphilis

Because syphilis swept through Europe shortly after Columbus returned from the New World, syphilis has been called the first American export. The theory is controversial, but there is no doubt about the severity of the sixteenth century European epidemic that earned it the name meaning "great plague." Syphilis has also been called the great mimic because it infects so many organs outside the genital tract. The first manifestation is an ulcerated *chancre* at the site of sexual contact, but it doesn't appear until ten to twenty-one days after the exposure. Even without treatment, the ulcer resolves, but four to eight weeks later the infection is back in force, with fever, a rash, swollen lymph glands, sore throat, and other manifestations. Again the infection goes into hiding but it is hibernating, not dead. In some patients, the disease returns three to thirty years later, producing devastating damage to the brain, spinal cord, or blood vessels and heart.

Doctors can diagnose syphilis with a blood test. Penicillin injections will cure the infection in its early stages but not in its late form; good alternatives are available for penicillin-allergic patients.

Syphilis has produced many tragic illnesses throughout its 400-year history. It has been up and down in the United States over the past fifty years. At present, it is down to just over 6,000 cases a year, but if history is any guide, down is not out.

Non-Gonococcal Urethritis

It is an unfamiliar name, but an all too familiar illness; with more than 400,000 cases reported annually, nongonococcal urethritis (NGU) is the most common STD in the United States.

In men, NGU causes a urethritis that is similar to gonorrhea except for a longer incubation period (one to three weeks), less burning, and a thinner, more watery discharge. Like patients with gonorrhea, men with NGU can also develop epididymitis (see Chapter Nine). In most cases, NGU is caused by a tiny bacterium called *Chlamydia trachomatis,* a first cousin of the chlamydia pneumoniae bacteria that produce pneumonia and may contribute to atherosclerosis (see Chapter Three). Although chlamydia trachomatis is troublesome for men, it is much worse for women, who can develop a high fever and painful inflammation of the pelvic organs that can cause infertility. The responsible bacterium is too small to see through a microscope and too fragile to grow in ordinary cultures, but it can be detected with DNA testing of urine specimens. *Azithromycin* (an antibiotic in the erythromycin family) or *doxycycline* (a tetracycline antibiotic) is the recommended treatment.

Genital Herpes

Gonorrhea, syphilis, and NGU are caused by bacteria that can be killed by antibiotics. Herpes is different; it is caused by a virus (*Herpes simplex virus* or HSV), and although it can be suppressed by special antiviral medications, it will lurk permanently in nerve roots where it can reactivate at any time.

About 45 million Americans are infected with HSV; many do not know it. After an incubation period of two to seven days, a newly infected man develops tiny blisters on his penis along with fever, fatigue, and swollen lymph glands in his groin. Headache and stiff neck can signal herpes meningitis, which resolves on its own and is not as threatening as it sounds. Without treatment, genital herpes settles down in about a week, but it can recur from within, even without additional sexual exposures. In most men, recurrences tend to become milder and less frequent over the months and years. Antiviral medications such as *acyclovir* (Zovirax) can speed the resolution of symptoms but will not cure the infection. Men who have frequent recurrences can take medication on a daily basis to prevent outbreaks. Because men with HSV can transmit the infection even if they do not have symptoms of active disease, they should always use condoms to protect their partners.

Venereal Warts (condylomas)

A virus, *human papilloma virus* (HPV), is responsible for this infection, which strikes about 1 million Americans annually. Some men develop penile warts, but others have no visible signs of the disease. Men who have warts on the skin can treat themselves by applying *podofilox* (Condylox) twice a day for four days; the therapy can be repeated up to four times with a four-day rest period between treatments. Doctors can use a variety of other techniques to treat genital condylomas. HPV is not serious in men, but it increases the risk of cancer of the cervix in women. Because men who have had HPV can transmit the virus even without visible warts, they should always wear condoms to protect their partners.

Hepatitis

Although the viruses that cause hepatitis B and hepatitis C do not produce genital lesions, they belong among the STDs. That's because these viruses remain in the patient's blood and body fluids for years and can be spread sexually. They can also be spread by blood products; testing has made America's blood supply very, very safe, but that is not true in many countries—and even in America, hepatitis B and C can ravage drug abusers who share needles.

Unlike the mild but more common hepatitis A, hepatitis B and C can be very serious, even producing liver failure or liver cancer. An excellent vaccine is available for hepatitis B; it should be administered to all children long before they become sexually active. Unfortunately, there is no vaccine for hepatitis C.

HIV AND AIDS

AIDS is the poster child for the prevention of STDs. Since it was first identified in five men in Los Angeles in 1981, HIV has become a global catastrophe that affects tens of millions of people and kills more than 3 million a year. In the world as a whole, the infection is equally prevalent in men and women, but the United States has three to four times more HIV-infected men than women.

HIV is an extremely deadly virus because it has a particularly nasty ability to infect the body's *helper T-lymphocytes,* the immune cells that stimulate and coordinate much of the immune system. HIV incorporates itself into the cells' most intimate machinery, but instead of lurking quietly (like HSV often does), it destroys the immune cells. That opens the floodgates to an enormous range of microbes that cause the devastating infections that transform an HIV infection into full-blow AIDS. It also allows tumor cells that ordinarily would be contained by the immune system to gain the upper hand, adding a variety of malignancies to the terrible burden of AIDS.

Reliable, inexpensive, widely available blood tests can detect the presence of HIV and determine the extent to which the virus has damaged the immune system. Who should be tested? Everyone who is at risk for HIV infection because of risky sexual behavior (gay or straight), drug abuse (by injection), transfusions (if the blood was not tested for HIV), or other exposures to potentially contaminated blood or body fluids. Prompt diagnosis of HIV can help limit the spread of infection, and it can lead to the combination drug therapy that has transformed the face of HIV, keeping most patients alive and active for many years.

In countries that can afford it, anti-HIV therapy can usually control, but never cure, the infection. Because the drugs are so helpful, many Americans are becoming complacent about HIV; it is a grave error.

CONTROLLING STDs

The HIV epidemic illustrates two key points about STDs: sex travels fast, and safe sex is the only way to prevent infection from following in its path.

All people with STDs should report their sexual contacts to public health authorities, who will track down contacts while preserving confidentiality. Because STDs travel in packs, everyone who is exposed to one STD should be tested for the others.

Sexual Dysfunction

Because they are the most sexually active (and the most reckless) segment of the population, young men are particularly vulnerable to STDs. Some older men may almost wish they had such problems, since maturity brings an increased risk of impotence (see page 298). But a variety of other problems involving sexuality, erections, and ejaculation can strike men of all ages.

Many sexual problems are compounded by myths about male sexuality, misinformation about male physiology, and a general male reluctance to talk about personal matters. Here are ten common myths:

- A real man should want sex all the time.
- Men should always initiate and orchestrate sexual activity.
- Manliness equals a large penis and a rigid erection.
- Real men never fail.
- Performance counts for everything, feelings for little.
- Sex should always culminate with intercourse and ejaculation.
- Sex should be spontaneous and natural, with lots of action but little planning and less talk.
- Sex should always be satisfying for both partners.
- Intimacy requires sex, and sex requires a rigid erection.
- Nobody believes these things anymore, which is the biggest myth of all.

Sexual myths are part of the common culture and are perpetuated by both men and women. (Woody Allen, in *Sleeper*: "My brain is my second favorite organ." Mae West: "A hard man is good to find," and "Too much of a good thing is . . . wonderful.") There is nothing wrong with having a good laugh about sex, but for many men it is not a laughing matter. Sexual mythology can affect mind and body; one example that is not a joke is the rising popularity of cosmetic surgery intended to enlarge the penis (*phalloplasty*).

The most important type of male sexual dysfunction is an impaired ability to attain or sustain an erection. Doctors call it impotence, but men rightly stay away from the term because it implies a general loss of power, thus perpetuating another myth that equates sex with power. But the politically correct phrase, erectile dysfunction, also has shortcomings, since it appropriates a term that could describe many types of erectile problems and applies it to just one. In fact, there are other types of male sexual dysfunction, many of which involve erection or ejaculation. Here is a quick review:

Lack of Desire

Sex is part of life, and many life events can affect sexual drive. Doctors think first of hormones and they have a point, since low levels of testosterone or high levels of the pituitary hormone *prolactin* can reduce or abolish libido. But these endocrine abnormalities are really quite uncommon. Much more often, a diminished sex drive reflects fatigue, stress, depression, or interpersonal conflicts. Faced with these problems, many men turn to alcohol, which is a mistake, since drinking can add to sexual woes. And since sex depends on a healthy body as well as a receptive mind, virtually any physical illness can sap desire, at least temporarily. Moreover, some of the most widely prescribed medications can reduce libido. Various drugs used to treat anxiety, depression, high blood pressure, heart disease, and allergies are among the suspects. Except for the antianxiety drugs, most can impair erection as well as desire (see Table 10.1, page 301). In fact, any condition that makes sex difficult or painful can reduce a man's interest in sex.

Premature Ejaculation

Premature ejaculation is a common problem affecting men of all ages, and it is a cause of frustration and discontent for both sexual partners. Because the duration of normal, mutually satisfying intercourse varies widely, a premature ejaculation cannot be defined simply in terms of the duration of a man's erection. Instead, a premature ejaculation is one that occurs before it is desired. Sometimes it is early in foreplay, even before a full erection occurs, but it can also occur later, after penetration but before mutual gratification is achieved. In either circumstance, it's a problem that can be treated.

Until recently, behavioral therapy was the only treatment for premature ejaculation. Perhaps the most widely used approach is the "pause and squeeze" technique developed by Masters and Johnson. A man who feels an orgasm developing prematurely temporarily interrupts sexual activity. Then the man (or his partner) squeezes the shaft of the penis between a thumb and two fingers. After applying gentle pressure just below the head of the penis for about twenty seconds, the squeeze is released and sexual activity is resumed. The technique can be repeated as often as needed. If all goes well, the man will eventually learn to delay ejaculation without the squeeze.

Behavioral therapy is safe and simple, and it helps 60–90 percent of men with premature ejaculations. But it requires the cooperation of both partners and relapses are common. As a result, drug therapy is gaining a role in treating premature ejaculation.

Drug therapy did not begin with a reasoned scientific attack on the problem of premature ejaculation, but with an unintended side effect. Some men taking antidepressant medications complained of delayed ejaculation. From there, it was a logical step to use antidepressants to treat premature ejaculation, and the results have been favorable, both with the popular *selective serotonin reuptake inhibitors* (SSRIs) and with the older *tricyclic antidepressants*. One of the most effective of these medications is *sertraline* (Zoloft); it can be taken four to six hours before intercourse or on a daily basis. Because antidepressant medications can produce unpleasant side effects of their own, most men with premature ejaculation should try behavioral therapy first. Still, it is reassuring that effective medications are also available.

DELAYED EJACULATION

Whereas premature ejaculations are never caused by disease, delayed ejaculation can result from either psychological or physical problems. Alcohol, medications (including antidepressants and some antihypertensives), and diabetes are among the most frequent causes of delayed or inhibited ejaculation. When drugs are responsible, the problem will usually respond to a change in medication. Psychological problems often respond to behavioral techniques or sex therapy.

RETROGRADE EJACULATION

During normal ejaculation, semen flows out of the penis because muscles at the neck of the bladder contract, preventing the semen from traveling up into the bladder. In retrograde, or dry, ejaculation the bladder muscles fail to do their job, so semen flows into the bladder and no emission occurs. It is a common complication of prostate surgery, occurring in 50–75 percent of men following *transurethral resection of the prostate* (TURP; see Chapter Eleven). Retrograde ejaculation can also be caused by diabetes or, much less often, by medication. Although retrograde ejaculation impairs fertility, it does not necessarily abolish the pleasurable sensation of orgasm.

PRIAPISM

Priapism is more than a long-lasting erection. It is a prolonged and painful erection that is unrelated to sexual desire and does not resolve following ejaculation. Whereas ordinary delayed ejaculation is a sexual problem, priapism is a medical problem, and it can be a medical emergency.

Priapism results from abnormalities of the blood vessels that control erections. *Veno-occlusive* or *low-flow priapism* occurs when narrowing of penile veins prevent blood from leaving the penis; *arterial* or *high-flow priapism* results when the arteries of the penis are abnormally dilated, allowing excessive amounts of blood to enter the penis. In either case, the penis is engorged, and without treatment it remains erect for six to twenty-four hours. Despite the similarities between the two types of priapism, the differences are critical.

Arterial priapism usually results from trauma. It is best diagnosed by *duplex ultrasound* and is usually treated by *arterial embolization*, which blocks the abnormal arterial channel that is responsible for carrying excessive blood to the penis. In the more common veno-occlusive variety, the tissues are deprived of oxygen so the penis is very painful, and it can be permanently damaged if prompt treatment is not available. Veno-occlusive priapism has many causes, including sickle cell anemia, oral medications (*trazadone, chlorpromazine, hydralazine* and many others), medications that are injected into the penis to treat impotence (*alprostadil, papaverine, phentolamine*), alcohol, cocaine, and tumors of the penis, which are rare. Often, however, the cause is unknown and may be related to sexually stimulated or nocturnal erections that escape normal control mechanisms. No matter what the cause, veno-occlusive priapism must be treated promptly to prevent scarring and impotence.

Men with priapism should treat themselves with ice packs and pain relievers en route to urgent medical care. Urologists can usually control the problem by aspirating blood from the engorged corpora cavernosa and injecting vasoconstricting drugs such as *phenylephrine* or *adrenaline* directly into these tissues.

Although priapism is the most serious erectile problem, it is also the least common. Still, it is a reminder that erectile function is a topic that is better suited to doctors than stand-up comics.

PEYRONIE'S DISEASE

In 1743, Francois de la Peyronie described a patient who had "rosary beads of scar tissue to cause an upward curvature of the penis during erection." The disease that bears his name produces penile deformities and erectile dysfunction. It is an uncommon problem that affects about 1 percent of men, usually between the ages of forty-five and sixty. Although its cause is unknown, Peyronie's disease is thought to result from trauma or inflammation in the *tunica albuginea* that produces a plaque of scar tissue in this otherwise thin structure that supports and surrounds the corpora cavernosa.

The plaque of scar tissue produces a curvature of the erect penis. The plaque can be painful, and the curvature can interfere with sexual intercourse. In most cases, the disease begins gradually and progresses slowly over one to two years. In many cases, the process stabilizes and in a few it appears to resolve spontaneously. Oral therapy with vitamin E is commonly recommended, and *aminobenzoate potassium* (Potaba) is sometimes prescribed; injections of *verapamil,* a calcium channel-blocker, or *dexamethasone,* a steroid in the cortisone family, have also been advocated. The only proven treatment, however, is surgery. Surgery should be reserved for men with significant pain or sexual impairment, and it should never be undertaken until the plaque is mature and the disease has stabilized.

BLOODY EJACULATION

Most men have never heard of *hematospermia,* and few understand what the medical term actually means. But every man who develops hematospermia recognizes at once that something is wrong, and most are extremely worried by the sight of blood (*heme*) in their semen (*spermia*).

In hematospermia, the blood may be fresh and bright red or it maybe brownish, suggesting that the bleeding occurred at least several hours before ejaculation. There may be just a few drops of blood, or the whole ejaculate may be discolored. Blood may be the only symptom, or ejaculation may have been accompanied by discomfort or pain. But whether it is fresh or old, scant or copious, painless or painful, a bloody ejaculate is frightening to men and their spouses. Cancer, venereal disease, sexual abnormalities, and infertility are the most common fears. These fears are understandable, perhaps inevitable, but are they medically appropriate? Is hematospermia as serious as it seems?

Semen contains fluid from three principal sources; sperm-rich fluid from the vas constitutes about 10 percent of the total volume, fluid from the prostate 20 percent, and fluid from the seminal vesicles 70 percent. Blood can enter the semen with any of these fluids. Physicians have identified many causes of the condition:

Functional Abnormalities. In many cases, hematospermia appears to result from disordered function of the ejaculatory apparatus without corresponding anatomical abnormalities. Sometimes, for example, hematospermia is attributed to prolonged sexual abstinence that results in excessive filling of the seminal vesicles.

Inflammation and Infection. Most men with inflammation of the prostate (*prostatitis,* see Chapter Eleven) or epididymis (*epididymitis,* see Chapter Nine) complain of pain in the pelvis or scrotum, fever, or slow and painful urination. But some men develop hematospermia, with or without the more characteristic symptoms of inflammation. Bacterial infections are usually responsible, but in rare cases viral infections, tuberculosis, or even parasitic infestations are to blame.

Stones and Cysts. Small stones can form in the prostate or seminal vesicles, and cysts can develop in the accessory glands and ducts of the reproductive organs. Hematospermia can result from any of these problems, alone or with other symptoms.

Vascular Abnormalities. When most men think of varicose veins, they think of their legs. Some also understand that hemorrhoids are varicose veins in the rectum. And some men with hematospermia learn that their problem stems from swollen veins in the seminal vesicles or prostate.

Tumors. It's the possibility that worries men most, but it is actually low on the list of things that cause hematospermia. Still, cancer of the prostate is a rare cause of bloody semen; rarer still are cancers of the seminal vesicles, urethra, or testicles.

Medical Treatment. With its increased use to diagnose prostate cancer, *transrectal prostate biopsy* is now the most common cause of hematospermia. Various other urological tests and treatments may also cause bleeding during ejaculation.

Is hematospermia serious? It depends who you ask. Most men with the problem think it is very serious and their sexual partners agree. Many doctors who have just seen a case or two are not sure what to think, and the medical literature contains a wide range of answers.

The best information comes from urologists at the Mayo Clinic. They evaluated 200 men with hematospermia, and were able to observe 150 of them for five to twenty-three years. The men ranged in age from twenty to seventy-four; most were between forty and seventy. In 85 percent, hematospermia was a recurrent problem, while the remainder had only a single episode.

Detailed urological studies were entirely negative in 63 percent of the patients. A variety of abnormalities were detected in the other men, including *benign prostatic hyperplasia* (BPH) in 17 percent, prostate stones in 7 percent, and abnormal veins in 8 percent. None of these disorders appeared serious, however, and the Mayo urologists were not sure if they were actually causing the bleeding or were just unrelated, coincidental problems.

Although 29 percent of the men had recurrent hematospermia during the follow-up period, most remained free of genitourinary disease. BPH did develop in 18 percent and prostate cancer in 4 percent; bladder cancer occurred in one man, kidney stones in another. But even in these men, there was no proof that the initial bleeding was related to the urological diseases that developed years later.

In this study, as in others, hematospermia proved to be a remarkably benign disorder. Most men with hematospermia rush to the doctor expecting aggressive tests and treatment, but elaborate tests are rarely necessary. Doctors should perform digital rectal exams, and they should examine the patient's testicles and scrotum. If there is any doubt about the source of the bleeding, men may be asked to ejaculate into a condom to see if the semen is in fact bloody. In any case, a urinalysis and urine culture are always important.

If the physical exam and urine are normal, testing can stop there. But if there is any hint of serious disease, other tests may prove helpful, including a measurement of *prostatic specific antigen* (PSA) in the blood and a *transurethral ultrasound* (TRUS) or *magnetic resonance imaging* (MRI) study to visualize the prostate and seminal vesicle. In a few cases, other studies may be in order.

There is no specific treatment for hematospermia. Since prostatitis is a treatable and relatively common problem, many physicians prescribe an antibiotic that can penetrate into the prostate, at least for the first episode of hematospermia. But the most important treatment of all is also the simplest: reassurance. In most cases, after all, hematospermia is a benign disorder, smoke without fire.

PAINFUL INTERCOURSE

It is much more common in women, but pain during sex (*dyspareunia*) can also bother men. Inflammation or infection of the prostate, epididymis, or bladder may be responsible. Even more frequently, pain results from inflammation of the penis itself. *Balanitis* is inflammation of the head of the penis or glans; it is most common in uncircumcised men, particularly diabetics. A related condition, *phimosis,* results from tightening of the foreskin over the glans, preventing it from retracting normally during an erection. Both conditions usually respond to good penile hygiene augmented by antifungal or antibacterial ointments. Gentle stretching of the foreskin may help relieve phimosis, but circumcision is the ultimate remedy (see Chapter Nine).

Erectile Dysfunction: Impotence

For many years, doctors have called it impotence, a term derived from the Latin for "loss of power." Then in 1992, a consensus panel convened by the National Institutes of Health, suggested the term erectile dysfunction. The goal was to remove the stigma of sexual dysfunction, freeing men to talk about the problem and seek help. It was a good idea but it did not work; male sexual problems stayed under the covers. But in 1998, Viagra and Bob Dole succeeded where the scientists failed, and male sexuality came in from the cold. The new acceptance of old sexual realities makes either name acceptable today.

What is Impotence?

In simple terms, impotence is the failure to achieve a normal erection. But nearly every man experiences erectile failure from time to time. Doctors restrict a formal designation of impotence to cases in which a man is unable to develop and sustain an erection adequate for intercourse in at least 25 percent of attempts. Even with this strict definition, impotence is very common, affecting many millions of American men.

Risk Factors

Age is the strongest risk factor; only 2 percent of forty-year-olds experience impotence, but the prevalence increases steadily with age. The Massachusetts Male Aging Study tells the story. It reported impotence in 25 percent of sixty-five-year-olds, 55 percent of seventy-five-year-olds, and 65 percent of eighty-year-olds. The severity of the erectile dysfunction also increased with age. In all, 35 percent of men aged forty to seventy experienced moderate to severe impotence, while 52 percent of all men reported at least some degree of erectile dysfunction.

Although erectile dysfunction increases with age, normal aging is not the culprit. It is true that testosterone levels tend to decline with age (see page 314), but they still remain within the normal range in most older men. It is also true that tissues become less elastic with age, that nerve conduction slows, and that mental stress mounts. But none of these events account for the staggeringly high prevalence of impotence in older men. Instead, the problem seems to be the gradual development of diseases that damage blood vessels and nerves; diabetes, hypertension, and atherosclerosis are the leading examples. Because they damage arteries, smoking and high cholesterol levels are also important risk factors. The medications used to treat chronic illnesses are another explanation. The treatments used for prostate disease also explain why older men are at risk. Similarly, pelvic radiotherapy or surgical removal of the bladder or rectum also contribute, since like prostate disease, cancers of the bladder and rectum occur mostly in older men.

A recent report by the Health Professionals Study provides additional insight, telling us that lifestyle also counts, that the way a man lives affects the way he loves. Agreeing with earlier research, the study found that age and high blood pressure were important risk factors—but it also found that obesity increased risk, while exercise and low-dose alcohol consumption were protective. The effects were substantial. For example, a man with a forty-two-inch waist is nearly 50 percent more likely to be impotent than a man with a thirty-two-inch waist, even after age, diabetes, and other risk factors are taken into account. Similarly, men who exercise for thirty minutes a day are 41 percent less likely to have erectile dysfunction than sedentary men. The effect of alcohol is more complex; a man who averages one to two drinks a day is 33 percent less likely to be impotent than a nondrinker, but men who drink more are at higher risk.

How can being lean, exercising, and drinking a little (but not too much) improve a man's sex life? It is not simply a matter of attracting partners, but a question of protecting the arteries (see Chapters Four, Five, and Seven). In terms of erectile function, the penis acts like one big artery. Things that damage blood vessels impair erectile function, while interventions that protect vascular health preserve sexual function.

Since so many parts of the body must be working just right to produce an erection, it is hardly surprising that many diverse problems can interfere with the process:

Medications. One of the most common culprits is not disease, but medication. Many drugs can produce impotence as a side effect. Older men are particularly vulnerable. Unfortunately, older men often take more than one drug that might cause erectile dysfunction, and they may also have medical disorders that cause impotence.

There is no simple way to test a man to see if his medications are to blame. Instead, it's a trial-and-error process of removing a medication, then waiting two to six weeks to see if potency returns. Many suspect medications, however, are important for health. Only a physician should juggle prescription drugs, but the patient has an important role, too. His first task is to report erectile dysfunction; then he should present the doctor with a list of all his medications, both prescription and over-the-counter. It sounds obvious, but many men just do not bring the subject up, and many doctors neglect to ask.

It has been estimated that up to 25 percent of all impotence is drug-related. Even if this figure is high, medication is always the first cause to consider, particularly since it is the most easily corrected. Table 10.1 contains a partial list of medications that have been reported to cause impotence. This side effect is more likely with some drugs on the list (such as beta-blockers) than others (such as ACE inhibitors).

Alcohol, Smoking, and Substance Abuse. Some men with erectile dysfunction may be tempted to turn to alcohol to help things along. It's a bad idea. In large amounts, alcohol can depress sexual reflexes; with prolonged use, it can damage the liver, raising estrogen levels and causing impotence. Street drugs, such as cocaine, heroin, barbiturates, and amphetamines, can all cause sexual dysfunction. Smoking, too, can contribute to impotence, probably by causing vascular disease.

Vascular Disease. Since erections depend on the arteries that supply blood to the penis, arterial diseases are the most common causes of impotence. Atherosclerosis ("hardening of the arteries") heads the list; high blood pressure, abnormal cholesterol levels, diabetes, and smoking all increase a man's risk of developing atherosclerosis and impotence.

Neurological Impotence. Disorders of the nervous system are frequently responsible for erectile dysfunction. Diabetes is the most common cause of this type of nerve damage. In addition, the nerves can be harmed by alcoholism, multiple sclerosis, and spinal-cord injuries. Because the seat puts pressure on the nerves and arteries that connect to the penis, prolonged bicycle riding can also produce erectile dysfunction.

Table 10.1: SOME MEDICATIONS THAT CAN CAUSE IMPOTENCE

TYPE OF MEDICATION	EXAMPLES
ACE inhibitors*	Captopril (Capoten) and many others
Alpha-blockers*	Prazosin (Minipress) and many others
Antidepressants	Amitriptyline (Elavil), Fluoxetine (Prozac), and many others
Antifungals	Ketoconazole (Nizoral)
Antiulcer drugs	Cimetidine (Tagamet) and others
Beta-blockers	Propranolol (Inderal) and many others
Calcium channel blockers*	Diltiazem (Cardizem) and many others
Cholesterol-lowering drugs*	Niacin, lovastatin (Mevacor), and others
Diuretics	Chlorthiazide (Diuril), spironolactone (Aldactone), and many others
Nitrates*	Isosorbide dinitrate (Isordil) and many others
Tranquilizers	Diazepam (Valium), thioridazine (Mellaril), and many others
Miscellaneous	Finasteride (Proscar), estrogens, antiandrogens, antihistamines, anticholinergics, and anticancer drugs

*Less likely to cause erectile dysfunction.

Diabetes. A very common cause of impotence, diabetes can interfere with erections by damaging blood vessels or nerves. Up to 50 percent of men with diabetes experience erectile dysfunction at some time. That's the bad news; the good news is that tight blood sugar control can help protect diabetics from erectile dysfunction.

Prostate Cancer and the Treatment of Prostate Diseases. Although the prostate itself has no role in producing erections, it is located near the nerves that are essential. Advanced prostate cancer can invade these nerves, causing impotence. In addition, impotence is a common side effect of surgery or radiation treatments for prostate cancer (see Chapter Twelve). Less often, it can result from surgery for *benign prostatic hyperplasia* (BPH, see Chapter Eleven).

Endocrine Disorders. Many impotent men blame their hormones, but few are correct. Endocrine disorders account for no more than 15 to 20 percent of all cases of impotence. *Hypogonadism,* or testicular failure, produces lower testosterone levels and is the most important endocrine cause of erectile dysfunction. An abnormally high level of *prolactin,* usually caused by a tumor of the pituitary gland, occupies second place. Less often, diseases of the thyroid or adrenal glands account for impotence.

Psychological Causes. Until recently, most impotence was blamed on anxiety or depression. Indeed, many impotent men experience psychological disorders, but it is now clear that mental distress usually results from impotence, rather than the other way around. Still, psychological factors are primarily responsible for about 15 percent of all impotence. Men who develop impotence very suddenly or who are impotent with one partner but not others are likely to have psychological impotence. An even more important clue is the presence of erections at night or on first awakening. Most healthy men experience three to five erections at night; the "organic" or "physical" causes of impotence impair nocturnal erections, but the psychological causes do not.

EVALUATION

Doctors can learn a lot about impotence from a thorough medical history and physical exam. Men should report when and how their sexual dysfunction began, and whether it involves loss of desire, erectile dysfunction, or difficulties with ejaculation and orgasm. Patients should review their previous illnesses and operations as well as their current medications. It is particularly important to note the presence or absence of nocturnal erections, which are most prominent when a man first awakens. Men should also report any symptoms of stress or depression.

Many men with impotence have normal physical exams, but others may display clues to underlying causes. Doctors should check blood pressures with the patient lying and standing. They should evaluate the circulation to the legs, often a clue to vascular diseases. Abnormally small testicles or enlarged breasts are among the possible hints of hormonal abnormalities. A digital rectal exam (DRE) should be performed to check the prostate. Neurologic testing should include simple checks of the sensation and reflexes in the legs as well as tests of rectal sensation and reflexes involving the muscles that support the scrotum.

Laboratory tests can also help track down potential causes of impotence.

Doctors can order blood tests to check for diabetes and to measure levels of testosterone, prolactin, and cholesterol.

If these studies fail to explain why a man is impotent, more elaborate testing may be indicated. *Nocturnal penile tumescence* (NPT) monitoring requires a man to wear a small gauge during sleep to check for nocturnal erections. Visual sexual stimulation is a simpler but less established way to test for psychological impotence. Men who get erections at night or after sexual stimulation are unlikely to have an organic cause for their sexual dysfunction.

Urologists can check for vascular impotence by injecting a drug that dilates arteries directly into the *penile corpus cavernosum*. A man with a normal penile circulation will develop a full rigid erection within ten to fifteen minutes. If the injection test is abnormal, or if the patient prefers a less invasive test, a color duplex Doppler ultrasound can be used to evaluate the penile arteries, the corpora cavernosa, and the penile blood flow.

Impotence can lead to lots of testing. All men deserve a thorough history and physical exam and basic blood tests, but few men benefit from elaborate or invasive tests, particularly since new treatments have become available.

TREATING IMPOTENCE

The best way to treat any medical problem is to correct its underlying cause. In the case of impotence, unfortunately, it is a difficult task. When medications are to blame, they can, and should, be changed or discontinued. If psychological factors account for impotence, psychological counseling or sex therapy can address the underlying cause. Hormonal abnormalities can also be corrected. Men who are impotent because of low testosterone levels can receive injections or apply a patch or gel to replace the missing hormone (see page 316). Men should always be checked for signs of prostate cancer before starting testosterone therapy, and periodic monitoring should continue during therapy. Men with normal testosterone levels will not benefit from hormone replacement, and they are still subject to potentially serious side effects from the therapy. Men with high prolactin levels or thyroid abnormalities can receive specific treatment for those problems.

In at least half the cases of impotence, however, the underlying problem cannot be corrected. Vascular and neurological impotence, diabetes, and impotence caused by prostate surgery or radiation therapy fall into this category. But men with these problems should not abandon hope; new advances in therapy have made several options available.

Men should consider all the alternatives; many will also benefit from frank discussions and counseling, including information about how he and his partner can obtain mutual satisfaction even without firm erections. But for a significant number of men (except those taking nitroglycerin or any other nitrate medications), Viagra will be the way to start.

VIAGRA

In April 1998, America's sexual horizons were transformed forever, as *sildenafil* (Viagra) burst on the scene. Within days, the little blue pill was the number-one subject for talk radio and late-night TV. Within weeks, Senator Bob Dole was a household name again, not for his political acumen but for his commercial discussion of erectile dysfunction. Within a month, 364,857 prescriptions for Viagra had been filled in the United States, making it the fastest-selling drug in history. And by the start of the new millennium, the sales of Viagra had topped $1 billion.

How Viagra Works. Viagra's success testifies to the enormous number of men with erectile dysfunction, and to the medication's effectiveness. Normal erections require a receptive state of mind, adequate levels of testosterone, and healthy arteries, veins, and nerves. But they also require a tiny chemical messenger called *nitric oxide* (NO) that serves two crucial functions, transmitting the impulses of arousal between nerves and relaxing the smooth muscle cells in the arteries, allowing them to widen and admit more blood to the penis.

Nitric oxide is essential for a normal erection, but it does not act alone. Instead, it signals the arterial cells to produce *cyclic guanosine monophosphate* (cGMP), the chemical that actually increases the flow of blood to the penis. But the tissues of the penis also produce *phosphodiesterase-5* (PDE5), an enzyme that breaks down cGMP.

In normal circumstances, the penis generates enough cGMP to produce a rigid erection and enough PDE5 to end the erection when ejaculation is complete. But in many men with erectile dysfunction, this intricate system is out of balance. In such cases, Viagra can often get things right. It inhibits PDE5, increasing the supply of cGMP. In many men, the extra cGMP will allow erections to develop in response to sexual stimulation.

Success Rates. Although studies vary, most suggest that about 70 percent of men respond favorably to Viagra. It works best in men with no identifiable organic cause of impotence (90 percent response), less well in diabetics (50 percent response). Men who have been treated for prostate cancer present special problems. That's because all forms of treatment are likely to damage the nerves that travel along the prostate to the penis (See Chapter Twelve). Doctors are still testing Viagra in these circumstances, but preliminary results are mixed. Men who have had standard *radical prostatectomies* rarely if ever respond to Viagra, but a quarter to a half of those who have had *nerve sparing radical prostatectomies* respond to Viagra. Improvement, though, is rare in the first nine months after surgery in men older than sixty, in men with complete impotence, and in men whose nerves have been preserved on only one side of the prostate. Viagra may help some men with impotence resulting from *external beam radiotherapy* and *brachytherapy*, but more research will be needed to determine which patients are most likely to benefit.

Side Effects. In men without cardiovascular disease, Viagra is very safe. The most common side effect is headache, which occurs in up to 16 percent of men. Other adverse reactions include facial flushing, nasal congestion, indigestion, and diarrhea. About 3 percent of Viagra users have visual disturbances, typically in the form of impaired color vision or a bluish haze. Like the other common side effects, such visual abnormalities are mild and temporary—but they are the reason the Federal Aviation Administration has prohibited pilots from using Viagra within six hours of flying. Men with *retinitis pigmentosa*, a rare eye disease, should check with their ophthalmologists before using Viagra.

Headaches and blue vision are one thing, cardiac abnormalities, quite another. Is Viagra safe for the heart?

The drug is safe for healthy hearts, but all men with cardiovascular disease require special precautions, and some cannot use Viagra under any circumstances. The reason for concern is Viagra's effect on arteries. All arteries, not just those in the penis, generate nitric oxide, so any artery can widen in response to Viagra. It does not happen often because Viagra specifically targets PDE5, which is concentrated mainly in the penis. But other arteries contain some PDE5, which is why Viagra temporarily lowers the blood pressure of normal men by a small amount, typically 5 to 8 mmHg (millimeters of mercury).

Organic nitrates are drugs that widen arteries by increasing their supply of nitric oxide; that is how they open the partially-blocked coronary arteries in patients with angina. But because the nitrates and Viagra both act on nitric oxide, the drugs do not mix. Normal volunteers given Viagra followed an hour later by nitroglycerin drop their blood pressures by 25 to 51 mmHg, a potentially dangerous amount. All the experts agree that men who are taking nitrates cannot use Viagra. This includes all preparations of *nitroglycerin* (short-acting under-the-tongue tablets or sprays), long-acting nitrates (*isosorbide dinitrate* or Isordil, Sorbitrate, and others, and *isosorbide mononitrate,* Imdur, ISMO, and others), nitroglycerin patches and pastes, and amyl nitrite or *amyl nitrate* (so-called "poppers" that are used for sexual stimulation by some men).

The American Heart Association and the American College of Cardiology have issued recommendations for the use of Viagra in men with cardiovascular disease. The key points are:

1. Men who are taking nitrates in any form (see above) cannot use Viagra. No one should take Viagra within twenty-four hours of taking a nitrate.
2. Men with mild stable angina who have been given prescriptions for nitroglycerin but rarely need the medication should discuss the potential risks of Viagra with their physicians. Even if men with mild coronary artery disease rarely need nitroglycerin, the stress of sexual activity could precipitate angina, thus creating the need for nitroglycerin. An exercise stress test may be helpful for such men. Men who can exercise vigorously without developing cardiac abnormalities can usually engage in conventional sex with a familiar partner without developing a need for nitroglycerin. However, if a man who has taken Viagra develops angina during sexual activity, he should not take nitroglycerin; instead, he should interrupt sexual activity at once and contact his doctor if the pain does not resolve promptly.
3. Patients who require complex, multidrug regimens to control high blood pressure may be at risk for Viagra-induced low blood pressure. Doctors may consider monitoring blood pressure in an office setting after a test dose of Viagra to identify men at risk.
4. Caution is also required in men taking other drugs that prolong the activity of Viagra; *erythromycin, cimetidine, diltiazem,* and *verapamil* are examples. Men with liver or kidney disease should exercise similar caution, because these abnormalities can also boost the effects of Viagra.

Faced with worry about Viagra and the heart, the FDA has also beefed up its warning, urging caution in patients who have suffered heart attacks, strokes, or serious disturbances of the heart's rhythm with six months, in men with a history of congestive heart failure or unstable angina, and in men with low blood pressure or uncontrolled high blood pressure (above 170/110).

Although these precautions are both wise and important, they should not scare men away from Viagra. In fact, the drug is quite safe for men who observe these simple guidelines.

Doctors from the University of Pennsylvania provided reassurance when they gave Viagra to fourteen men with severe coronary artery disease who were undergoing cardiac catheterization; the drug did not reduce blood flow to the heart, even in the most diseased arteries. And a 2000 analysis of 1,137 men taking medications for high blood pressure found no evidence that Viagra was harmful. Needless to say, none of the men in either study were taking nitrates.

Using Viagra. Faced with all these warnings, should any man use Viagra? Indeed, no one should use the drug needlessly or recklessly, but 30 million American men are plagued by impotence, and most can use Viagra safely.

Viagra comes in three strengths; most doctors prescribe 50 milligrams initially, reducing to 25 milligrams if the drug works well or increasing to 100 milligrams if it does not. Men with potential problems should always start with 25 milligrams, and every man who takes Viagra should be alert for potential side effects. Viagra works best on an empty stomach, and men should avoid consuming alcohol before taking the drug.

By itself, Viagra will not produce an erection, but it will improve the erectile response to erotic stimulation. Viagra starts to work in about thirty minutes and its effects can persist for up to four hours. For best results, though, it should be taken about an hour before sexual activity. Viagra should not be used more than once a day. It is not an aphrodisiac, and it should be used only to correct impotence, not enhance sexual performance. Men who do not respond to a 100 milligram dose on two or three different occasions should move on to other treatments; higher doses may be tempting, but they are both risky and ineffective.

Viagra is expensive; each strength costs about $10 a pill. As a result, men who respond to 25 or 50 milligrams can save money by cutting 50 or 100 milligram pills in half. Some insurers will pay for Viagra, many have restrictions, and others will not cover the drug at all. But for many men Viagra is worth the price—as long as the price is measured in dollars, not illness.

Although Viagra has earned its status as the favored treatment for impotence, many other options are available for men who cannot use the medication or fail to respond to it.

Injection Therapy

As far back as 1983, urologists began to treat impotence by teaching men to inject their penises with *papavarine* and *phentolamine,* drugs that induce erections by widening the arteries in the penis. Although these drugs helped some men, they have been replaced by a newer medication, *alprostadil* (Caverject, Edex, and Prostinur). Although the idea of injecting oneself seems daunting at first, most men can learn the technique, which uses a very small needle to inject medication directly into the corpus cavernosum. About 70 percent of men respond to the injections. When they do, an erection develops in ten minutes and lasts for thirty to sixty minutes.

The major side effect is penile pain, which is usually mild but causes about 10 percent of the men to discontinue injection therapy. Prolonged erections occur in 5 percent of men and about 1 percent develop priapism, painful prolonged erections that require emergency therapy to prevent irreversible penile damage (see page 294). Other side effects include bleeding and scarring. Alprostadil injections cost about $25 each.

Pellet Therapy

Alprostadil can also be administered by inserting tiny pellets directly into the urethra; the Medicated Urethral System for Erection (MUSE) was approved for clinical use in 1997. A man inserts a slender tube containing a pellet into his urethra, advancing it about an inch from the tip of the penis. When he presses a button on the applicator, the pellet is propelled into the urethra. Alprostadil is rapidly absorbed from the pellet and enters the corpora cavernosa, where it dilates arteries. About 40 percent of men with organic impotence respond to MUSE. The major complication is penile pain, which occurs in about 30 percent of men, but is usually mild. Painful prolonged erections are much less common with MUSE than with injections. However, about 3 percent of MUSE patients develop low blood pressure and dizziness.

MUSE is available in four strengths from 125 to 1,000 micrograms of alprostadil; as with the injections, physicians must determine the minimum effective dose and check for low blood pressure before prescribing it for home use. Each application costs about $25. Men should not use more than two pellets in 24 hours.

Since alprostadil bypasses nerves and produces erection by acting directly on arteries, it does not require sexual stimulation to do its work. Without proper erotic activity, however, some men may fail to achieve orgasm despite having strong erections. Because of the risks of low blood pressure and priapism, alprostadil should not be used with Viagra, except under very careful medical supervision. In some men who do not respond to alprostadil alone, combination injections of papavarine, phentolamine, and aprostadil (Trimix) may be effective, but the combination has not been approved by the FDA Combination therapy with alprostadil and an alpha-blocker such as *prazosin* (Minipres) is also experimental.

VACUUM PUMP THERAPY

Men who prefer to avoid medications can often achieve erections by using vacuum constriction devices. The penis is placed in an airtight plastic cylinder attached to a hand-operated pump. Air is pumped out of the cylinder to create a vacuum, which increases penile blood flow. When the penis is erect, a special band is secured around its base to retain the blood after the cylinder is removed. After intercourse is completed, the band is removed and the penis becomes flaccid. Vacuum devices are 80 to 90 percent effective in producing satisfactory erections within five minutes. They are cumbersome, however, and require some manual dexterity. About 10 percent of men experience adverse effects, including penile bruising, pain, and impaired ejaculation. Vacuum devices vary in price from $150 to $450. They are available without a prescription.

SURGERY

Surgical implants are another treatment for erectile dysfunction. Two approaches are available. One implants silicone rods that produce a permanent erection. Because the rods can be bent up and down, the erect penis can be concealed under clothing. The alternative is an inflatable device that produces an erection when it is filled with fluid pumped from a reservoir placed in the abdomen. Inflatable implants function more naturally, but they have a higher rate of complications and failure than rigid implants. More than 200,000 American men have had penile implants, but fewer are choosing this option now that less invasive treatments are available.

EXPERIMENTAL THERAPY

A cream or ointment that could be applied to the penis to induce an erection has obvious appeal. Researchers have tested creams containing nitroglycerin, alprostadil, and a combination of *aminophylline, isorbide dinitrate,* and *codergocrine mesylate* with mixed results. A cream containing alprostadil and SEPA, a chemical that enhances drug penetration through the skin, appears promising, but is still experimental.

Phentolamine tablets (Vasomax) are also under study. In early trials, 37 to 45 percent of men responded favorably. Side effects include headaches, facial flushing, and nasal congestion.

Apomorphine (Spontene) is a medication that is placed under the tongue. It produces erections in about half the men who have tested it. Nausea, which can be severe, is the most common side effect, but at high doses apomorphine can also lower the low blood pressure and cause fainting.

Ineffective Therapy

Despite the understandable appeal of pills and powders promoted as aphrodisiacs, men should be discouraged from experimenting with unapproved folk remedies or herbs. One traditional folk drug can be prescribed by doctors; *yohimbine* (Yohimex, Yocon) is an alpha-blocker derived from certain trees; although it is widely prescribed for impotence, it appears to help only men with psychological impotence. *Caveat emptor!* Buyer beware!

Sex and the Heart

It is a familiar scenario that has become all the more common since effective treatment for erectile dysfunction became available. A man who has had a heart attack is eager to return to normal sexual activity, his wife is worried and reluctant, and his doctor is caught in the middle. It is a familiar situation, but the next act has been harder to predict, as doctors have struggled to formulate the best response. To help reconcile conflicting approaches to this sensitive situation, an International Consensus Conference on Sexual Activity and Cardiac Risk has issued useful guidelines for men.

Sex as Exercise

Disappointingly, perhaps, people seem to spend more energy thinking and talking about sex than on the act itself. During sexual intercourse, a man's heart rate rarely gets as high as 130 beats a minute and his systolic blood pressure (the higher number, recorded when the heart is pumping blood) nearly always stays under 170. All in all, average sexual activity ranks as mild to moderate intensity exercise, similar to doing the foxtrot or raking leaves. Sex burns about five calories a minute; that is four more than a man uses watching TV, but it's about the same as walking the course to play golf. If a man can walk up two or three flights of stairs without difficulty, he should be in shape for sex.

SEX AS SEX

Raking leaves may increase a man's oxygen consumption, but it probably will not get his motor running. Sex, of course, is different, and the excitement and stress might well pump out extra adrenaline. Both mental excitement and physical exercise increase adrenaline levels and can trigger heart attacks and arrhythmias, abnormalities of the heart's pumping rhythm. Can sex do the same? In theory, it can. But in practice it is really very uncommon, at least during conventional sex with a familiar partner.

Careful studies show that fewer than one of every 100 heart attacks are related to sexual activity, and for fatal arrhythmias the rate is just one in 200. Put another way, for a healthy fifty-year-old man, the risk of having a heart attack in any given hour is about one in a million; sex doubles the risk, but it is still just two in a million. For men with heart disease, the risk is ten times higher, but even for them, the chance of suffering a heart attack during sex is just twenty in a million. Those are pretty good odds, but the new guidelines suggest that it may be possible to make the odds even better.

RATING THE RISK

The Consensus Conference arrived at a classification system based on a man's cardiac risk factors as well as his personal history of heart disease. In addition to age, the major risk factors for men included high blood pressure, diabetes, obesity, cigarette smoking, abnormal blood cholesterol levels, and a sedentary lifestyle. Based on these considerations, men can be stratified into one of three risk categories.

Low Risk. Most men will be in this group. Included are men with fewer than three major cardiac risk factors, men with well-controlled hypertension or mild, stable angina, men who have had successful angioplasties or coronary artery bypass operations, and even men who are as little as six to eight weeks out from heart attacks. Men with mild heart valve disease or mild congestive heart failure are also considered low risk.

According to the Consensus Conference, sex should be safe for low-risk men. As a result, they do not need special testing or extra precaution.

Moderate Risk. This category includes men with three or more major cardiac risk factors, men with moderately severe but stable angina, and men who are two to six weeks out from heart attacks. Also included are men with moderately severe congestive heart failure and those with evidence of atherosclerosis beyond the heart, such as previous strokes or peripheral vascular disease.

The Conference recommends caution for moderate risk men, suggesting that they avoid sex until they have had a detailed cardiovascular evaluation, usually including a stress test and an echocardiogram. Men who pass these tests with flying colors can be reclassified as low risk, but if problems show up, they may indicate high risk.

High Risk. Men who have had heart attacks within two weeks head the high risk group, which also includes those with severe or unstable angina, men with uncontrolled hypertension, and patients with severe congestive heart failure, dangerous arrhythmias, moderate to severe heart valve disease, and heart muscle disease.

The Consensus Conference suggests that high risk men refrain from sexual activity, at least until their medical conditions have improved substantially. Even then, full cardiovascular evaluation and individualized advice is necessary before giving the go-ahead.

Safe Sex

Sex is a normal part of human life. For all men, whether they have heart disease or not, the best way to keep sex safe is to stay in shape by avoiding tobacco (see Chapter Eight), exercising regularly (see Chapter Five), and eating a good diet (see Chapter Four). Other measures that reduce the risk of heart attacks are also important; low-dose aspirin heads the list (see Chapter Six). Needless to say, men should not initiate sexual activity if they are not feeling well, and men who experience possible cardiac symptoms during sex should interrupt the sexual activity at once.

With the new guidelines and simple precautions, sex is safe for the heart, but it should be safe for the rest of the body, too. Sexually transmitted diseases pose a greater threat than sexually induced heart problems. When it comes to sex, men should use their heads as well as their hearts.

Sex, Hormones, and Age

As usual, Shakespeare got it right: "Is it not strange that desire should so many years outlive performance?" In many men, sexual performance does decline over the years, but in most, age-related diseases are to blame, not age itself. Still, the clock ticks for all men and strikes more than just sex. By the time he is eighty, an average men loses twelve to twenty pounds of muscle, 15 percent of bone density, and almost two inches of height. The levels of testosterone and several other hormones also decline with age. Are falling hormone levels responsible for the negative aspects of aging, and can hormone replacement help?

Aging and Male Sexuality

Things change. For most men, sexuality is one of the things that change over time. For healthy men it is a gradual, almost imperceptible process that begins in middle age. Whereas most older men retain an interest in sex, it is generally a far cry from the preoccupation with sex that is so common in youth. Although interest is retained, desire tends to wane; many older men think about sex but do not have the drive to put theory into practice. And even when the spirit is willing, the flesh may be weak; male sexual performance typically declines more rapidly than either interest or desire. Most men experience decreased sexual responsiveness with increasing age. Erections occur more slowly and they become more dependent on physical stimulation than on erotic thoughts. Even when erections develop, most men in their sixties report that their penile rigidity is diminished and harder to sustain. The ejaculatory phase also changes with age. The muscular contractions of orgasm are less intense, ejaculation is slower and less urgent, and men experience a longer refractory period following intercourse, when they cannot respond to sexual stimulation. Semen volume and sperm counts also decline, but most men remain fertile.

Many surveys report that the frequency of sexual activity declines with age, but they disagree as to how often older couples have intercourse. In round numbers, 50 to 80 percent of healthy couples over seventy report sexual activity on a regular basis, including weekly intercourse in about one-half.

Sexual intercourse requires a partner. But male sexuality demonstrates age-related changes that are not dependent on interpersonal factors. Nocturnal erections diminish with age; men between age forty-five and fifty-four average 3.3 erections per night; between age sixty-five and seventy-five, average 2.3

erections. Nocturnal erections also tend to become briefer and less rigid as men age.

TESTOSTERONE

Testosterone makes the man. Production of the hormone begins early in fetal life and continues for a man's lifetime—but there are ups and downs. Testosterone levels fall just before birth and except for a few brief blips, they stay low until puberty, when they surge. Most men attain their highest levels shortly before age twenty, and levels stay high for another twenty years. But at about age forty, testosterone levels begin to fall. In women, sex hormone levels drop precipitously at menopause, but in men the decline is gradual, averaging 1 percent a year. It is an almost imperceptible process, but by age eighty, a man's testosterone level is about half of what it was at age eighteen. Still, in most older men, testosterone levels remain in the normal range, which is why healthy octogenarians can father children.

What's Normal? It's a simple question with a complex answer. Instead of a single normal level for testosterone, normal men exhibit a wide range. In most cases, healthy adult men have testosterone levels between 270 and 1,070 ng/dl (nanograms per deciliter). But, like so many biological functions, testosterone production waxes and wanes over a twenty-four-hour cycle; production is highest at 8 A.M. and lowest at 9 P.M. For measurements to be meaningful, they should be obtained at a standard time, usually first thing in the morning. Timing is particularly important for testing older men; because age takes a greater toll on the morning peak of testosterone production than on the afternoon plateau, a late-day level can look deceptively normal, but a feeble morning surge can still leave a man's twenty-four-hour total production low.

The aging process introduces a final complexity. Testosterone travels in the blood in one of two forms, either bound to protein or free and unbound. Only the free hormone is biologically active. The sex hormone binding protein rises with age, so an older man may have a normal total testosterone but still be low where it counts, in free testosterone.

It may not be important for a man to understand all the ins and outs of testosterone metabolism, but he should understand that these complexities account for important flaws in much of the medical research on testosterone replacement therapy. If you need to know where you stand, you should ask to have both your total and your free testosterone levels measured, preferably early in the morning.

Can Testosterone Help? There is no question about it: Testosterone can help men with *hypogonadism,* abnormally low testosterone production due either to testicular failure or to disorders affecting the pituitary gland. Hypogonadism, though, is uncommon (see Table 10.2).

Table 10.2: MAJOR CAUSES OF HYPOGONADISM

PROBLEMS ORIGINATING IN THE TESTICLES (*PRIMARY HYPGONADISM*)
Genetic errors such as Kleinefelter's Syndrome
Mumps (when it affects both testicles)
Severe trauma
Alcoholism
Cancer chemotherapy
Radiation
PROBLEMS ORIGINATING IN THE PITUITARY GLAND IN THE BRAIN (*SECONDARY HYPOGONADISM*)
Tumors (usually benign)
Brain trauma
Surgical treatment of pituitary disease
Medication
Hereditary disorders
Severe malnutrition
Chronic illness

Adult men with true hypogonadism lack libido, but they have problems that go far beyond sexual dysfunction; they have smallish muscles, reduced bone density, diminished body and facial hair, and increased body fat, particularly around their hips. Men with hypogonadism also have small penises and small, soft testicles and prostate glands.

Testosterone can correct all these manifestation of hypogonadism, but doctors should reserve treatment for men with truly low testosterone levels and clear evidence of hypogonadism. To be sure, your doctor should check pituitary hormone levels (FSH, LH, and prolactin) as well as liver and thyroid tests;

he should also measure morning free and total testosterone levels on several occasions.

In addition to treating hypogonadism, doctors are already using testosterone and other male hormones to treat a variety of serious medical conditions. Examples include the wasting syndrome of advanced AIDS and the pronounced muscle wasting sometimes associated with prolonged cortisone therapy and debilitating illnesses, such as severe emphysema, cirrhosis, and burns. Androgens can also be helpful for men and women with rare conditions that cause severe anemia (*aplastic anemia, Fanconi's syndrome*) or life-threatening tissue swelling (*hereditary angioedema*). Finally, some women with severe *endometriosis* benefit from androgen therapy, but side effects limit the duration of treatment.

Testosterone Preparations. Testosterone therapy is far from new; testosterone extracts were first used in 1889, and the hormone itself was synthesized in the 1930s, winning the Nobel Prize for the scientists who accomplished the feat.

Much has changed in the past seventy-five years, but one thing has not: Testosterone is not suitable for long-term use in pill form. That is because it is rapidly removed by the liver, where it impairs cholesterol metabolism and may lead to tumors, both benign and malignant. Scientists are working on new oral preparations that may be safe and effective. Chemists have already produced many related androgens that are effective in pill form but are not so safe. Unfortunately, many athletes abuse such *anabolic steroids,* risking health in the quest for enhanced muscular strength and athletic performance.

Until recently, injectable preparations have been the mainstays of testosterone replacement therapy. Several forms are available, including *testosterone propionate* (100 milligrams every week), *testosterone enthanate* (200 milligrams every two weeks) and *testosterone cypionate* (200 to 400 milligrams every three weeks).

Injections have two disadvantages: They are injections, and they produce roller-coaster testosterone levels that are abnormally high at first but undesirably low later on. To eliminate these problems, researchers have developed *transdermal* testosterone preparations that deliver steady levels of the drug through the skin. Four patches are now available in the United States; they are applied once a day, mimicking the daily fluctuation in blood testosterone levels that occur in healthy young men.

Two brands are designed to be placed on the upper arm, thigh, back, or abdomen each evening. Testoderm TTS delivers 5 milligrams of testosterone, Androderm delivers half as much, so men usually apply two patches at once. Men should pick a new location for the patch each day to reduce irritation, which is the major side effect. The third brand, Testoderm, comes in 4 milligram and 6 milligram strengths. It is less irritating to the skin, but since it will only deliver the medication through porous skin, it must be applied to the scrotum, which requires shaving. The scrotal patch produces higher levels of DHT, the testosterone derivative that stimulates the prostate, but doctors do not yet know if this will be harmful. All the patches are expensive, costing dollars a day instead of the pennies a day that injections cost.

The newest preparation is a testosterone gel (Androgel), which is applied once a day to the shoulders, upper arms, or abdomen. It raises blood testosterone levels within thirty minutes to four hours, and levels remain steady during the course of a day as the hormone is slowly absorbed from the gel. Androgel is convenient and it allows doctors to adjust the testosterone dose, but it is very expensive, costing about 50 percent more than the testosterone patches.

Testosterone for Aging? It is an important question, but doctors cannot yet answer it. That's because scientists have not conducted long-term studies of testosterone in healthy men. Small, short-term studies, though, illustrate the potential for testosterone therapy as well as its possible perils. For example, researchers in Seattle administered weekly injections of 100 milligrams of testosterone enthanate to thirteen healthy fifty-seven to seventy-six-year-old men with low or borderline testosterone levels. Three months of treatment produced an increase in muscle mass and red-blood-cell counts.

Testosterone produced an increase in the men's subjective feelings of well-being, but it did not reduce body fat. Surprisingly, perhaps, it seemed to improve blood cholesterol levels. But there was also a dark side to this brief trial: *prostate specific antigen* (PSA) levels rose, indicating stimulation of prostate cells. PSA levels also rose slightly in fifty-four healthy men over the age of sixty-five who used the testosterone patch for a three-year period. There was no overall improvement in bone density during the trial, but men whose initial testosterone levels were low appeared to benefit.

Testosterone has potential advantages: It can increase muscle mass and strength, improve bone density, and boost red blood cell counts. It is far from clear, however, if it will improve libido, erectile function, or sexual performance in older men; several small studies have been disappointing thus far. Long-term testosterone therapy has potential risks, including abnormal cholesterol levels and possibly heart disease, abnormal liver function, excessive red-blood-cell counts (*polycythemia*), sleep apnea, and prostate stimulation that could increase the risk of BPH and prostate cancer.

Despite the obvious appeal of testosterone replacement for aging men, most doctors advise against it, at least until new research weighs the risks and benefits. But that does not mean men have to accept the negative consequences of aging. Far from it. In fact, there are simple ways to get many of the benefits of testosterone without its risks. Along with a healthy amount of dietary protein, resistance exercises and other forms of strength training will help preserve muscle mass and strength, bone density, and musculoskeletal function. A reasonable intake of calcium (1,200 milligrams a day) and vitamin D (400 to 600 units a day) will help prevent osteoporosis. Above all, perhaps, a program of regular exercise and a low-fat, high-fiber, vegetable- and fruit-rich diet will help prevent atherosclerosis, hypertension, and diabetes—the three major causes of illness, disability, and impotence in older men (see Chapters Three through Five).

It is never too late to start living young, and it is never too early, either.

Testosterone for Athletes? It is a problem of epidemic proportions. In the United States alone, at least 1 million people are current or former androgen abusers. Most are competitive athletes or bodybuilders, but some use the drugs simply to "look good." Despite attempts to ban the abuse of "performance enhancing" steroids, the illicit practice appears to be increasing, both in men and women. Most individuals take very large amounts, sometimes 100 times the doses used for testosterone replacement therapy.

Some androgens can increase muscle mass and strength but others, like *androstanedione* (Andro), do not appear effective. But all illicit androgens can have major side effects including cosmetic changes (acne, abnormal hair growth, premature male pattern baldness), liver disorders (inflammation, benign and malignant tumors), sexual dysfunction (shrunken testicles, infertility), breast enlargement, behavioral problems (aggression, mood disorders), and abnormal cholesterol levels (high LDL, low HDL). High blood pressure, heart attacks, strokes, liver cancer, and psychosis have all been linked to androgen abuse.

Victory at any cost? Not when the price is health.

DHEA

It was first discovered in 1934. It is the most abundant hormone in the blood of young men. It is one of the best-selling nonprescription supplements, widely promoted to prevent or correct conditions ranging from Alzheimer's disease and impotence to aging itself. Yet despite its abundance and popularity, scientists know surprisingly little about its true function in humans. It's *dehydroepiandrosterone* (DHEA), the "mystery hormone."

What is DHEA? DHEA is a *steroid hormone*. Like cortisone, it is produced from cholesterol by the *adrenal glands* that are located above the kidneys. DHEA enters the bloodstream, where it circulates largely in the form of its sulfate derivative, DHEAS. Because both types of the hormone behave similarly and can be interconverted, it is reasonable to think of them together as DHEA.

Both men and women produce DHEA; in young adults, DHEA levels are 10–20 percent higher in men than women. Despite years of study, scientists have not yet been able to identify a direct role for DHEA in humans. The hormone's greatest importance may depend on the fact that it is converted into *androstenedione,* the steroid hormone that became notorious as Mark McGwire's Andro supplement. But the metabolism of DHEA does not stop with Andro; instead, the body converts it to biologically active androgens and estrogens, male and female hormones.

DHEA and Aging. Perhaps the most important reason that DHEA has attracted so much attention is its dramatic and puzzling relationship to aging. DHEA production begins during fetal life; in fact, fetal adrenal glands produce more than 200 milligrams daily, nearly ten times more than the amount produced by adults. After birth, though, DHEA synthesis slows to a crawl, and blood levels are very low. That changes at about the time of puberty, when levels begin to rise again. In both men and women, DHEA levels peak between age twenty and thirty, after which they decline steadily; in 1992, the Physicians' Health Study documented a decline of 3 percent a year.

DHEA levels fall as the unwelcome effects of aging develop. That's why DHEA has been touted as the "antiaging hormone." But does the decline in DHEA actually contribute to the changes of aging, or is DHEA merely a fellow traveler, drifting down as part of the normal aging process without affecting that process one way or another? It is the key question. If DHEA has a role in aging, supplements might be helpful, but if it does not, supplements would be useless at best.

Can DHEA Help? Until recently, well-designed human studies have been few and far between. In one small trial, 67 percent of subjects reported an increase in "well-being," but objective measurements found no change in body fat or sugar metabolism. In another study, DHEA treatment was associated with an increase in muscle strength and mass in the thigh, but only eight men participated in the trial. More recently, doctors in New York administered DHEA in a dose of at least 50 milligrams a day to ten men with an average age of sixty. After eighteen months, there were no changes in blood testosterone or prostate specific antigen (PSA) levels, but the study did not evaluate body composition or function.

Careful clinical studies of DHEA are badly needed, and a recent study from the University of Missouri Medical School represents a giant step in that direction. The participants were thirty-nine men aged sixty to eighty-four. Because all were long-time members of the ongoing Longitudinal Aging Study, the researchers were able to evaluate DHEA against a backdrop of careful clinical measurements dating back nearly thirty years.

All the volunteers were in good health when the nine-month DHEA trial began. The men were randomly assigned to take either DHEA or an identical-appearing placebo; neither the participants nor the researchers know which men were taking the hormone and which the dummy pill. The DHEA dose was 100 milligrams a day, a typical "replacement dose" that was calculated to boost DHEA blood levels into the youthful range.

Each man underwent careful evaluations before and after treatment. When the results were tallied, the researchers found no evidence that DHEA produced any beneficial changes. The men who took the hormone did not exhibit either a decrease in body fat or an increase in muscle mass; body weight did not change appreciably. Insulin levels and blood sugar levels were also unchanged. DHEA failed to produce an improvement in sexual function. Similarly, there were no changes in overall subjective well-being. Hormone therapy was associated with small alterations in red-blood-cell counts, cholesterol levels, and kidney function tests, but all of these results remained within the normal range.

The Missouri scientists also checked for potential adverse effects of DHEA, but they detected none. In particular, PSA levels did not rise, and urinary function did not change for better or worse.

All in all, DHEA produced little change for good or ill. Both proponents and critics of the hormone might argue that the dose was simply too small, but the researchers measured blood levels and found that DHEA increased dramatically during the trial; DHEA itself more than doubled, and DHEAS increased more than fivefold. As further evidence of a hormonal effect, the scientists reported that DHEA therapy produced a sharp increase in both male (free testosterone) and female (estradiol) hormone levels.

DHEA is also touted as a way to keep the heart healthy and the mind youthful. But the Physicians' Health Study found no link between DHEA and the risk of heart attack, and studies from Johns Hopkins and McGill University found no effect on cognitive function in older men.

Drug or Nutrient? DHEA is a controversial chemical. Despite the heated debate, two facts about DHEA are incontrovertible: It is a hormone, and it is not part of the human diet.

Facts notwithstanding, DHEA is freely available in health food stores and drug stores as well as on the Internet. It is sold as a nutritional supplement, not a drug, but it is aggressively promoted as a "super hormone," and "antidote for aging" that can strengthen the immune system, slow memory loss, prevent heart disease and cancer, and help with Alzheimer's disease and Parkinson's disease. However, no evidence exists to support those claims. Even so, there is little hope that recent research will stem the tide of popular enthusiasm for DHEA or limit its availability. It wasn't always that way. When the DHEA craze began to build in 1985, the FDA banned over-the-counter sales of the drug. DHEA is still outlawed by the International Olympic Committee and the National Collegiate Athletic Association, but the FDA has fallen silent. That's because Congress passed the Dietary Supplement Health and Education Act in 1994, removing nutritional supplements from the jurisdiction of the FDA. In a matter of months, DHEA was back, this time as a "nutrient."

Since DHEA is available without a prescription, it is up to each man to decide if it is right for him. The same is true for all supplements, and in deciding about any of them, men should use common sense and caution. Remember that supplements are not subject to FDA standards for purity, potency, efficacy, and safety. Remember, too, that neither booming sales nor gushing testimonials prove that a product is really effective, and that "all-natural" origins do not prove that a substance is safe.

Even with the new data in hand, more research on DHEA is needed to learn its normal function as well as whether supplements can be helpful or harmful. For now, men would be wise to consider two ancient dictums, one from medicine, the other from the marketplace: *primum non nocere* (first do no harm) and *caveat emptor* (buyer beware).

MELATONIN

Like DHEA, melatonin is readily available in the United States without a prescription. Like DHEA, it has been widely touted as an antidote to aging, to say nothing of insomnia, jet lag, impotence, cancer, and many other problems.

Melatonin is manufactured by the pineal gland, which is located in the brain. It has been aptly called the dark hormone because it is produced only at night. In humans, the hormone sets the body's clock, regulating the timing of the sleep-wake cycle. In some experimental models, melatonin has antioxidant, anticancer, and immunological-enhancing properties, but in others, it produces just the opposite effects. In a widely cited study, melatonin prolonged the life of elderly mice. But mice are not men, and melatonin's effects on all these aspects of human health are unknown.

Aging is associated with diminished melatonin levels. The youthful cycle of nighttime melatonin production can virtually disappear in old age. Sleep disturbances are common in older men; more than one-third of people over sixty-five complain of insomnia.

Can melatonin help? It is a possibility that deserves serious scientific study. Until research discloses the benefits and hazards of melatonin, men should not take it for aging or other unsubstantiated purposes. Limited, cautious use for insomnia or jet lag is reasonable with the understanding that its dosage, possible benefits, and potential toxicities have not been established.

Melatonin is a hormone, but because it is marketed as a dietary supplement instead of a drug, it is not regulated by the Food and Drug Administration. In Britain, however, melatonin is available only by prescription; prudence is a good prescription for American men considering it.

GROWTH HORMONE

Growth hormone is produced by the pituitary gland in the brain. It enters the bloodstream and travels throughout the body. Among its many important functions, growth hormone increases muscle mass and strength, and decreases body fat. Growth hormone levels are low in childhood, but rise dramatically during puberty; levels begin to fall as men enter their thirties and continue to decline throughout adult life.

As men age, they lose muscle mass and strength; on average, by the time a man is seventy years old, he will have lost half his muscular strength. Body fat also tends to increase as men age. Can replacement doses of growth hormone slow these trends?

A 1985 study raised our hopes. Elderly men who received growth hormone injections for six months demonstrated increased muscle mass and skin thickness as well as decreased body fat.

But a 1996 study of fifty-two healthy seventy- to eighty-five-year-old men offers perspective. All the men had low growth hormone levels; half received three injections of growth hormone each week while the others received an inert placebo. The groups were compared at the end of six months. Growth hormone treatment had increased muscle mass by more than 4 percent and reduced body fat by over 13 percent. But the men given the hormones were no stronger than the untreated men, and they did not display any improvement in endurance, mental function, or mood. Moreover, side effects were common, occurring in 77 percent of the treated men. This discouraging result has been confirmed in other recent studies of normal men, but a 2000 study found that the hormone can improve cardiac risk factors in men with growth hormone deficiencies.

Growth hormone can improve body composition in older men, but treatment does not improve functional capacity or subjective well-being. Side effects are common and, at $12,000 per year, the injections are very expensive. At present, growth hormone replacement is not the answer to the problem of male aging. More study is needed to identify just which men are deficient in growth hormone, to define the risks of deficiency, and to examine the long-term benefits and risks of varying doses of growth hormone therapy.

BEAT THE CLOCK

"Every man desires to live long," wrote Jonathan Swift, "but no man would be old." He was right, but the fountain of youth has proved illusory. Although more study is needed, hormones are not likely to be the answer for today's men. At present, it does not appear that the prescription medications (testosterone, growth hormone) and supplements (DHEA, melatonin, Andro) that are so popular in the early twenty-first century will be any more successful than the monkey testicle transplants that raised false hopes in the early twentieth century.

There is no way to stop the clock, but there are ways to slow the pendulum. To find out how, review Part II of this book, which summarizes the things men can do to stay healthy and young.

CHAPTER ELEVEN

The Prostate: Benign Disorders

Men and women differ in many ways, ranging from body size and muscular strength to hormones, behavior, social roles, and reproductive functioning. Although most men prefer their male attributes, there are two they would trade in if they could. One is longevity, since women consistently outlive men. The other is the prostate.

Prostate disorders are the most common health issues unique to men. They produce problems ranging from the pain and fever of *prostatitis* to the discomfort and bother of *benign prostatic hyperplasia* (BPH) to the threat of prostate cancer. But although men worry about their prostates, few understand the little gland that gets so much publicity. It's a shame, since men can do a lot to reduce their risk of prostate problems and to facilitate early diagnosis and effective treatment when disease strikes.

The Normal Prostate

The prostate is a walnut-shaped gland at the base of the bladder (see Figure 11.1). In healthy young men, it is about an inch and a half long and weighs about two-thirds of an ounce. It does not start out that way, of course. In boys, the prostate is small and rudimentary. At the time of puberty, the brain and pituitary gland signal the testicles to begin producing *testosterone,* the male hormone. Like the other reproductive organs, the prostate enlarges under the influence of testosterone. It also contains its own special enzyme, *5 alpha-reductase,* which converts testosterone to *dihydrotestosterone* (DHT). DHT is the androgen (male hormone) that has the greatest effect on the prostate.

The prostate is a reproductive organ: It produces fluid that enters the semen at the time of ejaculation. A normal ejaculate contains 2 to 6 milliliters of fluid, about one-third to one teaspoonful. The seminal vesicles deliver about 70 percent of the ejaculate, including the sperm, but the prostate contributes about 20 percent. Prostatic secretions contain calcium, potassium, zinc, and citric acid. The clear, colorless fluid also contains various enzymes, including

FIGURE 11.1. NORMAL PROSTATE

The prostate contains glandular cells, muscle cells, and stromal (supporting) cells that are organized into zones. The transition zone surrounds the urethra and is the site of BPH. The peripheral zone contains most of the glandular cells and is the most common site of prostate cancer.

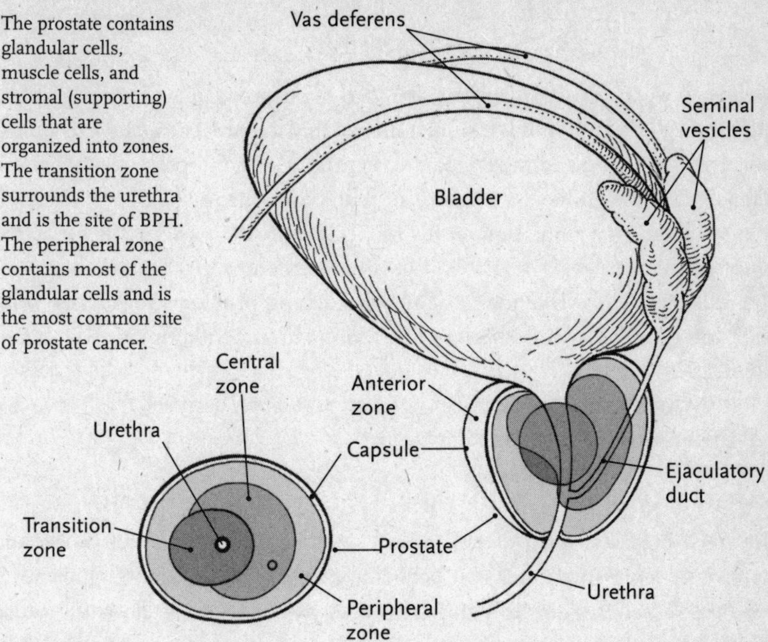

the famous protein called *prostate specific antigen* (PSA), which liquefies semen so that sperm can swim to their target, the woman's egg (see Chapter Ten).

Despite its modest size, the prostate is a complex organ that contains three major types of tissue. *Glandular cells* produce and secrete the various components of prostate fluid. *Muscle cells* contract at the time of ejaculation, propelling the fluid into the semen. *Stromal cells* provide structural support for the entire gland. The prostate also contains nerve cells, which tell the muscles when to contract so that they go into action at the same time as the other muscles involved in ejaculation.

The cells of the prostate are organized into four major zones (see Figure 11.1). Two zones are particularly important for disease. The *transition zone* surrounds the urethra and is the area affected by BPH (see page 330). The larger *peripheral zone* contains most of the glandular tissue and is the most common site of prostate cancer. In addition, the *central zone* holds the remaining glands, and the *anterior zone* contains muscular and structural cells. The entire gland is surrounded by a *capsule* of fibrous tissue.

Prostatitis

Most men worry about prostate cancer, and many are plagued by benign prostatic hyperplasia (BPH). But few men realize that the prostate gland can also be the site of infection and inflammation. Prostatitis is a forgotten disease, but it is far from trivial. In fact, an American man has a one in ten chance of developing prostatitis at some time in his life. In all, prostatitis accounts for 2 million medical office visits a year, half of them in men younger than fifty.

Prostatitis can strike men at any age, causing problems that range from acute infection with high fever to smoldering chronic inflammation with persistent pain.

Prostatitis is not one disease, but four (see Table 11.1); of these, two are well-understood, but two remain obscure.

Acute Bacterial Prostatitis (ABP)

The most dramatic form of prostatitis, ABP requires prompt diagnosis and therapy. As the name implies, it begins abruptly with high fever, chills, joint and muscle aches, and profound fatigue. A bad case of the flu could cause identical complaints, but men with ABP also experience symptoms that point to the prostate: low back and rectal pain, a strong urge to urinate, and frequent, painful urination. The urinary stream is usually slow and weak, and in some cases of ABP, the prostate is so swollen that it completely blocks the flow of urine.

Doctors can confirm a diagnosis of ABP quite easily. A digital rectal exam (DRE) shows the prostate to be swollen and soft, and pressure on the gland is very painful. A urine specimen discloses the presence of white blood cells, further confirming the diagnosis of ABP.

ABP is caused by infection. Bacteria creep up the urethra, ascending along the entire length of the penis to enter the prostate through the tiny ducts that normally allow prostatic fluid to travel in the other direction, from the gland into the ejaculate. The usual bacterial culprits are colon-dwelling bacilli such as *E. coli* and *klebsiella*, the same bugs that cause bladder and kidney infections in women.

Bladder infections in women respond promptly to antibiotics; in many cases, just a single dose of medication can do the job. But ABP is a different matter. The prostate has established a barrier that prevents most antibiotics from entering, rendering them all but useless for treating prostatitis. Fortunately, several antibacterials can penetrate the prostate including *trimethoprim-*

Table 11.1: MAIN FEATURES OF PROSTATITIS

	TYPE OF PROSTATITIS			
	ABP	**CBP**	**NBP**	**PD**
Onset	Abrupt	Gradual	Variable	Variable
Symptoms				
Fever	+++	+/–	–	–
Pain	++	+/–	+/–	++
Abnormal Urination	++	+	+	+/–
Digital Rectal Exam	Abnormal	Usually Normal*	Usually Normal*	Normal*
White Blood Cells in Prostatic Secretions	+	+	+	–
Cause	Bacteria	Bacteria	Unknown	Unknown
Treatment	Antibiotics	Antibiotics	Symptomatic	Symptomatic
Outcome	Excellent	Very Good	Fair	Variable

*Even when the prostate feels normal to the physician, the patient may experience abnormal discomfort.

sulfamethoxazole (Bactrim, Septra) and the newer fluoroquinolones such as *norfloxacin* (Noroxin), *ciprofloxacin* (Cipro), *ofloxacin* (Floxin), and *levofloxacin* (Levaquin). Nearly all men improve promptly with one of these medications—but even if the symptoms disappear in three to five days, it is important to continue the medication for at least two to four weeks to insure cure. In the first few days, sitz baths and stool softeners can help soothe rectal pain; aspirin or acetaminophen will also promote comfort early on, and a high fluid intake is important throughout the illness.

Without effective treatment, many men with ABP develop chronic infection; even with therapy, ABP can relapse or recur.

CHRONIC BACTERIAL PROSTATITIS (CBP)

Like ABP, CBP is caused by bacterial invasion of the prostate gland; unlike ABP, however, CBP is a subtle, smoldering infection that begins insidiously and persists for weeks or even months. The typical man with CBP has no fever, but is troubled by intermittent urinary symptoms, such as urgency, frequency, painful urination, and the need to urinate at night. Some men with CBP have low back or rectal pain. Others experience pain after ejaculation. In some cases, the semen can be bloody even in the absence of pain (see Chapter Ten). The symptoms can wax and wane without apparent explanation.

Because the symptoms are subtle, variable, and intermittent, many men with CBP don't know they have it. Since the prostate is not swollen or soft on examination, doctors may also miss the diagnosis, assuming that the urinary complaints are simply the result of BPH. But CBP is an active infection, and the clue to diagnosis is the presence of significant numbers of bacteria in the urine, usually in the company of white blood cells. CBP is caused by the same range of bacteria responsible for ABP, but doctors do not know why identical bugs produce acute infection in some men but chronic infection in others.

The treatment of CBP has been revolutionized by the availability of antibiotics that penetrate the prostate. In the past, ordinary antibiotics usually failed, and some men with CBP even underwent surgical removal of the prostate to control the symptoms. Trimethoprim-sulfamethoxazole and the fluoroquinolones have made surgery unnecessary. Most men respond to one of these drugs; it is not clear if one is better than another, but because it is an older drug, we have more experience with trimethoprim-sulfamethoxazole. It is also much less expensive than the others—not a small consideration since most men with CBP require one to three months of continuous antibiotic therapy. Even with prolonged treatment, the infection can relapse. When it does, it can usually be controlled by low-dose antibiotic treatment that is continued for months or even years.

NONBACTERIAL PROSTATITIS (NBP)

If CBP is a puzzle, NBP is a mystery.

NBP (also known as the *inflammatory chronic pelvic pain syndrome*) is the most common form of prostatitis, occurring eight times more often than ABP and CBP combined. The symptoms of NBP resemble those of CBP, and in both conditions the doctor's examination may not disclose anything abnormal. In both disorders, white blood cells are present in the urine and prostate fluid. The difference is that bacteria are also present in CBP but are absent in NBP. CBP is a bacterial infection, NBP is not.

Inflammation is present in NBP, but infection is not its cause. What, then, triggers NBP? No one is sure. Early theories implicated specialized microbes such as *mycoplasma, ureaplasma,* and *chlamydia,* but recent studies appear to exonerate these bugs. To the frustration of patients and physicians alike, we still have no good explanation for NBP.

It is not a surprise, therefore, that treatment is often unsatisfactory. It is reasonable to begin with a trial of antibiotics. Many physicians turn first to one of the drugs that are so beneficial in ABP and CBP, and then try doxycycline or erythromycin because of their superior activity against the atypical microbes putatively involved in NBP. If a course of antibiotics fails, as it usually does, additional antibiotic trials should not be administered. Instead, various symptomatic treatments should be used in a trial-and-error fashion.

Many men with NBP feel better after taking sitz baths. Emptying the prostate gland of its secretions can also help. Doctors can accomplish this by repeatedly massaging the prostate, but most men prefer to do it themselves by ejaculating frequently. Aspirin or other nonsteroidal antiinflammatory drugs (NSAIDs), which fight inflammation and pain, may also be very helpful. Doctors may also prescribe a trial of anticholinergic medications that relax the bladder muscles such as *oxybutynin* (Ditropan), alpha blockers such as *tamsulosin* (Flomax), or *finasteride* (Proscar) in an attempt to reduce the urinary symptoms. Some men report benefits from herbs such as *saw palmetto. Allopurinol* (Zyloprim), a medication ordinarily prescribed for gout, may possibly help some men with NP by reducing the amount of uric acid in the urine.

PROSTATODYNIA (PD)

If NBP is a mystery, PD is an enigma.

Although it can occur at any age, PD (also known as *noninflammatory pelvic pain syndrome*) is most common in young to middle-aged men, sometimes developing before age twenty. You may suspect that the fancy name assigned to the disorder is just a cover-up for medical ignorance about PD, but it is actually a literal description of the condition's major symptom: PD is a pain in the prostate. The pain is usually low-grade, nagging, and persistent; it is centered in the rectum and low pelvis but can radiate to the testicles, penis, groin, and low back. Although pain is the major complaint, urine flow can also be abnormal, with hesitancy, dribbling, a weak or interrupted stream, frequency, and urgency.

PD is a chronic condition that is often accompanied by depression, anxiety, or sexual dysfunction. It is not clear, however, if psychological factors cause PD, or if emotional distress is simply the result of a chronic, debilitating disorder. In either case, the patent's frustration is understandably compounded by his physician's inability to explain the cause of PD.

Doctors are stymied by PD because the prostate feels normal on examination, the urine is clear and free of infection, and the prostatic fluid does not contain white blood cells. Symptomatic treatment, such as that prescribed for NBP, is worth a try, but it often fails. The medications most likely to reduce symptoms of PD are the alpha-blockers such as *tamsulosin* (Flomax), *terazosin* (Hytrin), or *doxazosin* (Cardura). These medications relax muscles at the bladder neck, easing the flow of urine, but they must be used with care to prevent excessive reductions in blood pressure. Emotional support is extremely important for all men with PD; antidepressants, tranquilizers, or muscle relaxers may help.

Asymptomatic Prostatitis

Prostatitis is a complex problem. The existing four types have challenged doctors and patients for decades, and now the National Institutes of Health Consensus Conference on Prostatitis has added a fifth category. Men do not know they have asymptomatic prostatitis because it does not produce any complaints, but doctors recognize the problem if they discover inflammation in a semen specimen during a fertility work-up (see Chapter Ten) or in a prostate biopsy specimen they obtain while investigating some other problem. Most often, that problem is an elevated PSA test (see Chapter Twelve). Since it is a new entity, doctors do not know if they should treat asymptomatic prostatitis. If infertility is the problem or if inflammation seems to be responsible for an elevated PSA level, it is reasonable to prescribe a two-week course of antibiotics, then recheck the semen or PSA after six to eight weeks.

Benign Prostatic Hyperplasia (BPH)

In younger men, prostatitis is the most frequent cause of prostate problems; in older men, that dubious distinction belongs to BPH.

Despite its importance, doctors still cannot answer many basic questions about BPH. They have learned, however, that in most cases the all-important question about the choice of treatment is best answered by the patient. Paradoxically, perhaps, it is a question that may become more difficult for men to answer as their options increase.

Growing Pains

Like other reproductive organs, the prostate is small in childhood, then has a growth spurt during adolescence. Like the others, its growth slows and its size plateaus in early adulthood. Unlike other organs, however, the prostate has a second period of growth. It starts slowly in midlife, then accelerates and continues into old age; on average, the prostate enlarges by 1.6 percent a year beyond age forty. The result is BPH.

BPH begins in the transition zone of the prostate (see Figure 11.1). In young men, this zone constitutes just 2 percent of the prostate, but since it encircles the long axis of the urethra, enlargement here can pinch the urethra, slowing the flow of urine. Although the prostate is a reproductive organ, BPH does not usually affect sexual function or fertility. Instead, its symptoms involve the urinary tract.

BPH affects both glandular and structural tissues and begins with small nodules in the transition zone. At first, the nodules are so small that they can only be identified if prostate tissue is examined under a microscope. Over time, the microscopic nodules enlarge into macroscopic nodules that distort the normal anatomy of the gland. Finally, the abnormalities become pronounced enough to produce clinical BPH, the stage when men begin to feel the distressing symptoms of the disease.

The first microscopic nodules of BPH begin to develop surprisingly early in life, occurring in 10 percent of men by the time they are thirty. They become progressively more common with advancing age, so that 90 percent of eighty-five-year-old men have microscopic nodules. But only about half the microscopic nodules become macroscopic, and only about half of these become markedly symptomatic. These developments, too, become more common with age. By age eighty, in fact, about one-fourth of all men will develop BPH severe enough to require treatment, and many others will have milder symptoms that they can "live with." In all, an estimated 5.5 million American men have clinically significant BPH, and about 2 million seek medical help for their symptoms every year.

WHAT CAUSES BPH?

It's one of the great mysteries of modern urology. Doctors know that two things are essential for BPH to develop: age and testosterone. But they don't know why some men develop severe BPH as they age while others do not. Testosterone is not the whole answer; BPH will not develop without it, but men with BPH do not have higher hormone levels than men with normal prostates. It seems likely that various growth factors stimulate the prostate cells in men with BPH. In addition, a deficiency of normal programmed cell death, *apoptosis,* may contribute. There is also a slight tendency for BPH to run in families, but scientists have not yet identified the genes that control the prostate's growth.

RISK FACTORS

Although scientists have not yet discovered the ultimate cause of BPH, researchers have identified some important risk factors; much of the new data comes from the Health Professionals Study.

Race has been implicated as a possible determinant of BPH, but the Health Professionals Study found no difference between African Americans and whites. The study did find that Asians were less likely to require BPH surgery than whites, but the difference may not be genetic. In an interesting recent report, Australian researchers compared Chinese men living in China with Chinese men living in Australia and white Australians. The Chinese men living in China had smaller prostates and fewer prostate symptoms than either of the other groups, suggesting that an environmental factor comes into play. That factor may be nutrition. Traditional Asian diets contain lots of soy, which appears to reduce the growth of prostate cells (see Chapter Twelve). The Asian diet also contains less fat, and a recent European study found that butter and margarine are associated with an increased risk of BPH, while fruits were linked to a reduced risk.

The Health Professionals Study has investigated other lifestyle factors that influence BPH. It found a link between abdominal obesity and the severity of BPH symptoms. The study also reported that smoking, at least in large amounts, increases the risk of BPH; men who average thirty-five cigarettes a day are nearly 50 percent more likely to develop BPH than nonsmokers. In contrast, exercise appears protective; men who walk for two to three hours a week are 25 percent less likely to develop BPH than sedentary men.

The effects of alcohol are more complex. The Health Professionals Study tracked 29,238 men who were free of prostate disease when the study began in 1986. Over an eight-year period, 1,813 men required surgery for BPH and another 1,786 developed moderate to severe symptoms of the disorder. When the researchers evaluated the effect of drinking, they found that alcohol appeared to protect against BPH, even after age, ethnicity, obesity, and exercise were taken into account. It's a surprising finding, since alcohol is a diuretic and an increased urine flow should increase the bothersome symptoms of BPH. Perhaps that is why moderate amounts of alcohol were more protective than large amounts. The consumption of up to 50 grams of alcohol a day (roughly the amount in fifteen ounces of wine, thirty-six ounces of beer, or four and one-half ounces of spirits) was linked to a 41 percent reduction in the risk of BPH.

All in all, it appears that the prostate follows the same lifestyle rules as the rest of the body. Obesity is deleterious and exercise helpful. Men who choose to drink alcohol should drink in moderation, and men who choose to smoke are making a grave mistake.

SYMPTOMS

Until recently, doctors thought that the symptoms of BPH were strictly related to the enlargement of the gland. But new research shows that it is not so simple. In fact, the size of the gland is not a good predictor of the distress it causes; some men with very large prostates have few if any symptoms, while others with minimal enlargement have maximal discomfort. It is clear that the severity and the type of symptoms depend on many factors, including increased contractions of the muscles at the outlet of the bladder, narrowing of the urethra (the tube that carries urine out from the bladder), decreased strength of the bladder wall, increased activity of muscles in the prostate itself, and the size of the gland. Important, too, are a man's subjective responses to changes in his urinary function. Some men—particularly in the older age groups—perceive modest changes in urine flow as very bothersome, while others hardly seem to notice that their flow is very slow. Surprisingly, perhaps, doctors now believe that a man's own evaluation of his symptoms is the best tool for predicting the course of BPH, and the most important criterion for determining if treatment is needed.

The symptoms of BPH, collectively called *prostatism,* vary from man to man. One group of symptoms is caused by the obstruction of the urethra by the enlarged gland, much the same as an index finger and thumb can slow the flow of fluid through a straw. The other group is due to irritation of the bladder, caused by increased contraction of its muscles.

A weak, slow urinary stream is a typical obstructive symptom. Others include hesitancy of urination and straining to initiate and maintain voiding. Prolonged voiding and dribbling at the end of the urination also suggest obstruction. Most serious, perhaps, is incomplete emptying of the bladder with retention of urine. In many cases, retention does not produce any distress, but some men have a persistent sensation of bladder fullness; others leak urine at unpredictable times, so-called overflow incontinence.

Irritative symptoms are no less bothersome. They include an urgent, sometimes uncontrollable, need to void and the frequent passage of small amounts of urine. Nocturia, the need to void at night, is also an irritative symptom, but unless other irritative symptoms are also present, men should consider other causes of night-time irritation instead of simply assuming that BPH is the culprit (see Chapter Thirteen).

The American Urologic Association (AUA) has devised a simple method for evaluating the symptoms of BPH (see Table 11.2). Although the test is not specific for BPH, it does provide an accurate way to quantify symptoms, and it can help predict the need for treatment. You can take the test yourself to see where you stand; simply circle one answer to each question, then add up the numbers to determine your score.

Your AUA score compares your symptoms to those of other men. But can it tell you if your BPH is likely to get worse? The Health Professionals Study suggests it can. It followed 6,100 men for three years and found that the risk of complications increased with a rising symptoms score; men with scores above 8 and a clinical diagnosis of BPH had the highest risk of developing acute urinary retention.

Complications

The major consequence of BPH is discomfort. But the disorder can be more serious: It can cause a complete or nearly complete blockage in urine flow that requires emergency treatment. It can cause urine to back up toward the kidney, reducing kidney function. Or it can cause bladder stones, bleeding, or urinary tract infections. Fortunately, serious complications are rare. For example, only 3 percent of men with the highest AUA scores will develop urinary retention in the course of a year. In most men, BPH progresses quite slowly, so it is safe to monitor developments without rushing to therapeutic judgments.

BPH does not increase a man's risk of prostate cancer. However, it can complicate the diagnosis of prostate cancer, since BPH often raises the blood PSA to levels considered suspicious for cancer (see Chapter Twelve).

Medical Evaluation

Most men with BPH do not require elaborate medical tests. Most important is a simple evaluation of symptoms using the AUA index or similar questions. Doctors should also check the medical history for evidence of other conditions that can produce urinary symptoms, such as diabetes and neurological disorders that affect bladder function (see Chapter Thirteen). Men should also be asked about medications that can slow urine flow; decongestants and antihistamines are the most common. The doctor should perform a digital rectal examination to evaluate the size of the prostate and then check for abnormalities

Table 11.2: AUA SYMPTOMS INDEX FOR BPH

Circle one answer for each question. For questions 1–6, 0 = Not at all; 1 = Less than 1 time in 5; 2 = Less than half the time; 3 = About half the time; 4 = More than half the time; 5 = Almost always.

1. During the last month or so, how often have you had a sensation of not emptying your bladder completely after you finished urinating?

   0 1 2 3 4 5

2. During the last month or so, how often have you had to urinate again less than two hours after you finished urinating?

   0 1 2 3 4 5

3. During the last month or so, how often have you found that you stopped and started again several times when you urinated?

   0 1 2 3 4 5

4. During the last month or so, how often have you found it difficult to postpone urination?

   0 1 2 3 4 5

5. During the last month or so, how often have you had a weak urinary stream?

   0 1 2 3 4 5

6. During the last month or so, how often have you had to push or strain to begin urination?

   0 1 2 3 4 5

7. During the last month or so, how times did you typically get up to urinate from the time you went to bed at night until the time you got up in the morning?(For question 7, 0 = None; 1 = 1 time; 2 = 2 times; 3 = 3 times; 4 = 4 times; 5 = 5 times.)

   0 1 2 3 4 5

AUA scores of 0–7 are considered mild, 8–19 indicate moderate symptoms, and 20–35 suggest severe BPH.

suggesting cancer or infection. A urinalysis should be performed, and a kidney function should be evaluated with a simple blood test to measure the creatinine level. Many men also choose to have a PSA blood test, which does not help evaluate BPH but can be used to screen for prostate cancer (see Chapter Twelve).

It's not very different from a routine annual physical, and men with low AUA scores (0–7) and normal test results do not need additional tests or treat-

Table 11.3: INTERPRETING UROFLOWMETRY

Peak Rate of Urine Flow (ml/second)	Severity of Obstruction
15–20	None to Mild
10–14	Mild to Moderate
Below 10	Moderate to Severe

ment. But more advanced symptoms may merit further evaluation. The best way to measure urine flow objectively is by *uroflowmetry,* a noninvasive test that uses electronic monitors. After receiving instructions and waiting until his bladder feels full, the man simply urinates into the device, standing or sitting in private in his normal voiding position. Uroflowmetry records several functions, but the most useful is the peak flow rate (see Table 11.3).

Other tests may be helpful in certain circumstances. Ultrasound imaging of the kidneys and bladder is useful if obstruction is suspected. Comprehensive tests of bladder filling and emptying (urodynamics) can evaluate other causes of bladder dysfunction. The measurement of postvoiding residual urine can detect and monitor obstruction. Cystoscopy should be reserved for men who require surgical treatment. Although a set of X-rays of the kidneys and bladder obtained after the injection of dye (intravenous pyelography) was once part of the standard evaluation of BPH, it rarely is used today.

Treatment

The treatment of BPH is in transition. Until recently, men faced the stark options of having surgery or always knowing the location of the nearest bathroom. Now, however, they have many alternatives.

In a few men, the disease or its complications are severe enough to warrant speedy intervention. Recurrent urinary tract infections, urinary bleeding, bladder stones, persistent urinary retention, and kidney damage caused by BPH are among the problems that call for treatment. Fortunately, they are not common.

Because BPH progresses slowly, if at all, most men can decide for themselves when and if they should be treated; needless to say, their doctors should help decide how such treatment can be accomplished. A man should not decide to have surgery simply to prevent future complications or to improve a high AUA symptoms score. The key issue is quality of life. Men with BPH should ask themselves a question from the International Prostate Symptom Score (I-PSS) that is not part of the AUA index: "If you were to spend the rest of your life with your urinary condition just the way it is now, how would you feel about it?" Men who are unhappy with their symptoms should consider treatment, not because they are sick or at risk of becoming ill, but because they are bothered by BPH.

Many treatment options are available:

Watchful Waiting. It is really the only choice for men with low AUA scores, and it is a reasonable choice for many others who find that simple adjustments in lifestyle are able to take the BPH bother out of daily life. Here are a few tips:

- Reduce your intake of fluids, particularly after dinner.
- Limit your intake of alcohol and caffeine, and avoid them after midafternoon. Both are diuretics that increase urine flow.
- Avoid medications that stimulate muscles in the bladder neck and prostate. *Pseudoephedrine* (Sudafed) and other decongestants are the chief culprits.
- Avoid medications with anticholinergic properties that weaken bladder contractions. Antihistamines such as *diphenhydramine* (Benadryl) and many others are the most common offenders. Various antidepressants and antispasmodics have similar properties.
- If you are taking diuretics for high blood pressure or heart problems, ask your doctor to try to reduce the dose or substitute another medication that will work as well.
- Never pass up a chance to use the bathroom, even if your bladder does not feel full. Take your time, so you empty your bladder as much as possible. Plan to stop at regular intervals during auto trips. Request an aisle seat for air travel or at theatrical and sports events.
- When you are in new surroundings, learn the location of the bathroom before you really need it.
- Make your night-time trips to the bathroom easy and safe. Be sure the light is bright enough so that you can see where you are going, but avoid light so bright that it jolts you awake, making it hard for you to get back to sleep. Be sure no electrical cords, telephone wires, loose

rugs, or stray objects are between you and the bathroom; otherwise, a quick trip to the john can turn into an ambulance ride to have a broken hip repaired.

If you can live comfortably with BPH, do it. But if your symptoms are bothersome, you have several options to consider.

Medications

Prescription drugs can go a long way toward reducing the bothersome symptoms of BPH: Two types of treatment are available: the alpha-blockers, which relax smooth muscle cells in the prostate and bladder, and finasteride, which reduces the size of the gland.

The alpha-blockers were introduced in 1981 to treat high blood pressure, a task they accomplish by relaxing smooth muscle cells in the walls of arteries. Because the prostate and bladder neck also have smooth muscle cells, the alpha-blockers can act here too, relaxing the muscles to ease the flow of urine. Two of the alpha-blockers that are used for BPH, *terazosin* (Hytrin) and *doxazosin* (Cardura), are also used for hypertension. The third, *tamsulosin* (Flomax), is not effective for hypertension because it is much more active on urinary tract muscles than arterial muscles.

The three alpha-blockers are equally effective, producing mild to moderate improvements in the symptoms of BPH in about 70 percent of men. All act quickly, producing benefit in days to weeks; but the gains disappear quickly if the drugs are discontinued. All can be taken just once a day; tamsulosin is usually taken thirty minutes after dinner, terozosin or doxazosin at bedtime.

The usual dose for tamsulosin is 0.4 milligrams, but some men may benefit from an increase to 0.8 milligrams. Because the other alpha-blockers can lower the blood pressure, their dosage must be adjusted to attain the maximal benefit for BPH without lowering the blood pressure excessively. Doctors usually prescribe 1 milligram of either medication for starters, then gradually increase the dose as needed to a maximum of 10 milligrams for terazosin or 8 milligrams for doxazosin.

The major side effect of alpha-blockers is low blood pressure, which can produce lightheadedness, dizziness, or even fainting, usually triggered by standing up quickly; tamsulosin is less likely to produce these difficulties. Other side effects can include fatigue and nasal congestion. In most cases, doctors can minimize these problems by adjusting the dosage. In any case, they tend to diminish over time, and they resolve when the drug is stopped.

A recent trial has produced new concern about alpha-blockers, but the caution applies to men using the drugs for hypertension, not BPH. The Antihypertensive and Lipid Lowering Treatment to Prevent Heart Attack Trial (ALLHAT) was designed as a comparison of four different antihypertensive drugs. The subjects were 24,355 patients older than 55; all had high blood pressure and at least one other cardiac risk factor. Two of the drugs were doxazosin and *chlorthalidone* (Hygroton), a thiazide diuretic. These drugs were withdrawn from the study when a difference became apparent; over a three-year period, patients taking chlorthalidone were less likely to develop *congestive heart failure* (CHF) than patients taking doxazosin. However, there was no difference in nonfatal heart attacks or overall survival between the groups.

These data do not show that doxazosin causes CHF, but they do show that the drug is less beneficial than a diuretic in treating older adults with hypertension. Since diuretics are an effective treatment for CHF, it is not an altogether surprising finding. Still, confirmation will be important, but until other studies are in, ALLHAT will stand as strong evidence that alpha-blockers are less desirable than diuretics as first-line drugs for hypertension, at least in older people with cardiac risk factors.

To sum up, men with normal blood pressures can safely use alpha-blockers to treat BPH. Men with high blood pressure and enlarged hearts or other CHF risk factors should not rely on an alpha-blocker to treat both BPH and hypertension, but if they first use a cardioprotective drug such as a *beta-blocker* or an *ACE inhibitor* to lower their blood pressures, they can still take alpha-blockers to treat BPH. In that case, though, tamsulosin (Flomax) would be a better choice than doxazosin or terazosin, since it is less likely to make the blood pressure too low.

The other medication doctors can prescribe for BPH is entirely different. *Finasteride* (Proscar) acts to shrink the prostate by countering the effects of testosterone. But it does not stop the testicles from producing the male hormone, nor does it reduce the amount in the blood. Instead, finasteride inhibits *5 alpha-reductase,* the enzyme that normally converts testosterone to dihydrotestosterone, the key male hormone in the prostate (see Chapters One and Fourteen). This selective action explains why the drug affects some male traits without affecting others. Because DHT is the key to testosterone's action in the prostate and the hair follicles, finasteride is active in these regions. But since testosterone can act in other tissues without being converted to DHT, finasteride does not influence other male characteristics such as sperm production, musculature, or voice, and it affects libido and potency only infrequently.

Finasteride caused quite a stir in 1992, when it was marketed in a 5 milligram dose as Proscar. Until then, surgery was the only effective treatment for BPH; as the first alternative, finasteride was greeted enthusiastically. Some of that enthusiasm has worn off as it has become clear that it does not help all men with BPH and as alpha-blockers have proved their worth. Still, finasteride can help selected men with BPH.

Finasteride reduces DHT levels in the blood by about 70 percent and in the prostate by about 90 percent. As a result, the prostate shrinks, but the effect is slow and incomplete. On average, the drug takes three to six months to begin reducing the size of the prostate, and the gland may continue to shrink during the next twelve to eighteen months if treatment is continued. At its maximum, however, finasteride shrinks the gland by only about 25 percent.

Although finasteride reduces prostate size in most men who take it, the drug relieves symptoms for only about one-third of men with BPH. The men who benefit most are those with the largest prostates. Because prostate size can be estimated with a digital rectal exam (DRE) and more accurately measured with a transrectal ultrasound (TRUS), it is possible to predict which patients are likely to be helped. In general, men with glands smaller than 30 to 40 milliliters should not expect to improve on the treatment. In men with larger glands, though, the drug can reduce symptoms, control urinary bleeding caused by BPH, lower the risk of acute urinary retention, and diminish the chance of needing surgery.

To have these benefits, however, men with BPH and enlarged prostates must continue to take finasteride every day. That means years of therapy, which is expensive. Even in prolonged use, the drug appears safe. Impotence is the only major side effect, but it develops in just 4 percent of men and it improves when finasteride is discontinued.

Finasteride reduces *prostate specific antigen* (PSA) levels by about 50 percent, complicating screening for prostate cancer. Men who choose to monitor their PSAs should take the test before starting the drug and another after six to twelve months of therapy.

How does finasteride stack up against the alpha-blockers? A study of 1,229 men compared terazosin, finasteride, and a combination of the two with a placebo. At the end of a full year, terazosin was the clear winner. Combination therapy was no better than the alpha-blocker alone. Finasteride was no better than the placebo, but that does not mean the drug is worthless, since many men in the study did not have the large prostates that respond best to finasteride.

Because alpha-blockers act quickly, many doctors initially prescribe one of these medications for BPH, reserving finasteride or combination therapy for men with large glands who do not respond well to alpha-blockers.

HERBS

BPH is so common that it seems like human nature rather than a disease. Since BPH is a "natural" problem, it would be nice if there were a "natural" remedy. Perhaps that is why thousands of men are turning to herbs for BPH. Because they are sold as "dietary supplements" rather than medications, these herbs are not subject to the Food and Drug Administration's standards for efficacy, purity, or safety (see Chapter Six). There is much less scientific information about herbs than standard medications. Still, it is reasonable for men who do not respond to prescription medications (or would like to avoid them) to consider trying saw palmetto, the most promising of the many "natural" remedies touted for the prostate.

Saw palmetto or *Serenoa repens* is the American dwarf palm that was once used for food by various southwestern Native American tribes. The ripe berry is the source of an herbal extract sold under many brand names, some of which also contain extracts from other plants. When Consumers Union evaluated various preparations, it found that the amount of the herb in each tablet does not always correspond to the claims on the label—but one, the CVS brand, contained what it claimed and was also among the least expensive.

The active ingredient in saw palmetto is not known; the extracts contain a mix of fatty acids along with smaller amounts of sterols, flavonoids, and other compounds. In animal and laboratory experiments, saw palmetto displays several activities affecting the androgen and estrogen (male and female hormone) receptors on prostate cells. Despite earlier reports and popular beliefs, however, saw palmetto does not appear to share finasteride's action on 5 alpha-reductase, nor does it reduce prostate specific antigen (PSA) levels.

Does saw palmetto work? That is, of course, the crucial question, but it cannot be answered conclusively. Most studies of saw palmetto have been performed in Europe; they are encouraging, but there are flaws in the way they were conducted. When American scientists reviewed eighteen randomized controlled trials of saw palmetto in a total of 2,939 men, they concluded "the evidence suggests that [saw palmetto] improves urologic symptoms and urinary flow," but "further research is needed using standardized preparations . . . to determine its long term effectiveness and ability to prevent BPH complications."

Saw palmetto produces few side effects, but its long-term safety and its interactions with other medications have not been studied adequately. Preparations may vary in potency and purity as well as price. But if men who are bothered by BPH are not bothered by these uncertainties, saw palmetto may be worth a try. If it does not seem to help in one to three months, however, it is not worth continuing.

With sales topping $140 million annually, saw palmetto is the most popular herbal treatment for the prostate. But there are others, including extracts of the African plum (*Pyyeum africanum*), the stinging nettle (*Urtica dioica*), South African Star grass (*Hypoxis rooperi*) and rye pollen (*Secale cevale*). Chemicals including beta sitosterols and zinc have also been touted for "prostate health." None of these products have been studied carefully enough to warrant even a tentative recommendation for BPH. Similarly, although lycopene, vitamin E, soy, and selenium may have a role in reducing the risk of prostate cancer (see Chapter Twelve), none can be expected to prevent or treat BPH, either alone or in combinations.

Herbs for the prostate? Perhaps, at least in the case of saw palmetto. But as in the case of all unregulated supplements, the watchword is cautious skepticism.

SURGERY

Before the advent of alpha-blockers and finasteride and the renewed interest in saw palmetto, surgery was the only effective treatment for BPH—and even with these medical treatments, surgery remains the benchmark. When the Health Professionals Study compared the symptomatic benefits of alpha-blockers, finasteride, and surgery in 1,459 men with BPH, it found that surgery was the most effective. But because it also has the most complications, surgery is now usually reserved for men who fail to improve with medical treatment, particularly those with threatening complications such as urinary retention, recurrent infection, frequent bleeding, bladder stones, or kidney damage.

Developed fifty years ago, *transurethral resection of the prostate* (TURP) has been the "gold standard" of BPH therapy. In recent years, though, its luster has tarnished—not because of problems with the operation itself (it has actually gotten better), but because of new medical and surgical rivals. As recently as the early 1990s, about 400,000 American men underwent surgery each year; at a cost of almost $4 billion, TURP was second only to cataract surgery as the most common procedure reimbursed by Medicare. With our new understand-

FIGURE 11.2. TRANSURETHRAL RESECTION OF THE PROSTATE (TURP)

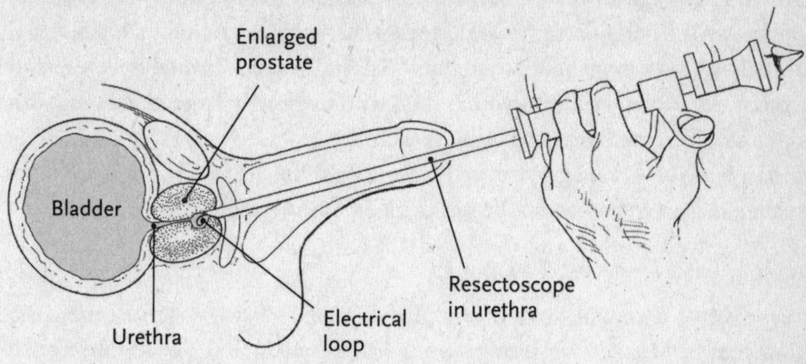

Transurethral resection of the prostate (TURP) is still the gold standard of therapy. The surgeon passes an electrical loop through a resectoscope, then uses it to cut away excess prostate tissue.

ing of BPH and new therapies, the number of TURPs has declined dramatically.

Although this trend is certain to continue, it is too early to put TURP on the endangered species list, since it is still a good choice for some men.

Although TURP does not require an incision through the skin, the ninety-minute operation does require hospitalization and anesthesia, either spinal or general. The surgeon passes a *resectoscope* through the patient's urethra, then uses an electrical loop to cut away prostate tissue that is impeding the flow of urine (see Figure 11.2). A Foley catheter is left in place to empty the bladder for a day or two, after which the patient can void on his own. If all goes well, he is home in two or three days.

Although results vary, TURP substantially reduces BPH symptoms in 80 to 90 percent of patients. But there can be complications. Early problems include infection or bleeding; pretreatment with finasteride appears to reduce the risk of bleeding. Late complications include retrograde (dry) ejaculation (50 to 75 percent), impotence (5 to 10 percent), and incontinence (1 to 3 percent). And since the prostate can regenerate, up to 20 percent of TURP patients require additional, less extensive, therapy within ten years. But new data from the United States and Europe have put to rest earlier concerns that TURP might be associated with an increased long-term death rate.

Although TURP is the standard operation for BPH, a few men may still require open surgery, which was first performed about 100 years ago. As the name implies, open prostatectomy involves an incision in the lower abdomen that allows the surgeon to see and remove the enlarged tissue that is blocking urine flow. It is a bigger operation than TURP and is performed only 5 percent as often, usually in relatively young men with extremely large glands that cannot be safely treated with less invasive techniques. Used only for BPH, it is not the same as the *radical prostatectomy* operations that are used to treat localized prostate cancer by removing the entire gland (see Chapter Twelve).

NEWER, LESS INVASIVE THERAPIES

It seems like acronym heaven or alphabet soup. Most men of a certain age know that BPH stands for *benign prostatic hyperplasia* and TURP for its traditional surgical remedy, *transurethral resection of the prostate*. But men who are considering new procedures to relieve symptoms of BPH are now confronted by a bewildering array of initials—such as TUMT, TUNA, TUIP, HIFU, TUBD, and, believe it or not, many others. That's because urologists have devised many new therapies for BPH, and more are on the way. Because these therapies are new, they are not available in all hospitals. Long-term results are not available, but most appear more effective than medication, though less successful than TURP. Still, if they are available in your medical center, they may be worth considering, since they generally have a lower risk of complications than TURPs and allow a quicker return to normal activities. Here is a chooser's guide:

Transurethral Incision of the Prostate (TUIP). Like TURP, TUIP is an established procedure that requires anesthesia and is performed through a resectoscope. But there is a difference. Instead of removing excess prostate tissue, TUIP involves only one or two small incisions in the prostate, which relieve pressure and allow the urethra to spring open. As a result, men can often go home on the same day as surgery, and they run a much lower risk of complications such as retrograde ejaculation (15 percent), impotence (2 percent), and incontinence (1 percent). Unfortunately, TUIP is effective only in men with prostates that are minimally enlarged to no more than 30 grams (one ounce).

Transurethral Electrovaporization of the Prostate (TVP). Like TURP, TVP is an electrosurgical technique. The difference is that TVP uses a roller electrode that vaporizes and also cauterizes tissue, so it appears to produce less bleeding than TURP. However, because tissue is evaporated rather than removed, it is not available for pathological examination. TVP seems best suited for moderately enlarged prostate glands of less than 50 grams. The anesthesia and hospitalization requirements and early efficacy of TVP and TURP are similar, but data on TVP are more limited.

Transurethral Microwave Thermotherapy (TUMT). Recently approved for clinical use in the United States, TUMT uses microwave energy to heat the prostate, destroying unwanted tissue. A tiny microwave antenna is introduced into the urethra through a catheter; a computer monitors the tissue temperature, delivering just enough energy to heat the prostate to 122 degrees F. TUMT takes about thirty minutes and can be performed without general anesthesia on an outpatient basis. TUMT is faster and less expensive than TURP and it has fewer complications. About 60 to 70 percent of men respond favorably, but up to two-thirds require additional treatment after four years. More time is needed to evaluate the results of this new therapy. Men with pacemakers, implanted defibrillators, or artificial hips cannot be treated with TUMT.

Transurethral Needle Ablation (TUNA). Like TUMT, TUNA uses heat to destroy unwanted prostate tissue, but in TUNA radio waves provide the energy. Two tiny needles are placed in the prostate through a catheter; radio frequency energy is delivered through the needles, destroying the tissue adjacent to the needles. Requiring only local anesthesia with sedation, TUNA is a rapid outpatient procedure. It has few complications and produces results comparable to TUMT's. Because TUNA has just been approved in the United States, the data are very limited and long-term results are not known.

Laser Surgery. It is a hot new area of minimally invasive prostate surgery, but several competing techniques are already available. Laser light energy can be beamed to the prostate under direct visualization through a cystoscope (*visual laser ablation of the prostate,* VLAP); another variation is *contact laser ablation of the prostate,* CLAP. Like TVP, laser energy heats, evaporates, and cauterizes tissue, removing obstruction with minimal bleeding. The Food and Drug Administration approved the first laser treatment system for clinical use in the United States in 1998. Early data suggest good efficacy and safety, but more information will be needed to determine the appropriate role for this promising new technique.

Transurethral Balloon Dilatation (TUBD). When it was first introduced in the mid-1980s, balloon dilatation was greeted with great hope and enthusiasm. It is a simple, low-risk procedure that can be performed with local anesthesia. The surgeon inserts a catheter into the urethra, then inflates a balloon that stretches the narrowed area. TUBD improves urine flow about 50 percent of the time. Unfortunately, BPH symptoms return in many men, sometimes in just a few months. It's a quick fix, but a short-lived one.

Prostate Stents. TUBD resembles *coronary angioplasty.* In both cases, a catheter is used to introduce a balloon that is inflated to widen a blockage; in both cases, however, recurrent blockage is common. Cardiologists get much better results when they introduce an expandable stent to keep the blockage open. Urologists, too, have been using stents to widen the urethra. Most are spring-like mesh cylinders made of titanium. They are easy to place under regional anesthesia and they improve urine flow in many men. Stents have been used mainly in older men who are poor candidates for surgery. They are new devices, and their long-term effects are not yet known.

Other Options. It is an embarrassment of riches, and despite all the choices that are available, urologists are experimenting with additional techniques, including hot-water balloon therapy and injecting the prostate with alcohol or enzymes. And older men who are not sexually active may choose another option, medical treatment with drugs ordinarily used for androgen-deprivation therapy of prostate cancer (see Chapter Twelve).

Benign Prostatic Possibilities

It is an interesting, rapidly changing time for BPH treatment. Paradoxically, perhaps, many new surgical treatments are being introduced just as medical therapies are taking hold. And all these treatment options are arriving at a time when new information about the natural history of BPH suggests that it is safe and reasonable for men who are not greatly bothered by their symptoms to choose watchful waiting rather than any active therapy. It's a brave new era that will allow well-informed men to take control of a vexing old problem.

CHAPTER TWELVE

Prostate Cancer

IT IS NO WONDER that men worry about prostate cancer. The disease is diagnosed in an American man every three minutes. With 189,000 new cases annually, prostate cancer is the most common internal cancer in American men, and with 30,200 deaths a year, it is second only to lung cancer among malignant causes of death in men.

The figures are worrisome, but they do not tell the whole story. The good news is that the prostate cancer death rate peaked in 1992 and has been falling by nearly 4 percent a year ever since. Credit for the progress goes to better methods of diagnosis, improved types of treatment, and growing evidence that lifestyle changes can help prevent the disease.

Doctors are encouraged by the progress, but they disagree about its true significance. In fact, scientists debate nearly every aspect of prostate cancer, from the value of early diagnosis to the best form of treatment. Faced with legitimate scientific doubts, each man must decide what is best for him. It is a difficult decision, but it should not be a lonely one; in this chapter, I will try to present a balanced account of what is known about prostate cancer and what is still debatable, hoping to guide each reader to sound decisions.

What Causes Prostate Cancer?

In a word, nobody knows. But like all malignancies, prostate cancer develops when the genes that govern a cell's growth and division lose control (see Chapter Three). Without proper checks and balances, malignant prostate cells multiply when they should not, then go where they should not as they invade normal tissues near the prostate and eventually spread to other areas of the body.

What causes the genes of a prostate cell to lose control? As in all malignancies, it is a combination of heredity and environment, of inborn genetic defects and acquired damage. How much is predestined and how much acquired? When scientists in Scandinavia evaluated the questions by studying 44,788 pairs of twins, they concluded that 42 percent of a man's risk of prostate cancer could be explained by hereditary factors, the other 58 percent by environmental influences. If the study is correct, heredity has a greater impact on prostate cancer than on all other common malignancies, including colorectal cancer (35 percent) and breast cancer (27 percent).

Scientists have not yet discovered the genetic abnormality responsible for prostate cancer, but they have made some progress. Two that increase risk have already been identified; one resides on chromosome 1 and is called HPC1, while the other is located on chromosome 17 and is called HPC2. But since these genes together account for less than 20 percent of all prostate cancers, others must also contribute to the disease. The Physicians' Health Study has identified one such candidate. It is the androgen receptor gene (AR) on chromosome 1; another is called ELAC2. Surprisingly perhaps, male relatives of women who have breast cancer have an increased risk of prostate cancer, particularly if the family carries a specific mutation of the breast cancer gene BRCA2.

Nature versus nurture—it's an old debate in human biology. Men should be glad that scientists are hunting down genetic abnormalities, but since they cannot trade in their parents and grandparents, they should pay particular attention to the personal factors they can influence with the hope of reducing risk.

Who Gets Prostate Cancer?

Almost everyone has a friend or relative with prostate cancer. And anyone who reads a newspaper or watches TV knows that fame and fortune do not protect a man from the disease; just ask FBI director Robert Mueller, former New York City Mayor Rudolph Giuliani, Yankees manager Joe Torre, Senator Bob Dole, General Norman Schwarzkopf, South Africa's Nelson Mandela and Bishop Desmond Tutu, golf legend Arnold Palmer, or entertainers like Harry Belafonte, Merv Griffin, Ed Asner, Sidney Poitier, and Jerry Lewis, to name a few. The disease strikes celebrities and statesmen, athletes and physicians, corporate chiefs and ordinary guys. Who gets prostate cancer? Any man can, but some men are at higher risk than others. Here is a summary of the major risk factors.

Age. Age is the strongest predictor of the risk of prostate cancer. The disease is very rare in men younger than forty, and quite uncommon in forty-to-fifty-year-olds. Above age fifty, however, a man's likelihood of developing prostate cancer begins to rise, and it goes on rising throughout life. The inci-

Table 12.1: AGE-RELATED RISK OF PROSTATE CANCER

AGE GROUP	RISK OF PROSTATE CANCER
50–59	10–42%
60–69	17–38%
70–79	25–66%
80 and over	Up to 90%

Modified from *Report of the U.S. Preventive Sciences Task Force: Guide to Clinical Preventive Sciences* 2nd ed., Williams and Wilkins; 1996: 121.

dence of prostate cancer, in fact, increases faster with age than any other major cancer.

What is the risk in specific age groups? Studies have produced a wide range of results, but all agree that as men age, their risk becomes astonishingly high (see Table 12.1).

It's a bit scary: If you live long enough, you probably *will* get prostate cancer. Remember, though, that most of the prostate cancers in these surveys are clinically unimportant—just a few malignant cells discovered in the course of complete autopsies on men who died from other causes. In all, an American man's lifetime risk of developing early microscopic prostate cancer is about 30 percent, but his risk of clinically evident prostate cancer is only about 9 percent, and his risk of dying from prostate cancer is about 3 percent.

Family History. Epidemiologists tell us that the risk of developing any given disease is relative. They also say that when it comes to prostate cancer, having relatives with the disease increases a man's risk.

Men who have a father or brother with clinically diagnosed prostate cancer are about twice as likely to develop the disease as men whose families are free of it; affected uncles and cousins have a much smaller impact than fathers and brothers. But a very strong family history of prostate cancer increases the risk even more. A man who has several close relatives with the disease, particularly if their prostate cancers were diagnosed before age fifty-five, is up to eight times more likely to develop prostate cancer himself.

Nationality. The incidence of prostate cancer varies enormously around the world. Even after correcting for age and diagnostic accuracy, it is 120 times more common in San Francisco than in rural China, and over four times more common in the United States than in Japan. Part of the difference may be genetic, but it is also due to environmental and lifestyle factors. For example, Japanese men who move to California acquire a much higher risk of prostate cancer, and the risk is higher still for the next generation born in America. That's why the Health Professionals Study found that Asian Americans have the same risk of prostate cancer as white Americans.

Race. Prostate cancer is about 30 percent more common in African Americans than in white Americans, even after accounting for age, socioeconomic factors, and access to medical care and testing. Genetics, of course, may account for racial differences, but lifestyle factors such as diet may also play a role. Most studies have estimated that black Americans have a 30 percent higher risk than whites, but in 2000 the Health Professionals Study reported a 73 percent higher incidence of the disease. African American men have a significantly higher rate of prostate cancer than black men living in Africa and Asia.

Diet. It is not clear just how lifestyle contributes to prostate cancer, but diet is the leading candidate. The Harvard men's health studies have had an important role in uncovering the link between diet and prostate cancer (see page 353).

Hormones. Testosterone and its derivative, *dihydrotestosterone,* promote the growth of prostate cells, both benign and malignant. Animals who are treated with testosterone are prone to develop prostate cancer, but men with prostate cancer do not have abnormally high levels of the hormone. The Physicians' Health Study, however, found that men with high-normal testosterone levels were more likely to develop prostate cancer than men with low-normal levels. In addition, the study reported that low levels of the female hormone *estradiol* were also associated with an increased risk of the disease. But the hormone issue is complex, and more study is needed. At present, it is not possible to calculate a man's risk of prostate cancer by measuring his hormone levels.

Smoking. Because smoking causes so many malignancies, it is a logical suspect in prostate cancer. The Health Professionals Study reported that recent heavy tobacco use has a substantial impact on the occurrence of fatal prostate cancer, but the excess risk dissipates within ten years of quitting. In contrast, the Physicians' Health Study found no link. Other studies are also mixed, with some reporting no association but others indicating that heavy cigarette smoking may boost a man's risk of dying from prostate cancer by up to 45 percent. The debate is likely to continue, but it is somewhat academic, since no man should use tobacco, regardless of smoking's impact on the prostate.

Alcohol. The evidence is mixed here, too. In 2001, the Alumni Study reported a link between moderate to heavy liquor consumption and prostate cancer, but a 2000 meta-analysis of thirty-three studies found no effect. All in all, concerns about prostate cancer need not affect a man's decision about drinking (see Chapter Seven).

Exercise. Can you run away from prostate cancer? It seems far-fetched, but exercise does reduce the risk of colon cancer (see Chapter Five) and of female breast and reproductive malignancies. For prostate cancer, though, the evidence is mixed. Studies from Finland, Norway, and the Cooper Clinic in Texas suggest that walking, but not heavy lifting, is associated with a reduced risk. But the Alumni Study set the bar much higher, finding protection only in men who exercise intensely enough to burn at least 4,000 calories a week; exercise was most protective in older men who sustained a high level of activity over many years. The Health Professionals Study is even less optimistic, finding no appreciable protection from exercise.

Body Size. Can a man's build predict his risk of disease? Obesity certainly increases the likelihood of developing heart disease (see Chapter Three), and it also increases the total risk of cancer. For prostate cancer, though, the evidence is mixed. A 1997 study of 135,000 Swedish men found that big men get more prostate cancer, whether bigness was measured in height, weight, or body mass index, which reflects obesity. The Physicians' Health Study found that being tall increases risk. The Health Professionals Study also identified height as a risk factor, but found that childhood (but not adult) obesity appeared protective. In contrast, a 2001 study of Chinese men implicated abdominal obesity as the only risk factor related to body size and shape.

Sexual Activity. The prostate's role is to contribute fluid to semen. Since it is a reproductive organ, men have asked if sexual activity has an impact on prostate cancer, either increasing risk or providing protection. Until recently, the answer has been no, but a 2001 study of 1,456 men from Washington State reported that men who had sex with thirty or more women during the course of a lifetime were 2.3 times more likely to develop prostate cancer than men with only one partner. Thirty partners may seem like a lot, but boasting did not seem to enter into a man's risk. Even a more modest exposure to two to four female partners was associated with a 1.7-fold increase in subsequent prostate cancer.

It is only one study, and confirmation is needed. If nothing else, it is likely to reopen one of the few questions about prostate cancer that scientists had considered to be resolved.

Growth Factors. Cell growth depends on a balance between hormones and proteins that stimulate growth and those that limit it (see Chapter Three). The Physicians' Health Study has identified a unique protein called insulin-like growth factor (IGF-1) as a prostate cancer risk factor.

IGF-1 is a hormone produced in large amounts by the liver and in smaller amounts by other tissues, including prostate cells. It is crucial for healthy development; it acts by stimulating normal cell growth and by inhibiting programmed cell death, or *apoptosis*. Because IGF-1 is so important for normal tissue growth, the body regulates it in several ways. Growth hormone, produced by the pituitary gland in the brain, boosts IGF-1 production, while various inhibitory proteins counter its actions.

To find out if high levels of IGF-1 could predict an increased risk of prostate cancer, the Physicians' Health Study obtained blood samples from 14,916 men in 1982, then followed the group for ten years. In fact, IGF-1 levels proved significantly higher in the men who developed cancer than in the men who did not. The association was surprisingly strong. In all, the 25 percent of men with the highest IGF-1 levels were 4.3 times more likely to develop prostate cancer than were the 25 percent of men with the lowest levels; men with intermediate levels had intermediate risk. The link between IGF-1 and prostate cancer held up even after the scientists analyzed other factors that might have influenced the results, including PSA levels, hormone levels (including the male hormones testosterone and DHT and the female hormone estrogen), key health habits (smoking and diet), and body size (height, weight, and body fat).

It is exciting research, holding out the hope that a blood test for IGF-1 may be able to predict a man's risk of prostate cancer years before the tumor is large enough to be detected. And if IGF-1 proves to have a role in the disease, drugs could be tailored to counter its effects, perhaps providing new ways to prevent or treat prostate cancer. But at present, IGF-1 is only a research tool, and it is far too early to know if these possibilities will be realized.

Other Factors. Even after considering all these known risk factors, many cases of prostate cancer remain unexplained. Epidemiologists are smart people, and they have looked for other explanations. What they have discovered, however, is a long list of factors that have little if any effect on prostate cancer, including infectious agents and occupation (though occupational exposure to cadmium may be a weak risk factor). Although the Health Professionals Study raised concern about vasectomy in 1993, newer research has exonerated it as a risk factor (see Chapter Ten). And whatever else you may think about prostate cancer, it is a democratic disease; socioeconomic status has no effect on risk. Finally, neither benign prostatic hyperplasia (BPH) nor prostatitis (inflammation of the gland) is linked to prostate cancer (see Chapter Eleven); no man enjoys these benign prostate problems, but at least he need not worry about a higher risk of developing cancer as well.

What do prostate cancer risk factors mean? Men cannot trade in their relatives, alter their genes, or halt the aging process. But if these major risk factors cannot be modified, others can. Diet, in fact, is the key to a healthy lifestyle that not only benefits the prostate, but protects against heart disease, hypertension, diabetes, and obesity. A healthy prostate, after all, needs a healthy body around it.

Diet and Prostate Cancer

You are what you eat.

It is an aphorism that has been applied to many parts of the body, from a man's heart to his haunches. And an ever-increasing amount of evidence suggests that it applies to the prostate as well.

Diet is complex, and so are its effects on prostate cancer. Here is a summary of the nutrients that matter most:

FAT

Dietary fat occupies first place among the lifestyle factors that add fuel to the fire of prostate cancer. The Health Professionals Study demonstrated the relationship in 1993, when it reported that men who eat the most fat are 1.79 times more likely to develop prostate cancer than men who eat the least. But not all fats are equally harmful. Animal fat was linked to cancer risk, but vegetable fat was not. Red meat was the food most strongly associated with advanced prostate cancer; men who ate the most beef, bacon, pork, or lamb were 2.6 times more likely to develop prostate cancer than men who ate the least. Men who ate chicken with the skin on were at increased risk, but men who ate it without the skin were not. Other foods linked to prostate cancer included butter, mayonnaise, and creamy salad dressings.

The Health Professionals Study does not stand alone in implicating dietary fat as a prostate cancer risk factor. International comparisons of dietary fat intake and the incidence of prostate cancer provide corroboration; men living in countries with a high consumption of fat have a much greater risk of developing prostate cancer than do men in countries with a low fat intake. The difference in risk is not genetic; men who migrate from a low-risk country trade the low risk of their fathers for the high risk of their neighbors.

For example, in Japan, fat provides 24 percent of an average man's calories, and as recently as 1955, the Japanese diet was just 10 percent fat. In the United States, fat intake averages 37 percent—very high, but still an improvement from the recent peak of 44 percent. Men in America, including those of Japanese descent, are nine times more likely to die from prostate cancer than are men in Japan.

Because there are so many differences between cultures, international comparisons are tricky, but even within individual countries from Italy and England to Canada and America, dietary fat is tied to risk, and animal fat from meat or dairy products is the leading offender. Animal experiments also demonstrate the link between fat and cancer.

How does dietary fat promote prostate cancer? Scientists do not know, but they have raised several possibilities. Fat could have a direct effect on prostate cells or it could act by enhancing testosterone action. Because fat is calorically dense, it could increase risk by promoting obesity; in animals, at least, caloric restriction slows the growth of prostate cancer. Finally, it is possible that men who eat lots of fat are not harmed by the fat itself, but because they are not getting enough of the vegetable foods that may reduce risk. Whatever the cause, a high intake of fat seems to increase a man's risk of developing prostate cancer by as much as 60 to 90 percent.

Are particular fatty acids to blame? The *saturated fatty acids* found in red meat and whole dairy products are the leading culprits, but another class of fats requires special consideration. The *omega-3 fatty acids* are *special polyunsaturated fats* that appear to reduce the risk of heart attack and stroke (see Chapter Four). Two of the most important, *eicosapentaenoic acid* and *docosahexanoic acid,* are found only in fish, particularly only fish from deep cold waters. The good news is that the marine omega-3s appear to protect against prostate cancer as well as cardiovascular disease. But another omega-3 comes from plants and presents a dilemma for men. *Alpha-lineolenic acid* appears to protect the heart, but both the Health Professionals Study and the Physicians' Health Study tied it to an increased risk of prostate cancer. In the years since these eye-opening reports of 1993 and 1994, studies from Norway, Spain, Uruguay, and Washington State have also detected an association between a high intake of alpha-lineolenic acid and prostate cancer—but studies from Canada, New Zealand, and the Netherlands have not.

Alpha-linolenic acid is most abundant in flaxseed oil (50 percent), canola oil (11 percent) and soybean oil (7 percent); lesser amounts are present in walnuts and wheat germ. Except for flaxseed oil (which has been gaining popularity in alternative medicine circles), these foods have all been considered healthful. More research is needed to learn if alpha-linolenic acid is a boon or a bane. Until then, men should get the bulk of their omega-3s from fish; nuts and soy are also reasonable. Clearly, men with heart disease or major risk factors might choose to use canola oil along with olive oil, but men who have special reasons to worry about prostate cancer might decide to forego the cardiac benefits of canola.

TOMATOES AND OTHER VEGETABLES

To find out if any foods can reduce the risk of prostate cancer, the Health Professionals Study analyzed forty-six different fruits, vegetables, and related foods. Although dark green leafy vegetables appear to reduce the risk of various malignancies, they do not protect against prostate cancer. Instead, tomatoes emerged as the only item linked to a reduction in prostate cancer. Products containing cooked tomatoes appeared even more protective than raw tomatoes; pizza headed the list, which is a bit embarrassing since it is hardly a health food, yet all 47,894 men in this study were dentists, pharmacists, veterinarians, and other health professionals.

An earlier study of Seventh-Day Adventists also linked tomato consumption to protection against prostate cancer. What makes tomatoes so special? Nobody knows, but one possibility is *lycopene,* the most potent antioxidant in the beta-carotene family. Cooking releases the lycopene, making it easier to absorb. A 1997 study, in fact, found that men absorb 2.5 times more lycopene from tomato paste than from fresh tomatoes.

In a recent report, the Physicians' Health Study identified lycopene as the carotenoid associated with a reduced risk of prostate cancer. A 1998 study from Maryland demonstrated that a high intake of tomato juice raises blood lycopene levels, and a 2000 study from Illinois went one step further, finding that high blood levels are linked to high lycopene concentration in the prostate itself.

If carotenoids in vegetables help—even a little—how about taking them in vitamin pills? The evidence is mixed, but it is not encouraging (see Chapter Six). In the ATBC trial of beta-carotene and vitamin E supplements in 29,133 Finnish male smokers, beta-carotene was actually linked to a 25 percent increase in prostate cancer. However, no such increase was observed in either the CARET Study of 18,314 American smokers or in the Physicians' Health Study of 22,071 American men, of whom only 11 percent smoked. In the Harvard study, in fact, beta-carotene supplements were linked to a 35 percent lower risk of prostate cancer in men with a low dietary consumption of carotenoids.

At this point, the best advice is to get your lycopene from tomatoes, not supplements. And don't neglect other vegetables. British researchers recently reported that a vegan diet appears to reduce levels of IGF-1, the growth factor that the Physicians' Health Study linked to prostate cancer (see page 352). In addition, a 2000 study from Seattle found that a high consumption of all vegetables was protective, and that cruciferous vegetables (broccoli, cabbage, brussels sprouts, cauliflower, and coleslaw) were most beneficial.

VITAMIN E

Like lycopene, vitamin E is an antioxidant. Does it have a role in protection against prostate cancer? Perhaps. The ATBC study of male smokers that reported a deleterious effect of beta-carotene pills found a protective effect of vitamin E. The men who took 50 milligrams of *alpha-tocopherol* a day (equivalent to about 75 units of vitamin E) enjoyed a 32 percent lower risk of developing prostate cancer and a 41 percent lower risk of dying from the disease. It's hopeful news, but the apparent protection may be confined to smokers. A study of 2,974 Swiss men found that low blood levels of vitamin E were associated with an increased risk of prostate cancer in smokers but not in nonsmokers, and the Health Professionals Study found that vitamin E supplements appeared protective only in smokers and recent quitters. A study from Washington suggested that supplements might help, but it did not take smoking into account.

The Health Professionals Study has cast doubt on the value of vitamin E, but it may not have the last word. Vitamin E is not a single compound, but a family of chemicals known as *tocopherols*. The most common member of the family is *alpha-tocopherol.* It is the form of vitamin E that's present in most supplements, and it's the compound that has been linked to a reduced risk of prostate cancer in smokers.

The alpha-tocopherol story is complex, and its benefits are far from certain. But even before the last chapter has been written, new research tells us that the situation is even more complex than it seemed.

The latest player is *gamma-tocopherol,* a form of vitamin E that is found in foods such as soybean and corn oil, but not in most supplements. A new study of 10,456 Maryland residents found that men with the highest blood levels of gamma-tocopherol were only one-fifth as likely to develop prostate cancer as men with the lowest levels. High levels of selenium and alpha-tocopherol also seemed to help, at least in men who also had high levels of gamma-tocopherol. And if this were not complex enough, there is another wrinkle: Vitamin E supplements that provide large doses of alpha-tocopherol (especially above 400 international units) may actually lower blood levels of gamma-tocopherol.

It will take time for scientists to sort this out. Until they do so, vitamin-rich foods continue to look pretty good.

GRAINS

Vegetables provide more than just vitamins; they also provide dietary fiber. Whole grains are also high in vitamins, minerals, and fiber—and a recent study offers a grain of hope that they may help ward off prostate cancer.

To explore the relationship between nutrition and prostate cancer, researchers in Massachusetts examined lifestyle factors and prostate cancer death rates in fifty-nine countries from around the globe. To accomplish this formidable task, the scientists used data collected over the years by the United Nations and the World Health Organization. In addition to food consumption, the data provided information on tobacco and alcohol use, reproductive factors, and socioeconomic status. The study focused on men forty-five to seventy-four years of age and on the years between 1985 and 1990.

The new research confirmed many of the previously known facts about prostate cancer. Death rates varied tremendously, from a low of just 0.53 deaths per 100,000 men to a high of 69.5 per 100,000. As in previous studies, the risk of dying from prostate cancer increased as men ate more of the Western foods associated with affluence. Dietary fat, especially animal fat from meat and whole dairy products, increased risk, as did alcohol, sugar, and total calories. As in earlier studies, vegetables (particularly cabbage and soy) had the opposite effect, reducing risk. But the new research adds an important dimension: Cereal and other whole grain products decreased risk, as did nuts, oilseeds, and fish.

How strong was the protective effect? It was substantial. Compared to men eating the fewest whole grain products, the men eating the most cereal suffered 19.5 fewer prostate cancer deaths per 100,0000. For perspective, the protective effect of cereal was even stronger than the deleterious effect of a high fat diet.

How might cereals and whole grains help reduce the risk of prostate cancer? Scientists are not sure, but they speculate that protection depends on traditional unrefined foods that contain rye, buckwheat flour, or flaxseeds. These foods are rich in *lignans,* chemicals that have antioxidant properties and also appear to partially block the interaction between testosterone and hormone-sensitive malignancies, such as prostate cancer. Because plant lignans are located in the bran layer of grains, they are lost when whole grains are processed into refined flours. Affluent industrial societies who consume refined flour have had a high risk of prostate cancer, while traditional societies that consume whole grains have a low incidence of the disease.

The international study also found that nuts and seeds appear to reduce the risk of prostate cancer. It is another new observation that has not yet been explained fully. Both nuts and seeds provide vitamin E. They are high in fat, but instead of the saturated fatty acids found in meat, whole dairy products, and other animal products, they contain polyunsaturated fatty acids, including the contentious omega-3, alpha-linolenic acid. Still, vegetable fats may exert a protective influence. Indeed, a 1998 study of 1,025 Canadian men found that men who ate the most vegetable fat were 60 to 67 percent less likely to develop prostate cancer than men who ate the least.

Selenium

Selenium is a mineral that has antioxidant properties. Two important studies suggest that it may have a role in reducing the risk of prostate cancer. In the first, a team of scientists based in Arizona administered either 200 micrograms of selenium or a placebo each day to 1,312 volunteers whose average age was sixty-three. After four and a half years, the men who took selenium enjoyed a 63 percent lower risk of dying from prostate cancer than those who took placebos. More recently, the Health Professionals Study evaluated 33,737 men, comparing their risk of prostate cancer with their selenium consumption as measured by the selenium content of their toenail clippings. The men with the highest selenium levels (a daily intake of about 159 micrograms) were only a third as likely to develop advanced prostate cancer as the men with the lowest levels (corresponding to a daily consumption of 86 micrograms).

Although the new international research appears to have little in common with these two American studies, there may be a link. In fact, grains and vegetables grown in selenium-rich soils are an excellent source of the mineral. Fish and Brazil nuts are also high in selenium, as are poultry, meat, garlic, and shellfish.

Only small amounts of selenium are needed for health; the Dietary Reference Intake for men is just 55 micrograms a day. It is too early to recommend selenium for prostate cancer protection, but men who are attracted to the possibility can consider supplements of up to 200 micrograms a day, the dose used in the Arizona study. Daily doses above 400 micrograms can be toxic, damaging the skin and hair.

SOY

Prostate cancer is uncommon in Asia, where the diet is high in soy products such as tofu, soy milk, tempeh, and miso. Soy contains *isoflavones* such as *genistein* and *daidzein*. These chemicals are *phytoestrogens,* plant compounds that can bind to hormone receptors on human tissues, perhaps explaining why a high intake of soy is associated with a low risk of hormone-responsive tumors including both breast and prostate cancers. Genistein may also act against prostate cancer by nonhormonal mechanisms. It appears to inhibit the growth of prostate cancer cells in test tubes, and it may reduce *angiogenesis,* the process that allows cancers to develop new blood vessels as they grow.

More research is needed to learn if soy can actually reduce the risk of prostate cancer. But even if it does not, soy is a healthful food. It provides fiber, vitamins, and high-quality protein, and in a daily dose of 25 grams it can reduce blood cholesterol levels by an impressive 13 percent.

VITAMIN D

Prostate cancer death rates are higher in North America and Northern Europe than in the Far East, Africa, and Central America. Men in northern climates get less sunshine than southerners. The ultraviolet rays in sunlight produce vitamin D in the skin. Perhaps, then, vitamin D is involved in prostate cancer.

It is an interesting possibility. In laboratory experiments, vitamin D compounds are able to slow the growth of prostate cancer cells. Early studies of blood levels of vitamin D suggested that men with low levels had an increased risk of prostate cancer. But a 1995 investigation of more than 20,000 men and a 1996 report from the Physicians' Health Study found no relationship. An observation from a 1997 study may help explain the varying results. Vitamin D acts on the prostate by binding to a special receptor; the study found that men with an abnormal vitamin D receptor gene have a greatly increased risk of developing aggressive prostate cancers. In 1998, the Physicians' Health Study reported a receptor effect only in men with low vitamin D levels. Additional research is required to clarify the interaction between sunlight, dietary vitamin D, and the vitamin D receptor gene. It is an important area, particularly in view of the new concern about calcium and prostate cancer.

Calcium

It's an article of faith, almost on a par with motherhood and apple pie: Calcium reduces the risk of osteoporosis and fracture, but the evidence of benefit is much stronger for women then men (see Chapter Four). For both sexes, calcium may help lower blood pressure.

Until 1998, nobody worried about calcium and the prostate. But in that year, the Health Professionals Study noted that men with a high consumption of calcium from either food or supplements had an increased risk of advanced prostate cancer; the risk was greatest in men who got more than 2,000 milligrams of calcium per day. At the same time, the researchers found that a large amount of fructose (fruit sugar) was protective; they also confirmed the link between dietary fat, especially animal fat and prostate cancer.

Although fat is a well-established prostate cancer risk factor, the worrisome news about calcium and the good news about fructose were new. But the Harvard scientists speculate that calcium and fructose are linked to the prostate through vitamin D. High levels of calcium can reduce the body's production of active vitamin D (calciferol); by lowering levels of phosphate, low levels of fructose can have the same result.

In the years since the Health Professionals Study raised concern about calcium, additional data have started to appear. The results are mixed. In 2001, the Physicians' Health Study reported that men who have a high intake of milk have low levels of active vitamin D and a 32 percent increase in the risk of prostate cancer. But three smaller studies from other centers in the United States and Italy disagree, finding no risk from calcium in supplements or foods.

It's a work in progress. More research is needed to clarify a possible relationship among calcium, fructose, and vitamin D. For now, men should follow the current guidelines for calcium (1,000 milligrams per day until age fifty, 1,200 milligrams thereafter) and vitamin D (200 international units per day below age fifty, 400 international units from fifty-one to seventy, and 600 international units thereafter). And, yes, men should eat plenty of fruit.

WHAT TO EAT

Prostate cancer is complex and incompletely understood, and so is nutrition. Scientists know that a man's diet affects his risk of developing prostate cancer, but the details are still being worked out. New research adds cereals and whole grains, nuts and seeds, and fish to the "good" list that already includes tomatoes, soy, and other vegetables. Although data are less convincing, vitamin D may help, and supplements of selenium and vitamin E (at least in smokers) appear promising. In contrast, animal fat leads the "bad" list, and there are preliminary concerns about a high consumption of alpha-linolenic acid and calcium.

It will take time for scientists to unravel the intricate interplay between nutrition and prostate cancer. While they are at work, though, it would be reasonable for men to pile on the whole grains and tomatoes and to seek soy where they can. Men who are attracted to supplements can consider a multivitamin for its vitamin D and reasonable doses of selenium (200 micrograms a day) and vitamin E (100 to 400 international units a day). Above all, skip the burgers.

The Natural History of Prostate Cancer

Although proof requires additional research, there are many reasons to suppose that a good diet and healthful lifestyle can reduce a man's risk of prostate cancer. But prevention is not perfect, and every man should understand what is likely to happen if prostate cancer strikes.

If there is a single word that describes the natural history of prostate cancer, it is variability. The course of the disease is hard to predict. In many cases, it is an indolent disease that grows slowly . . . so slowly that two of every three men with prostate cancer never develop any symptoms of the disease. Indolent prostate cancers take ten to twelve years before they are even large enough to be detected by sophisticated tests—and then they take another five or six years to double in size. Many indolent prostate cancers remain microscopic in size and are discovered only after a man dies of some other cause.

Although many prostate cancers are indolent, some are much more aggressive, which is why 30,200 American men will die from prostate cancer this year. It is a frightening statistic, but it's important to remember that only one of every ten men with prostate cancer actually dies from the disease.

Without effective treatment, aggressive prostate cancers enlarge within the gland itself, then penetrate through the capsule that surrounds the prostate to invade adjacent tissues such as the seminal vesicles. From local tissues, the tumors spread next to the lymph nodes in the pelvis, then to distant organs and tissues. Metastatic prostate cancer often invades bones, particularly in the spine and in the pelvis itself.

Because men with the disease in its early stages feel perfectly well, the only way to detect tiny prostate cancers is to screen men routinely (see page 363). But when prostate cancer enlarges and spreads, it can produce symptoms ranging from urinary and sexual dysfunction to bone pain, weakness, and weight loss.

In order to predict a man's prognosis and plan appropriate treatments, doctors should be able to distinguish indolent cancers from aggressive ones. Unfortunately, it is often impossible. The only available measure is the Gleason score, which relies on how the cells look under a microscope (see Staging Prostate Cancer, page 377). But two-thirds of all prostate cancers fall into a gray zone of mid-range Gleason scores, and doctors cannot tell if they will grow slowly or quickly. It is an urgent problem that cries out for new research.

Because prostate cancer is so variable and so unpredictable, it is hard to know if particular methods of diagnosis and treatment are beneficial. Men with indolent cancers might remain well without any treatment, while some with unusually aggressive tumors might succumb despite all therapy. It is one of the things that makes prostate cancer so puzzling and frustrating—and there are other barriers to understanding the unusual disease:

First, the disease grows slowly. In many other cancers, doctors can declare a cure after five years, but since most prostate cancer patients survive more than five years without any therapy, doctors have to wait ten or even fifteen years before they can be sure a treatment is effective. Studying cancer is always hard; studying prostate cancer is also slow.

Second, the method by which prostate cancer is diagnosed has changed dramatically. In the past, most prostate cancers were diagnosed when they were large enough for doctors to feel during a *digital rectal exam* (DRE), or when they had spread far enough to cause symptoms. Since the early 1990s, though, most have been detected much earlier as a result of the blood test for *prostate specific antigen* (PSA) (see page 363). Scientists cannot make valid comparisons between small tumors detected by PSA testing and those diagnosed by older methods.

Third, treatment has also changed (see page 381): Advances in surgical techniques have improved the *radical prostatectomy* operation; *3-dimensional conformal radiotherapy* and *brachytherapy* (seed implants) have revolutionized radiation treatment; new drug programs are changing *androgen-deprivation therapy,* and entirely new methods such as *cryotherapy* (freezing) are being introduced. It is always hard to compare treatment methods, and even harder when the methods are changing so quickly.

Faced with a frightening disease like cancer, many patients decide simply to follow the advice of their doctors instead of trying to figure out what to do on their own. In most cases, it is a good strategy, but men with prostate cancer are likely to get very different advice from different doctors. Researchers from Harvard, the University of Massachusetts, and the University of Connecticut highlighted the problem when they asked more than 1,000 physicians what they would recommend for a typical prostate cancer patient. Faced with exactly the same clinical profile, 93 percent of the urologists recommended surgery while 72 percent of radiation oncologists suggested radiotherapy.

It is a terrible dilemma that researchers at Harvard Medical School have described as "chaos." The only way out of the quagmire is with clinical trials (see Chapter Two). More than 100 trials of prostate cancer diagnosis and treatment are in progress, and many more are being planned. Many trials are now recruiting participants, but each has strict eligibility requirements. To find out what trials are available, you can call the National Cancer Institute at 1-800-4-CANCER (1-800-422-6237) or you can visit the National Institutes of Health website at www.clinicaltrials.gov and enter "prostate." Be sure to review all trials with your doctor before you take the plunge.

Until new research results are available, uncertainties about the diagnosis and treatment of prostate cancer will persist. Still, men confronted with the possibility of prostate cancer cannot wait five or ten years to find out what really is best. Instead, they have to use the best current information to decide on testing and treatment.

Diagnosing Prostate Cancer: The PSA

The *prostate specific antigen* (PSA) test is the most important recent development in men's health. It is also the most controversial. The test is important because it is the best way to detect prostate cancer at its earliest, most curable stage. But it is controversial because doctors do not yet know if routine PSA testing will save lives. It is a confusing situation that will only be resolved with clinical trials similar to the ones that proved that routine Pap smears help women—and the ones that discovered that routine chest X-rays do not have a role in preventing lung cancer deaths.

What Is PSA?

PSA is a *glycoprotein,* a sugar-containing protein. It is called prostate-specific since the only cells in a man's body that produce significant amounts of PSA are the epithelial cells of the prostate gland. In healthy men, PSA's job is to liquefy semen, allowing it to flow freely after ejaculation (see Chapter Ten); it works by digesting other proteins in semen. PSA is present in high concentrations in semen, and it can easily be detected in the ejaculate. In fact, it was discovered by forensic pathologists in search of an easy way to detect semen in cases of suspected sexual assault.

Blood PSA Levels

Although PSA is intended for semen, it finds its way into the blood as well. Blood PSA levels of 0 to 4 ng/ml (nanograms per milliliter) are considered normal. Levels between 4 and 10 are borderline, those above 10, clearly abnormal. The higher the PSA, the greater the likelihood of cancer. But there is no sharp dividing line between levels that are reassuring and those that are worrisome, and many things besides cancer can affect PSA levels.

Doctors and patients worry when they see high PSA levels, but low PSAs do not necessarily rule out cancer. Men with low testosterone levels tend to have low PSAs. Therapy with *finasteride* (Proscar), used to treat *benign prostatic hyperplasia* (BPH), also lowers PSA levels (see Chapter Eleven).

While cancer is the most important cause of high PSAs, it is not the most common cause of elevations. That dubious distinction belongs to BPH. PSA levels generally rise with age, since older men have larger prostates and more PSA-producing cells. Prostatitis (inflammation and infection) also boosts PSA levels. Despite earlier beliefs, digital rectal exams do not cause a significant rise in the blood PSA. Mythology notwithstanding, bicycle riding has also been exonerated. But ejaculation does seem to increase the blood PSA level. The rise is brief, peaking at one hour after ejaculation and returning to normal within twenty-four to forty-eight hours. Although not all studies agree that ejaculation boosts the PSA, men should abstain from ejaculation for forty-eight hours before having a PSA test. Even without ejaculation, PSA levels can vary considerably from day to day, sometimes by as much as 2 nanograms per milliliter. Because of this, abnormal results should always be confirmed before any action is taken, particularly if they fall in the borderline 4 to 10 range.

Although many factors can influence the PSA level, cancer is clearly the most important cause of elevations. When cancer is responsible for raising the PSA, levels below 10 usually reflect early disease confined to the gland itself, levels of 10 to 20 often signify local spread, and levels above 50 indicate widespread cancer involving lymph nodes, bones, and other tissues.

THE PSA IN MEN WITH CANCER

There is no debate about the value of the PSA in these circumstances. Every man with clinically suspected prostate cancer should have a PSA test. Most often, suspicion arises because of abnormal findings on digital rectal exams, but cancer may also be suspected if rapidly progressive bladder obstruction, impotence, bone pain, weight loss, or other symptoms raise concern. And every man with diagnosed prostate cancer should have his PSA measured, not just once, but at regular intervals. That's because serial PSA measurements are the best way to monitor the course of the disease and the efficacy of treatment (see page 381).

THE CASE FOR ROUTINE PSA SCREENING

The American Cancer Society (ACS), the American Urological Association (AUA), and the American College of Radiology recommend that doctors offer annual PSA testing to every man above age fifty. They also call for yearly testing to start at age forty (AUA) or forty-five (ACS) for men at increased risk, including African Americans and men with strong family histories of prostate cancer.

They have a point. Requiring only a single blood sample, PSA testing is quick, easy, and safe. With a typical cost of about $40, it is inexpensive, and covered by Medicare and most insurance plans. In addition, technical improvements have made it reliable in most labs. In the most favorable studies, PSA screening has a sensitivity of about 80 percent; the Physicians' Health Study reported a sensitivity of 73 percent. In other words, the PSA succeeds in detecting cancer in seven to eight of every ten men with the disease. Without PSA screening, about 40 percent of prostate cancers are not diagnosed until they have spread too far to be curable. Early detection is surely the best hope for curing prostate cancer, and PSA is the best way to find early disease. The American prostate cancer death rate has been falling steadily since 1992, and many experts give the PSA testing credit for the progress.

The Case Against Routine PSA Screening

The U.S. Preventive Services Task Force, the Canadian Task Force on the Periodic Health Examination, and the Canadian Urological Association recommend against PSA testing in men who seem healthy. The American College of Physicians and Academy of Family Physicians says that men should be counseled about "the known risks and uncertain benefits of screening for prostate cancer" before they undergo any testing.

They, too, have a point. Although an individual PSA test is inexpensive, it would be very expensive to test every American man above fifty and to follow up abnormal results with biopsies (about $12 billion). Still, testing would save money if early diagnosis could reduce the need for even more expensive treatment of advanced cancer. But critics of PSA testing go beyond economics to consider drawbacks of the test itself.

First, they consider sensitivity. Even if PSA screening were 80 percent sensitive, it would fail to detect two of every ten prostate cancers, and some studies peg the failure rate even higher. Still, if men with early disease benefited from the test, their gain would outweigh the false reassurance provided to the men whose disease had been missed. But what of the test's specificity? What of the men who have high PSA results but do not have cancer? In some studies, up to two of every three men with elevated PSA results turn out *not* to have cancer. That means they experience the worry of a possible cancer diagnosis, and the discomfort of a prostate biopsy without needing any of it.

Most men would gladly trade two false alarms for one life-saving early diagnosis. But here is where the debate really heats up. The value of an early diagnosis of cancer seems indisputable. Indeed, the early diagnosis of invasive breast cancer, cervical cancer, and colon cancer has saved millions of lives. But counter to expectations, prostate cancer may be different.

Unlike the other common malignancies, prostate cancer can have a long *latent phase*. Cancer cells can exist in the prostate gland for years, even decades, without causing harm. An American man's risk of developing prostate cancer at some time in his life is about 30 percent, yet his risk of developing clinically important disease is less than 10 percent. In other words, two of every three prostate cancers are harmless, even if untreated.

Early prostate cancer is usually treated with either surgery or radiation.

Both treatments carry risks, ranging from pain and diarrhea to urinary incontinence (1 to 3 percent for radiation, 1 to 27 percent for surgery) and impotence (40 to 67 percent for radiation, 20 to 85 percent for surgery). Even so, most men would trade continence and potency for life, but it's not that simple. About 9 million American men have prostate cancer right now, but only about 30,200 of them will die from the disease this year. Even if the PSA test was cost-free and 100 percent sensitive and specific, universal testing would lead to expensive, potentially harmful treatments for millions of men who would never need therapy. For some early prostate cancers, particularly in older men, no treatment ("watchful waiting") may be just as effective as aggressive therapy (see page 382). For example, in a recent study from Connecticut, men who were diagnosed with localized, low-grade prostate cancer between the ages of sixty-five and seventy-five but did not receive treatment lived just as long as men who never had cancer. And the prostate cancer death rate in England and Wales has declined in parallel with the death rate in the United States, even though PSA screening has not been adopted in Britain.

FUTURE DIRECTIONS

Experts disagree about the value of PSA testing, but they all agree that improvements are needed. Current research efforts focus on two goals: improving the accuracy of the PSA itself and evaluating the impact of early diagnosis on survival and quality of life.

Improving the PSA. Three refinements of the PSA are being evaluated:

- *Age-Adjusted Normals.* Since the PSA level rises with age in healthy men, perhaps age should be taken into account to decide if a man's PSA is normal. Here is a proposed adjustment:

Table 12.2: AGE-ADJUSTED PSA RANGES

AGE (YEARS)	NORMAL PSA RANGE (NG/ML)
40–49	0–2.5
50–59	0–3.5
60–69	0–4.5
70–79	0–6.5

Until age-adjusted reference ranges are validated by additional research, however, most doctors will still use the single value of 4.0 as the upper limit of normal.

- *PSA Velocity.* Although PSAs tend to rise with age, rapid increases are more suggestive of cancer. The PSA velocity reflects the rate of change: PSAs are measured yearly, and annual increases of more than .75 nanograms per milliliter are considered worrisome. PSA velocities are most accurate in men who have had at least three annual tests. Although interesting, this approach requires that a man with an elevated PSA wait a year before having additional tests. More study is needed before the PSA velocity can be recommended.
- *Free PSA.* PSA travels in the blood in one of two ways, either bound to other proteins or unbound and free. A large number of studies report that bound PSA rises in cancer, whereas a high free PSA is more likely to reflect benign enlargement of the gland. Free PSAs that are less than 25 percent of the total PSA increase the likelihood of cancer; values below 10–15 percent are particularly worrisome. In contrast, free PSAs amounting to a percentage above 25 are reassuring. The free PSA is the most promising refinement of PSA screening, but it does not eliminate the problem of false positive results, nor does it tell if screening saves lives.

Outcome Studies. The bottom line for any test is its ability to prolong and improve life. A computer analysis of the current PSA test produced the gloomy prediction that in the average man, a test at age fifty would prolong life less than a day, while slightly diminishing its quality. But mathematical models cannot replace observations of real men. Two American studies, the Prostate, Lung, Colorectal, and Ovarian (PLCO) screening trial and the Prostate Cancer Intervention Versus Observations Trial (PIVOT), are already under way, as is the five-nation European Randomized Study of Screening Prostate Cancer (ERSPC). But the all-important results will not be available for a decade or more.

What is a Man to Do? In ten years we may know if PSA screening is worthwhile. But that's a long time to wait. What should men do today?

Nobody really knows. There is considerable pressure for every American man over fifty to have an annual PSA test. The American Cancer Society and the American Urologic Association have been joined by distinguished Americans such as football legend Johnny Unitas, General Norman Schwarzkopf and Intel CEO Andrew Grove in urging the tests. Women who understand the value of PAP smears are perhaps even more influential. They may be right.

Despite its real value, however, the PSA is no "male PAP test." It can detect many cancers long before they can be diagnosed by any other means, but it will also miss many. About two of every three men who have abnormal PSAs will undergo frightening, invasive tests only to find that they are perfectly healthy. Above all, doctors do not yet know if the aggressive treatment of prostate cancers diagnosed by PSA screening will prolong life and some are concerned that such treatment may actually reduce the quality of life.

Should you have a PSA? There is no right answer to this all-important question, but there are two wrong answers, "no" and "yes." At present, the only truly honest answer is "maybe." Until new research is available, every man should discuss the decision with his doctor and his family then decide for himself. Men with higher than average risks (positive family histories, African Americans, high-fat diets) might be more likely to request it. Men who would elect aggressive treatment for early cancers are also likely to want a PSA tests. On the other hand, men over age seventy, men who are concerned about the discomfort of transrectal ultrasounds and prostate biopsies, and men with medical conditions that limit their life expectancy to ten years or less may reasonably decide against the test.

The U.S. Office of Technology Assessment said it best: "An informed and reasonable patient could equally well decide to have screening or forego it." Here is a summary of the four main facts you will need to make your decision:

1. Prostate cancer is common. Unlike most malignancies, the growth pattern and natural history of prostate cancer is highly variable. It may be aggressive and lethal, but it is more likely to be indolent.

2. The PSA is the best way to detect prostate cancer in its early, potentially curable stages.

3. PSA testing has false-negative and false-positive results. There is a substantial probability that annual testing will lead to invasive testing that does not detect cancer.

4. The early diagnosis and aggressive treatment of prostate cancer may save lives, but it can also have substantial adverse side effects. The benefits of PSA screening and aggressive treatment have not been proven. If screening has value, it is likely to diminish after age seventy and is less likely to help men with serious medical conditions.

In a sense, the PSA is a paradigm for much of modern medicine. It is a great technological advance, but it has provided *knowledge* about diagnosis before doctors have gained *wisdom* about treatment.

Diagnosing Prostate Cancer: The Digital Rectal Exam

The digital rectal exam (DRE) is a traditional part of the annual physical exam for men older than forty. Time-honored or not, many experts are now questioning the value of the routine DRE. That is because newer tests are much better at detecting early prostate and colorectal cancers, two of the principal goals of the DRE. In reviewing the evidence, the blue-ribbon U.S. Preventive Services Task Force concluded, "There is insufficient evidence to recommend for or against routine screening with [the] digital rectal examination."

Few men would regret the demise of the DRE, which is surely the least pleasant part of the annual physical exam. But is it really wise to abandon it? Has modern technology made your doctor's educated finger obsolete?

The Exam

Most men recall the procedure quite vividly, but few realize that there is a simple way that patients can make the exam much easier on themselves, and on their doctors.

The DRE is simplicity itself. The doctor inserts a well-lubricated, gloved index finger into the patient's rectum, and then feels the prostate gland in a process called *palpation*. At the same time, the physician feels for rectal masses that might indicate rectal cancer or other abnormalities. In most cases, the exam takes less than fifteen seconds, but immediately after the DRE, most docs will perform an additional step, using an inexpensive but very sensitive chemical test to check for traces of blood in a tiny fecal specimen. Because the test looks for amounts of blood too small to be visible to the eye, it is called the *fecal occult blood test* (FOBT).

Although the main purpose of the routine DRE in men who feel well is to examine the prostate and rectum, doctors will also evaluate the rectal opening itself. That is where you can make things much easier. The rectum is guarded by strong *sphincter muscles* that close the passage to keep you from soiling yourself. If you bear down as if to move your bowels, you will relax your sphincter muscles, facilitating entry and making the exam faster and less uncomfortable. You can also lend a hand by spreading your buttocks apart.

Although the exam is uncomfortable (and undignified), it should not be painful. DREs are quick and, and most cases, free of cost and side effects. To perform the exam, some doctors ask men to lie on their sides with their legs curled toward their chests, while others ask men to stand and bend forward with their arms resting on the exam table.

That's all there is to the DRE. But while they are in the vicinity, many doctors will also check their patient for groin hernias or enlarged lymph nodes and for abnormalities of the scrotum and testicles (see Chapter Nine).

THE DRE FOR SYMPTOMS

Although there is controversy about the role of the DRE in screening men who feel well, there is no doubt of its value when men have certain symptoms.

The DRE is essential to evaluate men with *prostatitis* or other infections of the genitourinary tract (see Chapter Eleven); urinary burning and frequency, rectal discomfort, fever, and cloudy or bloody urine are among the common symptoms. A DRE should also be performed in men who are found to have even modest numbers of red or white blood cells detected in a urinalysis.

Men with rectal or intestinal symptoms also should have DREs. The exam can be very informative in men who notice rectal discomfort or itching, constipation, painful bowel movements, narrow stools, protracted diarrhea, or the presence of blood or mucous in the feces. Doctors will also use the exam as a quick check for internal bleeding in men with anemia, ulcer symptoms, or unexplained *hypotension* (low blood pressure).

DRE FOR SCREENING

If you head into your doctor's office for an annual check-up, you're likely to be hitching up your trousers on the way out, even if you have no urinary or rectal symptoms. Does it really have to be that way?

Doctors use the routine DRE to screen for two major diseases, prostate cancer and colon cancer. Everyone agrees that they are common and serious diseases. Prostate cancer is diagnosed in about 189,000 American men annually and it is responsible for nearly 30,200 deaths; colon cancer is detected in about 50,000 men a year and is responsible for at least 23,000 deaths. Can the DRE detect either disease early enough to make a difference?

DRE for Prostate Cancer

Until the late 1980s, the DRE was the only way to screen for early prostate cancer. But it's an imperfect test. During DREs, doctors can feel only the rear and sides of the prostate and at least 30 percent of cancers occur in areas of the gland that are simply out of reach. Even when they are in range, prostate cancers are too small to be felt in their earliest stages, which is also when the potential for cure is greatest. On its own, the DRE will detect only a fraction of prostate cancers in asymptomatic men; although the figures vary, it is likely that routine DREs will miss at least 80 percent of prostate cancers. And the DRE has another shortcoming, since doctors may feel a nodule, hard area, or asymmetry of the prostate in many men who do not have prostate cancer. Of every ten men who have prostate biopsies because of abnormal exams, only three or four will turn out to have cancer.

Enter the PSA; despite disagreements about the test, even the severest critics agree that it is more sensitive and specific than a DRE. Does that spell the doom for the DRE? According to researchers in Rotterdam, the Netherlands, the answer is yes. As part of the European Randomized Study of Screening for Prostate Cancer, doctors performed both DREs and PSAs on 10,525 men who had no prostate symptoms. They also performed *transrectal ultrasounds,* but this imaging test is no longer recommended for cancer screening (see page 373). By itself, the DRE detected prostate cancer in 264 men, but PSA-based screening detected 473, nearly twice as many.

But this 1998 European report is not the end of the story, much less of the DRE. In fact, scientists in the United States have arrived at different conclusions. Researchers in St. Louis screened 22,513 men with both PSAs and DREs at six-month intervals. They found suspicious DREs in 2,703 men who had normal PSA results (below 4 nanograms per milliliter). Biopsies were performed in 1,905 of these men; 244 or 13 percent had cancer. And more than 75 percent of the men had early, potentially curable tumors.

Scientists in Minnesota evaluated the question in another way. They tracked the residents of Olmstead County to see if men who had DREs fared any better than men who did not. In all, men who had the exam were only half as likely to die from prostate cancer as men who did not.

Each of these studies has limitations, and none settles the issue. But in reviewing all the evidence, a multispecialty panel convened by the American Urologic Association concluded, "There is clearly strong evidence in favor of including both DRE and PSA in any program for early detection of prostate cancer." It is an entirely reasonable conclusion, but it does not answer the more important, still unresolved question of whether any form of prostate cancer screening saves lives.

Does the DRE have a role in following men who have had radical prostatectomies? (See page 387.) Probably not. Doctors in Miami tracked 501 men after the operation and reported that DRE was never helpful unless the PSA was elevated. Similar results have been reported in men who have had radiation therapy.

Men who choose to be screened for prostate cancer should have a DRE along with a PSA. But although every man above age fifty should be screened for colon cancer, the DRE is not the answer; it has been supplanted by much better tests, which are discussed in the Epilogue.

Diagnosing Prostate Cancer: Imaging and Biopsy

A picture is worth a thousand words. When it comes to the prostate, unfortunately, it's not so easy. The gland is small and located deep in the body at the base of the bladder. Like other soft tissue organs, it does not show up at all on ordinary X-rays. And even computed tomography (CT scanning) is unable to picture the prostate in sufficient detail. But in recent years, new techniques have been developed to provide images of this elusive organ.

ULTRASOUND

Ultrasound is used to image internal organs in many parts of the body. In all cases, the guiding principle is the same. High-frequency sound waves are beamed into the body; the sound waves echoed back from the target organ are processed by a computer, then projected onto a video screen and captured in photographic images. In most cases, the ultrasound probe is placed on the skin, but sometimes it is placed in a body cavity to get a closer look. For example, a probe can be placed on the chest wall to picture the heart, but more accurate pictures can be obtained if the probe is passed down the esophagus, positioning it just behind the heart.

Although prostatic ultrasonography was introduced some thirty years ago, it has improved substantially in recent years. Now, a small ultrasound probe is placed into the rectum, allowing sound waves to be aimed directly at the nearby prostate, in a procedure called *transrectal ultrasonography* (TRUS).

TRUS may be a bit uncomfortable, but it is not painful, hazardous, or time-consuming. However, it is expensive. The accuracy of the test depends on good equipment, a well-trained operator, and an experienced radiologist or urologist to interpret the images. When everything is right, TRUS can produce detailed pictures of the prostate, measuring it in three planes to allow an accurate calculation of its volume. As a result, TRUS can detect prostatic enlargement, establishing a diagnosis of benign prostatic hyperplasia (BPH). TRUS may also be able to detect infections of the prostate, including prostatitis and prostatic abscesses. But when it comes to cancer, TRUS has a mixed record.

Prostate cancers do not reflect sound waves as well as normal prostate tissue. As a result, lesions that are *hypoechoic* on TRUS are considered suspicious for cancer. TRUS can detect lesions as small as 5 millimeters (about the size of a pencil eraser), so it can identify some cancers that cannot be detected by DRE because of their small size or because they are located deep in the gland (see Figure 12.1). That's the good news. The bad news is that TRUS is not reliable for the diagnosis of early prostate cancer. That's because up to 30 percent of prostate cancers have the same echo patterns as normal prostate tissue, so they evade detection by TRUS. Conversely, inflammation and other benign lesions can have low echo reflections, which may look just like cancers. In all, only about 20 percent of hypoechoic lesions prove to be cancerous when they are biopsied. For the same reasons TRUS is not able to determine whether or not a tumor has penetrated through the prostate's capsule, a key factor in planning therapy (see Staging Prostate Cancer, page 377).

Even though TRUS has limited value in screening and staging, it has great value in managing prostate cancer. That's because it allows doctors to visualize the prostate when they perform a biopsy, and it is also essential for placing the radioactive seeds used to treat patients with *brachytherapy* (see page 395).

New technology is further refining TRUS—and advances in physics and biomedical engineering have produced a rival, *magnetic resonance imaging* (MRI).

Magnetic Resonance Imaging

MRIs have revolutionized many areas of medicine. They are particularly valuable for neurologic diseases because they are able to provide detailed images of the nervous system from the brain to the spine. In magnetic resonance imaging, a radio transmitter is used to beam photons into the patient's tissues, which absorb the photons. As a result, the tissues emit energy, which is cap-

FIGURE 12.1. TRANSRECTAL ULTRASOUND OF PROSTATE

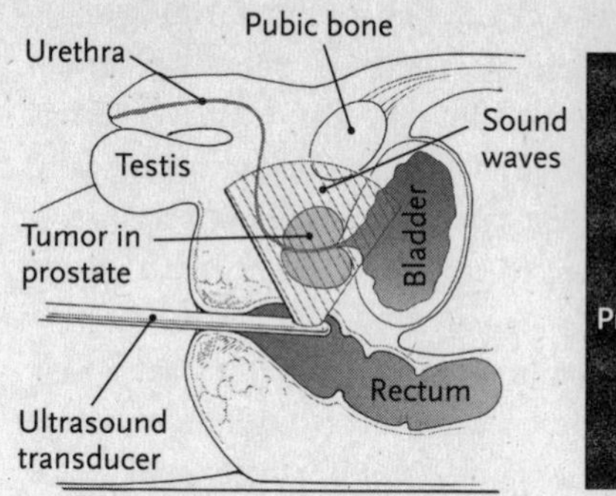

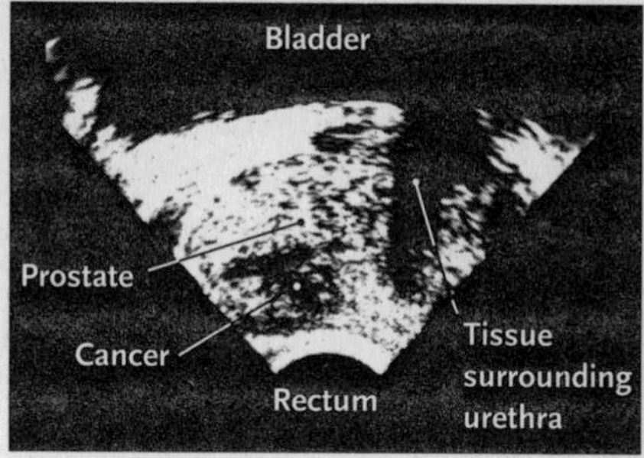

If prostate cancer is suspected, a transrectal ultrasound exam may be performed to provide an image of the prostate. In this procedure, the patient lies on his side and a small probe (the ultrasound transducer) is placed in the rectum. Sound waves are beamed at the prostate, and the waves that are reflected back are transformed by a computer into images on a video screen. In the sonograph above, the irregular dark area within the prostate is a cancer. The larger dark area on the right side of the image represents the tissue surrounding the urethra.

tured by a magnetic coil and processed by a computer to produce an image of the tissue. Like ultrasound, MRI does not use radiation and is extremely safe.

Either an external body coil or an internal rectal coil may be used to obtain MRIs of the prostate; the rectal coil is superior. MRI is more expensive than TRUS, and some patients may experience claustrophobic panic reactions in the MRI chamber. But despite its much more sophisticated and expensive technology, MRI has not been much more successful than TRUS for diagnosing early cancers and microscopic spread, though it can help detect advanced disease in patients with very high PSAs (see Staging, page 377). New techniques such as *proton spectroscopic MRIs*, *gadolinium-enhanced MRIs*, and *multi-coil MRIs* may eventually help doctors stage prostate cancer more accurately.

Biopsy

A tissue biopsy is the gold standard for the diagnosis of cancer. The rule applies to the prostate as much as any organ, but until 1989, prostate biopsies were difficult hit or miss affairs. That changed dramatically when doctors began to use ultrasound-guided, spring-loaded biopsy guns to biopsy the prostate.

It sounds brutal, but it's not. The patient lies on his side with his knees pulled up to his chest. Then the doctor introduces an ultrasound probe into the patient's rectum. So far it's exactly like any TRUS. But after performing an ultrasound, the doctor introduces a biopsy gun through the rectal probe, lines it up with the prostate, and fires a set of needles into the gland. Most men feel pressure but little pain, and the discomfort lasts only a second or two. Finally, the physician removes the biopsy gun and retrieves the tissue specimens, which are sent on to labs where pathologists examine them under a microscope.

Transrectal biopsies can be performed in a doctor's office and the whole process takes only ten to fifteen minutes from start to finish. Complications are uncommon; pain is the most frequent complaint, but it is usually mild, and a new study reports that preparing the rectum with a simple anesthetic gel can reduce discomfort. Many men note blood-tinged urine or semen and about 10 percent have blood in their feces, but the bleeding is mild and it stops on its own in nearly all cases; to reduce the risk of bleeding, patients should not take aspirin or similar medications that increase the risk of bleeding for seven to ten days before the procedure. Bacteria may enter the urine during the biopsy and they sometimes make their way into the blood, but only 2–3 percent of men develop fever and require antibiotics. Still, men with abnormal heart valves or artificial joints that could become infected should receive special antibiotic preparation for a biopsy.

Transrectal biopsies are simple and safe because the needles are so tiny, less than one-sixteenth of an inch in diameter. But the small size of the needle is the weakness of the test as well as its strength. Each biopsy specimen is a tiny thread of tissue about one-half inch long and no thicker than a fishing line.

If a TRUS or digital rectal exam reveals a specific abnormality, the doctor will target that area for biopsy. Most often these days, though, a biopsy is performed because of an elevated PSA and there is no specific target. In that case, the biopsy simultaneously samples cores of tissue from six to sixteen regions of the prostate.

Because the samples are so small, a needle biopsy will miss 15–30 percent of prostate cancers that are large enough to raise the PSA but too small to show up on a TRUS or DRE. It is one of the many, many paradoxes of prostate cancer: Though reassuring, a negative transrectal biopsy does not completely rule out cancer.

Many urologists have switched from the original 6-core technique to 8, 12, or even 16-core biopsies to improve the accuracy of prostate biopsies. Some repeat a biopsy if the first is negative, and still others follow the patient's PSA and DRE, repeating a biopsy only if things change.

New studies demonstrate that 12-core biopsies are as safe as the older 6-core procedures; some studies show they improve the diagnostic yield, but others disagree. And doctors don't yet know the answer to the sixty-four-dollar question: Will an aggressive program of screening men with PSAs and biopsies save lives?

Staging Prostate Cancer

"How bad is it, Doc?"

It is the question most men ask after they get over the shock of hearing that their prostate biopsy found cancer. It is a crucial question, but it is hard for doctors to answer, since prostate cancer is such a variable disease. Still, to plan therapy, doctors will have to estimate the extent and severity of a man's cancer. To do so, they evaluate the tumor's grade and its stage.

MICROSCOPIC GRADING

Pathologists diagnose cancer by examining biopsy specimens under a microscope. But they also evaluate how malignant the cells look; *well-differentiated* cells look the closest to normal; *poorly-differentiated* cells have a wilder, more malignant appearance; *moderately-differentiated* cells lie between the extremes. In general, well-differentiated cancers have the best prognosis, poorly-differentiated, the worst.

Like other malignancies, prostate cancers are classified according to their cellular differentiation. But since that system provides only a rough guide, pathologists also use the *Gleason grading system,* which is based on the architectural relationship among cells rather than the appearance of individual cells. Using this method, pathologists assign a grade between 1 and 5 to the tumor. Grade 1 tumors look the most normal, with individual cells lined up in a nearly normal glandular pattern; Grade 5 tumors are distorted and irregular, with cells clumped into cords and tubes; Grades 2, 3, and 4 lie between the extremes. But since cancer cells can look different in a single prostate biopsy, pathologists score the two most representative regions independently, then tally them to arrive at a single Gleason score between 2 and 10. Tumors with scores 2, 3, and 4 have the best outlook, tumors with scores of 8, 9, or 10, the worst. Tumors with Gleason scores of 5, 6, and 7 behave variably. Since two-thirds of prostate cancers are in this gray zone, it is very hard for doctors to predict if they will be aggressive or indolent. Scientists are working hard to develop better systems, but until they succeed, the Gleason grade will remain the best guide to a tumor's likely behavior.

Anatomic Staging

Diagnosing prostate cancer and assigning a grade to the tumor are relatively simple. To plan therapy, though, doctors must determine the stage of the disease. That is because prostate cancer begins in one area of the gland and then spreads, first within the prostate, then through its capsule to the *seminal vesicles* and neighboring tissues, then to lymph nodes and bones. Different stages of the disease require different treatments.

Most prostate cancers are diagnosed by means of an ultrasound-guided transrectal-core biopsy. In such cases, doctors will have three important pieces of information by the time they perform the biopsy that diagnoses prostate cancer: the results of a digital rectal exam, a blood PSA level, and the results of a transrectal ultrasound (TRUS). For most men with PSAs below 20, additional imaging tests are rarely positive—but even though they are not necessary, many doctors order them anyway. It is a waste of money and it can produce as much worry as reassurance. On the other hand, men should have more imaging tests if they have PSAs above 20, very high grade tumors with PSAs of 10 to 20, or worrisome symptoms such as back pain, weakness, or weight loss. In such cases, *magnetic resonance imaging* (MRIs) or *computed tomographic (CT) scanning* may be used to look for enlarged lymph nodes in the pelvis and abdomen. In addition a *bone scan* can be employed to look for metastatic disease.

Unfortunately, however, patients with negative scans may still have microscopic spread of the tumor through the capsule. It is a crucial distinction that determines if a man is eligible for surgery, but until new MRI techniques prove their mettle (see page 374), the only way to be sure is to remove the gland surgically and send it to a pathologist for evaluation.

There are two major systems for evaluating prostate cancer based on the location and size of the tumor: the older Whitmore-Jewett classification and the more widely used TNM system. Although the fine print varies, both methods convey similar information (see Table 12.3). The Whitmore-Jewett system assigns a letter from A to D to each cancer, with a number to indicate gradations within each stage. The TNM system also evaluates the primary tumor (T), the lymph nodes (N), and distant metastases (M). Before surgery, patients are

Table 12.3: STAGING PROSTATE CANCER

WHITMORE-JEWETT	TNM (TUMOR, NODE, MESTASTASES)
Stage A. Microscopic cancer confined to the prostate and too small to be felt by digital rectal exam (DRE) A1. Cancer well differentiated and confined to one site A2. Cancer moderately or poorly differentiated or present in more than one site	**Primary Tumor** T1. Microscopic cancer, too small to be detected as a nodule by DRE or imaging. T1a. Involves less than 5 percent of tissue obtained by transurethral resection of the prostate (TURP) T1b. Involves more than 5 percent of tissue obtained by TURP T1c. Identified by needle biopsy performed for high PSA
Stage B. Cancer large enough to be felt on DRE B1. Small nodule on one lobe of prostate B2. Large nodule, several small nodules, or a nodule containing poorly differentiated cells	**T2.** Larger cancers that are still confined to the prostate T2a. Involves half of lobe or less T2b. Involves more than half a lobe, but not both lobes T2c. Involves both lobes
Stage C. A large cancer involving nearly the entire gland C1. Cancer may have spread a small distance beyond the gland C2. Cancer has invaded the neighboring tissue	**T3.** Tumor extends through capsule T3a. Extends on one side T3b. Extends on both sides T3c. Involves seminal vesicles
Stage D. Widespread (metastatic) cancer. D1. Cancer in pelvic lymph nodes D2. Cancer in bone or other organs	**T4.** Tumor invades beyond seminal vesicles T4a. Invades bladder, sphincter muscle, and/or rectum T4b. Invades pelvic muscles **Lymph nodes** N0. No involvement N1. Small tumor in a single pelvic node N2. Medium-size tumor in one node or small tumors in several nodes N3. Large tumor in one or more nodes **Metastases** M0. No tumor detected M1. Distant spread present M1a. Distant lymph node, beyond the pelvic region M1b. Bone involved M1c. Other organs invaded

assigned to a stage based on clinical criteria; clinical staging can be noted by a "c" placed before the T stage. Patients who undergo radical prostatectomy are staged pathologically based on an examination of their tissues; a "p" before the T stage denotes pathological staging.

INTERPRETING THE RESULTS

If the behavior of prostate cancers could be predicted simply and accurately, there would be only one staging system. Since the disease is unpredictable, however, there are many factors to consider. In general:

- Low-volume tumors that are too small to be felt on DRE or seen in TRUS have a better prognosis than tumors large enough to form detectable nodules.
- Tumors that are present in only one region of the gland have a better outlook than those that are found in cores from several different regions of the prostate.
- Men with low PSAs (below 10 to 20) have a better prognosis than men with higher PSAs. PSAs below 10 usually reflect early, localized disease, whereas levels of 10 to 20 may signify local spreads, and levels above 50 usually indicate widespread disease.
- Well-differentiated tumors with low Gleason scores (2 to 4) are less aggressive than poorly differentiated tumors with high Gleason scores (8 to 10).
- Cancers confined to the prostate gland (stages A and B, or T1 and T2) have a better prognosis than tumors that have extended beyond the gland (stages C and D or T3 and T4).
- Men without lymph node, bone, or other organ metastasis (stage C or N0, M0) fare better than men with metastatic spread (stage D or N1-3, M1).

Knowing the grade and stage of prostate cancer is one thing, knowing what to do about it, quite another thing. Unfortunately, treatment decisions are like most areas of prostate cancer, uncertain and even contentious.

Treating Prostate Cancer: The Big Picture

Nearly 200,000 American men will be diagnosed with prostate cancer this year, and each will have an urgent need to know what treatment is best for him.

It's a crucial question and a fair one. To answer it, the American Urological Association (AUA) convened an authoritative Prostate Cancer Clinical Guidelines Panel, but after reviewing more than 12,500 studies, it was unable to establish standard-of-care recommendations. When the panel tried to compare the outcome of patients treated with watchful waiting, surgery, and radiation, they found they were comparing apples to oranges. The studies that have been completed to date differ so substantially in patient age, disease stage, and follow-up that direct comparisons are not possible. New studies to resolve these issues are already in progress, but they will not be completed for years. Until the results are in, the panel recognized that there are many acceptable options for the management of prostate cancer. They suggested that doctors inform their patients about the advantages and limitations of each treatment, enabling every man to choose among them for himself.

It's a sound position, but it puts men with prostate cancer in the very difficult position of making hard decisions about complex questions, often before the shock of the diagnosis has worn off. Fortunately, however, there is no need to rush into treatment. Instead, men with prostate cancer should take the time they need to gather information, digest the facts, and discuss them with relatives and friends. In many cases, the decision-making process will benefit from independent second and third opinions from doctors with unique perspectives; urologists, radiotherapists, and oncologists have their own views, and each can help. A diagnosis of prostate cancer calls for decisions that are difficult, but they should not be lonely.

THERAPEUTIC OPTIONS

"Who should decide," asked Alexander Pope, "when doctors disagree?" Here are some general guidelines to help men decide for themselves: Prostate cancer can be managed conservatively or aggressively. At present, the major choices include observation alone (watchful waiting), surgery (radical prostatectomy), radiation (external beam or brachytherapy with implanted radioactive seeds); hormonal manipulation followed by radiation (neoadjuvant therapy), and hormonal treatment (androgen deprivation therapy). Doctors are also investigating cryotherapy for localized disease and chemotherapy and for advanced disease.

To make a choice, a man must know the stage of his tumor and its Gleason grade. But other factors are just as important; a man must also consider his age, his general health and life expectancy, and the experience and skills of his medical team. Last but not least, every patient should include quality of life considerations, including the side effects of treatment, in his decision.

In general, men with early disease (stages A and B or T1 and T2) have the widest range of options; older men with small tumors and low Gleason scores often choose radiation or watchful waiting; younger men with higher Gleason scores often choose surgery or radiation. Most men with locally advanced disease (stage C or T3) receive radiation, with or without hormonal treatment. Men with widespread disease (stage D or T4) usually benefit from androgen deprivation therapy.

General guides, however helpful, do not apply to every man. Each man with prostate cancer should consider his options in detail.

Treating Prostate Cancer: Watchful Waiting

It is an approach that goes by many names, including observation, surveillance, expectant treatment, and deferred treatment. By any name, when a man elects watchful waiting he decides to forgo prompt, potentially curative therapy for prostate cancer.

Refusing treatment for a newly-diagnosed cancer sounds suicidal, but in the case of prostate cancer, it is not. That's because most prostate cancers grow slowly, and many never produce any symptoms. Men choose watchful waiting because they believe they may die from another disease before their prostate cancers become threatening.

Watchful waiting does not mean that a man's prostate cancer will go untreated. Instead, it means that doctors will start treatment only if symptoms develop or if tests suggest that symptoms are likely to occur. Although deferred treatment with androgen deprivation therapy and/or radiation is not curative, it can produce excellent results, with prolonged relief of symptoms.

Men who select watchful waiting should be watched, but doctors disagree on just how closely they should observe their untreated prostate cancer patients. Most patients return for a digital rectal exam and a PSA blood test every six months. If the PSA rises by more than a few points or if the doctor detects a new or enlarging lump in the prostate, additional tests such as transrectal ultrasounds, CT scans, or bone scans may be indicated.

Above all, men who elect deferred treatment should watch themselves, reporting to their physician if they develop pain, urinary symptoms, impotence, fatigue, or weight loss. Some men may also elect to follow a low-fat, whole-grain rich diet and take supplements of lycopene, vitamin E, selenium, vitamin D, or soy products. None of these has a proven role in prostate cancer, but each shows promise, at least for prevention (see Diet and Prostate Cancer, page 353).

SURVIVAL WITHOUT THERAPY

Because the clinical course of prostate cancer is so variable, doctors have to rely on the size and grade of prostate cancers to predict their behavior. Based on these criteria, an American College of Physicians task force offered estimates summarized in Table 12.4.

Table 12.4: THE IMPACT OF UNTREATED PROSTATE CANCER ON LIFE EXPECTANCY

	ESTIMATED LIFE EXPECTANCY		
	At Age 55	**At Age 65**	**At Age 75**
Men who do not have prostate cancer	21.4 years	14.5 years	9.0 years
Men with very small* low-grade prostate cancers	21.4 years	14.5 years	9.0 years
Men with small** low-grade prostate cancers	17.5 years	12.6 years	8.3 years
Men with medium-grade prostate cancers	17.5 years	12.6 years	8.3 years

*Tumor volume less than 0.5 ml
**Tumor volume above 0.5 ml

Source: Coley et al. *Annals of Internal Medicine*. 1997; 126, 468–479.

DOES WATCHFUL WAITING WORK?

This is, of course, the crucial question, but there is no absolute answer. That's because the criteria for diagnosing and staging prostate cancer vary from study to study, and the patients included in various investigations also differ. Still, there is enough information to identify some men for whom watchful waiting may be a good choice and to recognize the larger number of patients who would probably benefit from prompt treatment with either surgery or radiation.

Most of the information comes from Europe. In particular, doctors in Scandinavia tend to recommend watchful waiting much more often and surgery much less often than their American counterparts. Some recent examples of individual studies from both sides of the Atlantic:

- A 2000 study evaluated 813 Swedish men who had been diagnosed with localized prostate cancer (stage T1 or T2) between 1974 and 1986. The men were managed with watchful waiting and were followed for ten to twenty years. The prostate cancer survival rates were 85 percent at ten years, 80 percent at fifteen years, and 63 percent at twenty years. Men with low-grade tumors fared better than those with moderate or high-grade cancers (ten-year survival rates: 90 percent, 74 percent, and 59 percent respectively).
- A 1998 Connecticut study of 767 men with localized prostate cancer diagnosed between 1977 and 1984. The men were fifty-five to seventy-four years of age at the time of diagnosis; none received surgery or curative radiotherapy. During fifteen years of observation, men with low grade (Gleason score 2 to 4) tumors had only a low risk (2 to 7 percent) of dying from prostate cancer. In contrast, men with high grade (Gleason score 7 to 10) tumors had a 42 to 87 percent chance of dying from prostate cancer within fifteen years.
- A 1998 Swedish analysis of fifty men with an average age of seventy-one who were diagnosed with locally advanced prostate cancer between 1978 and 1982. Although all the men had T3 tumors that had spread beyond the prostate, none received aggressive treatment. During the first five years of watchful waiting, only 10 percent of the men died from prostate cancer; by twelve years, 30 percent had died from the disease while 44 percent had succumbed to other illnesses.
- A 1997 report from Sweden that analyzed 642 patients with an average age of seventy-two who were diagnosed with prostate cancer between 1977 and 1984. After fifteen years of follow-up, prostate cancer accounted for 37 percent of the 541 deaths in the entire group. But in the 300 patients with localized disease at the time of diagnosis, only 19 percent died of prostate cancer—and the percentage was identical for the 223 men who deferred treatment and the seventy-seven who were treated promptly.

- A 1997 report from Sweden that followed 133 men with an average age of sixty-eight who were diagnosed with low-grade, localized prostate cancer between 1978 and 1982. During the first five years of watchful waiting, only 29 percent required therapy but 57 percent of the men who survived ten years received treatment during that time. In all, only 10 percent of the group died from prostate cancer during ten years of observation, but by fifteen years, the prostate cancer death rate was 25 percent.
- A 1997 report from Denmark that evaluated 719 men with an average age of seventy-five who were diagnosed with prostate cancer between 1979 and 1983 and were managed with watchful waiting. Among the men with early disease, 26 percent died from prostate cancer within ten years, but this relatively poor outcome may reflect the fact that most of the men had symptoms by the time they were diagnosed and only a few of the men underwent diagnostic tests to accurately stage their disease.
- A 1995 report from Connecticut that evaluated 451 men with an average age of seventy-one who were treated with watchful waiting for localized prostate cancer that was diagnosed between 1970 and 1976. After fifteen years of follow-up, men with low-grade tumors (Gleason grade 2 to 4) survived as long as men who did not have prostate cancer at all, but men with higher grade tumors experienced a progressively decreased life expectancy.
- A 1992 report from Washington, D.C., that evaluated 233 patients who chose watchful waiting for localized prostate cancer diagnosed between 1967 and 1989 in a single private urology practice. The overall survival was not different from the survival predicted from life tables of men of similar ages who did not have cancer.
- A 1990 report from Wisconsin that evaluated 111 men diagnosed with early prostate cancer between 1967 and 1975. At the time of diagnosis, the patients were randomly assigned to receive watchful waiting or surgery (*radical prostatectomy*). After fifteen years of follow-up, the overall survival was identical. Men with low-grade tumors survived as long as predicted from life tables for men of similar ages, but men with high Gleason scores had a poorer survival, whether treated with watchful waiting or surgery. Because this was an early study, the pa-

tients did not have detailed staging tests; as a result, the disappointing results of surgery may not apply to men who are staged by current standards.

Each of these small studies has its limitations, and their findings may or may not apply to American men diagnosed with prostate cancer today. Although reports that pool individual studies also have limitations, they are also instructive. Recent examples include:

- A 1997 analysis of 59,876 prostate cancer registry patients age fifty to seventy-nine. For low-grade cancers, the ten-year survival from prostate cancer for men treated with watchful waiting was 93 percent, about the same as for surgery (94 percent) or radiotherapy (90 percent).
- A 2001 study of 2,311 men who were between the ages of fifty-five and seventy-four when they were diagnosed with prostate cancer in the years between 1971 and 1984. For men with low-grade cancers, the ten-year survival from prostate cancer was the same, 94 percent, for those treated with watchful waiting and surgery, and was 83 percent for the radiotherapy patients.
- A 1994 analysis of 828 men treated with watcful waiting for early prostate cancer. The ten-year survival from cancer for men with low- and moderate-grade tumors was 87 percent but only 34 percent for men with high-grade disease.
- A 1993 analysis of 586 patients treated with watchful waiting found a ten-year prostate cancer survival rate of 83 percent.

QUALITY OF LIFE

Most patients view a diagnosis of cancer as a matter of life and death, and most treatment trials agree, focusing on the length of survival as a measure of success. But the quality of life is important as well, particularly when the disease is as slow-growing as many prostate cancers.

Although the quality of life is harder to measure than the length of life, studies of prostate cancer suggest that watchful waiting has the edge over aggressive therapy. Watchful waiting has no side effects, while surgery and radiation have many, ranging from transient pain and diarrhea to permanent impotence and incontinence. A 1995 study from California, for example, found that men who were treated with watchful waiting for localized prostate cancer had a better disease-related quality of life than men treated with either surgery or radiation. Faced with therapeutic options, most men with prostate cancer will consider survival first, but all patients should also consider comfort and function as they arrive at a decision.

DECISIONS, DECISIONS

It is hard for doctors to interpret studies done at different times in different countries with patients diagnosed by different criteria. For a patient with prostate cancer, it is even harder to digest all the statistics. Still, a picture of the men who are most likely to benefit from watchful waiting emerges from these studies.

Watchful waiting is a reasonable option for men with early, low-grade (Gleason score 6 or less) localized prostate cancer (stages A and B, T1 and T2) who do not have symptoms from the disease. Men with larger or higher grade tumors are likely to develop symptoms that require treatment.

Watchful waiting is most appropriate for older men, particularly those above seventy to seventy-five. Older men are much more likely to die *with* prostate cancer than *from* it. Younger men with disease that limits their life expectancy to ten years or less are also good candidates for watchful waiting.

Watchful waiting is a reasonable option for men who understand the potential advantages and disadvantages of deferred treatment and who are comfortable with the approach. Many men, particularly Americans, expect that a diagnosis of cancer will be followed promptly by treatment; watchful waiting is not appropriate for men who "want to get it all out" or "get on with it." But men of a certain age who can live comfortably with a diagnosis of cancer should consider the option, providing they have early, asymptomatic disease. In fact, watchful waiting can enable many men with prostate cancer to live more comfortably without sacrificing life expectancy.

Treating Prostate Cancer: Surgery

It is the oldest treatment for prostate cancer, having been introduced by Dr. Hugh Young in 1905. But it has been improved greatly over the years as a result of the *retropubic* approach developed in the 1940s, the nerve-sparing operation pioneered by Dr. Patrick Walsh in the 1980s, and the improved techniques for postoperative care devised in the 1990s. The future may be even brighter, as surgeons work to perfect *minilaparotomy* and *laparoscopic* approaches, small-incisional operations that are not yet widely available. At present, though, most American urologists consider the *radical prostatectomy* the "gold standard" therapy for localized prostate cancer, which is why it will be performed in as many as 100,000 men this year. But despite its long history and popularity, the radical prostatectomy is a sometimes controversial operation that has attracted its share of skeptics as well as its passionate advocates.

Many men with prostate cancer choose surgical treatment for their disease, and with good reason. But every man should consider the advantages and disadvantages of surgery and the options that are available before arriving at that decision.

The Operation

Unlike the simple operations that treat benign prostatic hyperplasia by removing only the portion of the gland that blocks the flow of urine (see Chapter Eleven), the radical prostatectomy is designed to cure cancer by removing all the disease. As a result, the operation removes the entire prostate gland along with the seminal vesicles and surrounding tissues. It is not an easy task. The prostate lies deep within the body, wedged between the rectum and bladder, wrapped around the urethra, and surrounded by important nerves that are vulnerable to injury.

Surgeons can approach the prostate from either of two directions. Most favor the retropubic technique that uses an incision in the lower abdomen. It has the advantage of allowing the surgeons to remove pelvic lymph nodes to be sure they do not contain cancer before operating on the prostate itself. The older perineal prostatectomy uses an incision in the area between the anus and scrotum. It is now regaining some of its lost popularity because the PSA test can help determine if lymph node sampling is necessary, and surgeons can use a small abdominal incision to sample lymph nodes through a laparoscope before making the perineal incision itself.

If the surgeon suspects the cancer may have spread to the patient's lymph nodes, he will remove the nodes and rush them to the pathologist who is standing by to examine them through a microscope. If cancer is present, surgery will not be able to cure the disease, so the operation will go no further and the patient will be offered radiation or hormonal treatment. But if the lymph nodes are negative, the surgeons will carefully separate the prostate and seminal vesicles from the surrounding tissues. To actually remove the gland, the surgeons will have to cut through the urethra just above the bladder, but they sew the tube that carries urine out from the bladder back together once the prostate is removed. Once removed, the tissue will be sent to the pathology laboratory for microscopic evaluation. If the cancer is present only within the prostate, the operation has the potential to cure, but if the tumor has already extended through the capsule surrounding the gland, additional treatment is usually recommended.

The nerve-sparing prostatectomy is an important variation on the theme. It is designed to protect and preserve the fine network of blood vessels and nerves that run along both sides of the prostate. If the nerves are not damaged, there is a greater chance that the patient will preserve his potency, but the operation requires special skill, and some surgeons are concerned that a nerve-sparing operation is more likely to leave some cancer cells behind. It is an unresolved question, and newly-available treatments for impotence have introduced another variable. All in all, men who choose a radical prostatectomy should discuss the pros and cons of a nerve-sparing procedure with their urologists before deciding. And all men should keep an eye on new surgical developments; a few doctors are experimenting with nerve mapping and nerve transplants in an attempt to preserve potency, but it is far too early to know if these efforts will succeed.

Most radical prostatectomies are performed under general anesthesia, but spinal anesthesia is also an option. The operation is quite safe, with a mortality rate below 1 percent in most centers. After spending three to five hours in the operating room, the average patient will spend just two to four days in the hospital. Even so, he will need several weeks to recuperate at home, and he will have to urinate through a Foley catheter for one to three weeks while his urethra heals.

SURGICAL RESULTS

Even with advanced surgical techniques and improved postoperative care, a radical prostatectomy is a big deal. Knowing that, men choose to have the operation because they believe it offers the best chance to cure prostate cancer. Indeed, men with low-grade cancers confined to their prostates can expect excellent results. The ten-year-cancer-survival rates for such men may exceed 90 percent.

With such excellent results, why doesn't every man choose a prostatectomy? For one thing, low-grade localized cancers also respond very well to less invasive management strategies, including radiotherapy and even watchful waiting. In addition, the surgery carries a substantial risk of complications. As with any operation, pain is to be expected, but it usually responds well to treatment. Bleeding and infection are also possible, but they, too, can usually be corrected. But a radical prostatectomy has unique complications, including impotence, urinary incontinence, and fecal incontinence. The risk of these complications varies from surgeon to surgeon and hospital to hospital. That is why every man who chooses surgery should seek out an experienced urologist with a good track record and a top-notch surgical team. (See Selecting a Surgeon, page 391). The variability also makes it difficult to predict the risk of complications. In broad terms, the risk for impotence ranges from 20 to 80 percent and for urinary incontinence, 2 to 15 percent; a 2000 National Cancer Institute study of 1,156 prostatectomy patients reported that 79.6 percent were impotent and 9.6 percent incontinent two years after surgery. Fecal incontinence is less common, occurring in perhaps 2 to 5 percent of patients.

The Decision

Cure versus complications—it is a hard equation to balance, particularly since the predicted percentages vary so widely. But there is even more to the equation, since a man with prostate cancer must also consider the stage of his disease, the grade of his tumor, and his age and general health.

Radical prostatectomy is potentially curative only when prostate cancer is confined to the gland. Even with the best available staging procedures, though, it is impossible to detect microscopic spread before surgery itself. Hence, 14 to 54 percent of patients undergo the operation only to learn that the pathologist detected unsuspected tissue invasion that requires additional treatment. For these men, unfortunately, the operation represents pain without gain.

A second issue is the grade of a man's tumor. Even with disease confined to the prostate, radical prostatectomies are most successful for low-grade cancers (Gleason scores 2 to 4). In a broad review of 59,876 cancer registry patients, for example, 94 percent of men with such tumors did not succumb to prostate cancer for at least ten years after radical prostatectomy. But the corresponding figures for moderate (Gleason 5 to 7) and high-grade (Gleason 8 to 10) tumors were 87 and 67 percent, respectively. The 2001 study of 2,311 men produced similar results; the ten-year-cancer-survival figures for surgical patients were 94 percent for low grade, 88 percent for moderate-grade, and 64 percent for high-grade cancers.

But if surgery is least likely to cure a patient with more aggressive tumors, these men many actually be the best candidates for surgery. It sounds like a paradox, but it is not. That's because the results of the competing therapeutic

Selecting a Surgeon

Doctors have made important improvements in the radical prostatectomy operation, but it is still a tricky procedure that requires a highly trained surgeon with special skill and experience. While some general surgeons perform the operation, you are likely to get a better result from a fully trained urologist who is certified by the American Board of Urology.

Although most young urologists have steady hands and good judgment (and every surgeon has to start with his first case), experience is an asset. If possible, pick a urologist who has at least a hundred of these operations under his belt and who averages two to three radical prostatectomies a month. Remember, too, that a surgeon is only as good as his supporting staff. That is why men who need the operation should consider going to a top-notch medical center.

Credentials carry a lot of weight, but they do not tell the whole story. Look for a doctor you can relate to and trust. Favor urologists who encourage you to consult with radiation therapists and medical oncologists before you decide on your treatment. Talk with other patients who may give you insights into how the doctor takes care of his patients in the months and years after surgery. And just as secretaries may be the best judge of their bosses' characters, nurses may be able to provide special insights into how a doctor operates.

For more information on picking a doctor, turn to the Epilogue.

choices fall off even more sharply with advancing tumor grades. In the same two studies, the ten-year cancer survival rates for radiation were 90 and 83 percent for low-grade tumors, 76 and 72 percent for moderate-grade, and 53 and 43 percent for high-grade tumors. For watchful waiting, the drop-off was even sharper, falling from 93 and 94 percent to 77 and 75 percent to 45 percent (in both studies) with advancing tumor grade.

It is important to stress that these results from 1997 and 2001 are far from definitive. As pointed out by the AUA Expert Panel, direct comparisons between treatment modalities are not really valid unless they are generated by a randomized, prospective, controlled clinical trial. No such trial has been completed. Still, most authorities interpret the available data as suggesting that radical prostatectomy is most likely to benefit men with localized but moderate to high-grade prostate cancers.

The third factor is the patient's age and health. Because most prostate cancers grow slowly, aggressive therapy is most likely to help men with the longest life expectancies. Men with serious diseases that could cause death or major disability within ten years are not likely to benefit from radical prostatectomy. The same is true for men in their seventies and eighties, even if they are in fine general health. It is a tricky issue, since no man likes to contemplate his mortality. Many eighty-year-olds feel great and are tempted to choose a surgical option that is best suited to younger men. In general, it is a mistake.

AFTER SURGERY

Because prostate cancer grows slowly, it can recur years after treatment. That is why all prostate cancer treatments require surveillance, even after successful radical prostatectomies. In most cases, follow-up takes the form of a simple office visit once or twice a year. The doctor will ask about your general health and he will check your weight and perform a digital rectal exam. If everything is fine, the only test you will need is a simple blood PSA. Since a radical prostatectomy removes the entire gland, the PSA should fall to immeasurably low levels within a month of surgery. As long as your PSA remains undetectable, you can be sure that you are free of recurrent prostate cancer. On the other hand, a rising PSA indicates recurrent disease. But in most cases, that is not as bad as it sounds. Since the PSA is so sensitive and since prostate cancer often grows slowly, it will take eight years for the average man whose post-operative PSA rises to at least 0.2 nanograms per milliliter to progress to metastatic disease, even if no therapy is administered. Men whose original tumors were high-grade malignancies, men with early PSA relapses, and those with rapidly rising PSAs are likely to develop clinical problems early on. To check for recurrent disease, doctors may perform ultrasounds, CT scans, bone scans, or biopsies. Even if cancer is detected, radiation or hormonal treatment can be very helpful. According to a recent study of 3,494 Medicare patients, 35 percent of radical prostatectomy patients require additional treatment within five years of surgery.

Treating Prostate Cancer: Radiotherapy

Along with watchful waiting and surgery, radiotherapy has been one of the traditional options for treating early prostate cancer, and it also has a well-established role in the management of more advanced disease. It has been hard enough for a man with early prostate cancer to choose among these alternatives, and the decision is getting even harder. That's because radiotherapy is changing; it now offers several options of its own, including advanced methods for delivering external beam therapy, new techniques for providing internal radioactive seed therapy, and evolving strategies for combined radiation and hormonal treatment.

All forms of radiation contain energy; it's what boils water in a microwave oven and what burns your skin after an ill-advised day at the beach. Radiotherapy delivers much more energy, enough to kill cells. Because cancer cells are growing faster than normal cells and are less able to repair radiation damage, radiotherapy can be used to treat many forms of cancer. The trick is to focus the radiation on the tumor as precisely as possible, thus minimizing damage to healthy tissues in the vicinity. In the case of prostate cancer, doctors can focus the energy of radiation from outside the body (*external beam radiation*) or from the inside, by placing radioactive seeds within the prostate (*brachytherapy*).

EXTERNAL BEAM RADIATION THERAPY

It is the standard approach to radiotherapy, but although it has been in use for decades, it has improved greatly in the past few years. Doctors can thank their physicist colleagues for these improvements, called *three-dimensional conformal radiation*. After a man chooses external beam therapy, his first step is to undergo a CT scan. The CT image is relayed to a computer that constructs a precise three-dimensional map of his prostate and seminal vesicles. The map allows the radiation therapist to target precisely the cancerous tissues while shielding the healthy tissues nearby, including the vulnerable bladder and rectum. As a result, doctors can now deliver 15 percent more radiation with fewer complications (3 percent rectal bleeding vs. 15 percent). And new studies show that high-dose radiotherapy produces better survival than conventional-dose therapy.

Each radiation treatment is based on the initial computerized simulation. The therapist is responsible for placing the patient on the treatment table in precisely the right location and for being sure his bladder contains the same amount of urine each day. The next step is to position lead shielding blocks to protect normal tissues. Finally, the therapist activates the overhead *linear accelerator* that actually delivers the radiation. Each treatment is painless and quick, lasting just a few minutes. But because the therapeutic dose must be built up gradually, the treatments are repeated five times a week for seven or eight weeks.

Modern conformal therapy can be tricky, and the best results come from experienced centers with sophisticated equipment and skilled therapists. But if high-quality treatment is available, external beam radiation is a good choice for many men with early prostate cancer.

As with any form of treatment, the results are best for small, low-grade cancers that are confined to the prostate. Controlled trials have not compared radiotherapy to surgery or watchful waiting, but the 1997 cancer registry study of 59,876 men with prostate cancer suggests that the three approaches have similar results for men with the most favorable disease, and those results are excellent, with ten-year-cancer-survival rates above 90 percent. In the smaller 2001 study, radiotherapy patients fared a bit less well (83 percent) than the surgical or watchful waiting patients (94 percent for both). For moderate-grade (Gleason 5 to 7) and high-grade (Gleason 8 to 10) cancers that are confined to the prostate, radiation does not seem as successful as surgery, but it appears similar to watchful waiting. Among men with such tumors, perhaps 45 to 75 percent can expect ten-year survival following external beam radiation. The results of radiotherapy are less favorable for cancers that have spread beyond the prostate, but surgery is not an option for men with such advanced disease.

Until comparative trials are completed, it will not be possible for doctors to predict which form of treatment is best. But even now, it is clear that radiation produces fewer side effects than surgery. Most men will experience fatigue and weight loss as their treatment progresses, but most are able to continue working throughout therapy. About 15 percent develop rectal symptoms (discomfort, diarrhea, bleeding) during or shortly after therapy, but long-term rectal symptoms persist in only about 3 percent. Similarly, bladder symptoms (discomfort, bleeding, incontinence) occur in about 10 percent early on, but persist in only about 3 percent of patients. The reverse is true of impotence, which becomes progressively more common as time goes by. In general, 50 to 90 percent of men experience erectile dysfunction within two years of radiotherapy. A 2000 National Cancer Institute study of 435 radiotherapy patients reported that 61.5 percent were impotent and 3.5 percent incontinent two years after treatment.

Since radiotherapy does not destroy the entire prostate gland, the PSA falls slowly and only rarely to undetectable levels. In addition, the PSA can "bounce" up and down following radiation. On average, it reaches its lowest level about a year and a half after successful therapy. Men with PSAs that fall to 0.5 ng/ml can expect the best results. Conversely, if the PSA rises from its low point on three consecutive tests taken three to six months apart, relapse is likely.

Radiotherapy is a good option for men with prostate cancer. It is usually the treatment chosen by men older than seventy and by men with medical conditions that would make surgery hazardous or decrease life expectancy to ten years or less. But even younger, healthier men with low-grade prostate cancer can benefit from radiation, and they should consider the merits and drawbacks of this option.

BRACHYTHERAPY

External radiation for prostate cancer dates back to 1915, when it was attempted by Dr. Hugh Young, the urologist who had introduced surgical removal of the prostate ten years earlier. Because of poor results, external radiation was abandoned until the 1950s and 1960s, when better equipment made it possible. The year 1915 also marked the start of brachytherapy, when Dr. Benjamin Barringer of New York attempted to treat prostate cancer by placing radium needles within the gland. Because of many problems, internal radiation was abandoned until the 1970s when it was revived briefly, only to be discontinued again because of poor results. But in the 1990s, internal or interstitial radiation has been gaining momentum, because improved imaging techniques are allowing doctors to implant tiny radioactive seeds directly in the prostate without surgery.

Although it goes by many names, most doctors refer to implant therapy as *brachytherapy*. That is because the radioactive seeds or pellets emit radiation that only travels a short distance; "brachy" comes form the Greek word for short. But since the radiation does not travel far, the seeds have to be placed in exactly the right location. *Computed tomography* (CT) and *transrectal ultrasounds* (TRUS) now make that possible.

Brachytherapy is performed under general or spinal anesthesia. First, the doctor places an ultrasound probe in the patient's rectum and often a Foley catheter in his bladder (see Figure 12.2). Next he uses TRUS and a computerized map of the prostate to guide his placement of the pellets, which are inserted through needles placed in the *perineum* (the area between the anus and scrotum). The procedure is over in an hour or two. Most patients can return home as soon as the anesthesia wears off, but men with bloody urine may have to use a urinary catheter for a day or two. Most doctors advise men to abstain from sex for about two weeks, then use a condom for several weeks, but there are usually no other restrictions on the patient's activity.

The seeds are composed of radioactive palladium, gold, or iodine. Because

FIGURE 12.2. BRACHYTHERAPY

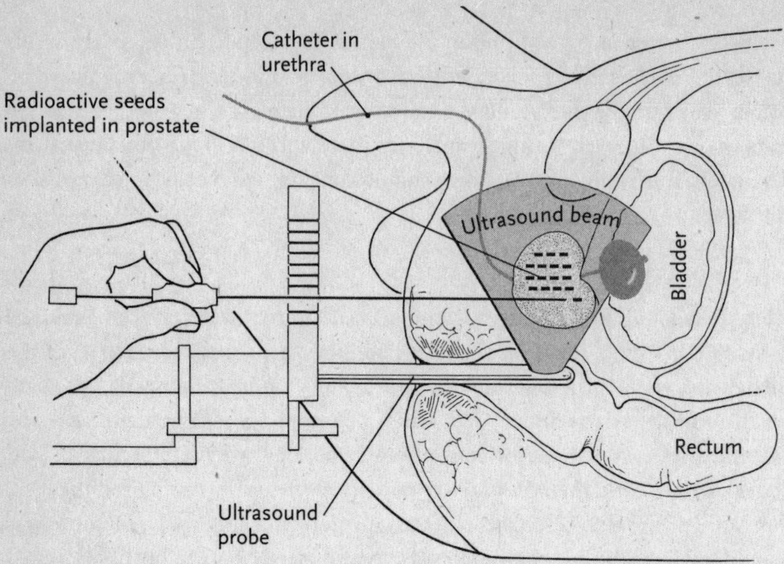

Brachytherapy is a new way to kill prostate cancer cells with radiation. Using ultrasound as a guide, the doctor inserts fine needles into the prostate, then places radioactive seeds directly into the gland. Unlike external beam radiation, brachytherapy requires only a single treatment, but anesthesia is necessary. More research is needed to compare the efficacy and side effects of the two forms of radiotherapy.

the pellets stop emitting radiation after several months, they can be left in place permanently. Because the radiation travels only a short distance, rectal and bladder complications are uncommon, but because some seeds are placed near the nerves and blood vessels that surround the prostate, erectile dysfunction often develops.

Compared to external beam radiation, brachytherapy has the advantages of requiring only a single treatment and of producing fewer complications. But it also has a major disadvantage: it is new. Preliminary data suggest that brachytherapy is about as effective as external beam radiation or surgery for low grade cancers, but less effective for higher grade tumors. However, it will take years for doctors to learn if these results will stand the test of time.

At present, doctors typically offer brachytherapy for men who choose radiation and have low-grade (Gleason scores less than 6) tumors and PSAs below 10. But more studies will be needed to learn if these seeds of hope will blossom into a major therapeutic option and to evaluate the new combination of external beam and implant radiotherapy.

COMBINED RADIATION AND HORMONAL THERAPY

Many forms of therapy are available for prostate cancer. Since no method is clearly superior to the others, patients and physicians must together choose among the available options. Since no form of therapy is uniformly successful, doctors are increasingly recommending combined treatments, especially for men with more advanced or high-grade tumors.

An example is the use of radiation following surgery. Surgery is the primary treatment. If a radical prostatectomy succeeds in removing all the cancer cells that can be identified, no additional treatment is necessary. But if the surgeon discovers cancer in the seminal vesicles, at the margin of the tissue that has been removed, or in nearby lymph nodes, the surgery will not be curative. In that case, doctors often recommend a secondary treatment, usually external beam radiation or hormonal therapy.

When the secondary treatment is administered shortly after the primary treatment, it is called *adjuvant therapy.* But sometimes the ancillary therapy is administered before the main therapy in an attempt to shrink or downstage the tumor before definitive treatment. When it is administered first, the secondary treatment is called *neoadjuvant therapy.*

Although combination therapy for prostate cancer is new, it holds real promise for men with locally advanced disease (stages B2 and C or T2C and T3; see Table 12.3). The goal is to shrink the tumor and make it more responsive to radiation by depriving it of *testosterone* and other *androgens* (male hormones). Although various approaches are under study, they all use androgen deprivation therapy before, during, or after radiotherapy. Preliminary results are encouraging, reporting improved control of the tumor, fewer recurrences, and improved survival. Combination therapy does produce more side effects than radiation alone, and further study will be needed to determine if it has long-term value. Unfortunately, neoadjuvant androgen deprivation therapy does not appear to improve the results of radical prostatectomy—but early androgen deprivation therapy after surgery may help men who have microscopic deposits of cancer cells in their lymph nodes.

Treating Prostate Cancer: Cryotherapy

Cryotherapy uses very cold temperatures to kill cancer cells. It is a hot new area of prostate cancer research, but it actually dates back to the 1970s. The early results of cryotherapy were poor, but major technical advances in the 1990s have revived interest in the procedure. Rescinding a 1996 decision, Medicare began paying for the treatment in 2000, and the American Urological Association has recently accepted cryosurgery as "one of the methods of management of adenocarcinoma of the prostate," but adds the important proviso that "the long-term curative efficacy of this treatment modality has not been established." Although some doctors would apply that proviso to all treatment methods, cryotherapy really is very new and should still be regarded as experimental.

From the patient's perspective, cryotherapy reassembles brachytherapy. It is performed under spinal or general anesthesia and requires only a brief hospital stay. As in brachytherapy, the doctor first places a rectal probe that allows him to use ultrasound to guide him as he places probes through the perineum. The fine probes are used to circulate liquid nitrogen through the gland, delivering freezing temperatures to the prostate. After the gland is frozen, the liquid nitrogen is shut off, allowing the gland to thaw. The best results are obtained when the freeze-thaw cycle is repeated a second time. A warming solution is circulated through the urethra to protect it from damage.

Because modern cryotherapy is so new, its long-term results are not known. Preliminary data suggest that about 15 percent of men who receive cryotherapy as the primary treatment for prostate cancer relapse in two years and about 45 percent have recurrences within five years. Unlike radiation or surgery, however, cryotherapy can be repeated to treat recurrent cancer, and it can be used as salvage therapy for men who relapse after radiation.

The complications of cryotherapy include rectal complaints and, more often, urinary incontinence. Impotence is very common after even one treatment, and the risk of urinary complaints increases when cryotherapy is repeated or when it follows failed radiation.

Cryotherapy is a new option that is currently available only at selected research centers, and more research is needed. But although further advances are surely needed, men with recurrent or advanced prostate cancer already have a tried and true treatment option: hormonal therapy.

Treating Prostate Cancer: Androgen Deprivation

Hormonal therapy for prostate cancer dates back to 1941 when Drs. Huggins and Hodges reported that *androgens* (male hormones) fuel the growth of prostate cancers and that androgen-deprivation therapy could slow or halt that growth. It was a seminal discovery, important enough to earn the Nobel Prize, and it remains the basis for the treatment of advanced prostate cancer more than half a century later. Despite the long and successful history of androgen-deprivation therapy, however, it shares two features common to all the newer therapies: uncertainty and debate. While all doctors agree that hormonal therapy has an important place in treating advanced prostate cancer, they disagree on which treatment is best and when it should be started. As in all areas of prostate cancer, the choice among options for hormonal therapy requires an individualized decision by the patient and his doctor.

HORMONES AND THE PROSTATE: A LENGTHY CHAIN

Doctors Huggins and Hodges discovered that androgens stimulate the growth of prostate cells, both benign and malignant, but those brilliant scientists might be surprised to learn how complex the process has turned out to be (see Figure 12.3).

It all begins in the brain, where the *hypothalamus* produces the hormone that starts things off. Although it is a single protein, it has two names, *gonadotropin-releasing hormone* (GnRH) and *luteinizing hormone-releasing hormone* (LHRH). Hormones are chemicals that are produced in one part of the body before traveling to another part, where they do their work. LHRH is a true hormone, but it does not have to travel very far to do its job. Instead it acts on another part of the brain, the *pituitary gland,* where it stimulates the release of two additional hormones, *follicle stimulating hormone* (FSH) and *luteinizing hormone* (LH).

FSH and LH were named by scientists who discovered that they stimulate the female ovary, but they are just as important for men. LH stimulates the *Leydig cells* in the testicles to produce *testosterone,* the primary androgen or male hormone. About 95 percent of a man's androgens are produced by his testicles, the remainder by his *adrenal glands,* which are not under the control of LH and FSH.

After testosterone enters the blood, about 95 percent of the hormone is bound to proteins while 5 percent circulates free. It is the free testosterone that acts on the prostate by diffusing into the gland's *epithelial cells.* Androgens from the adrenal gland also enter prostate cells, where they are converted to testosterone.

After testosterone enters the prostate cells, it is converted to *dihydrotestosterone* (DHT); the enzyme *5 alpha-reductase* is responsible for the conversion.

FIGURE 12.3. HORMONES AND THE PROSTATE

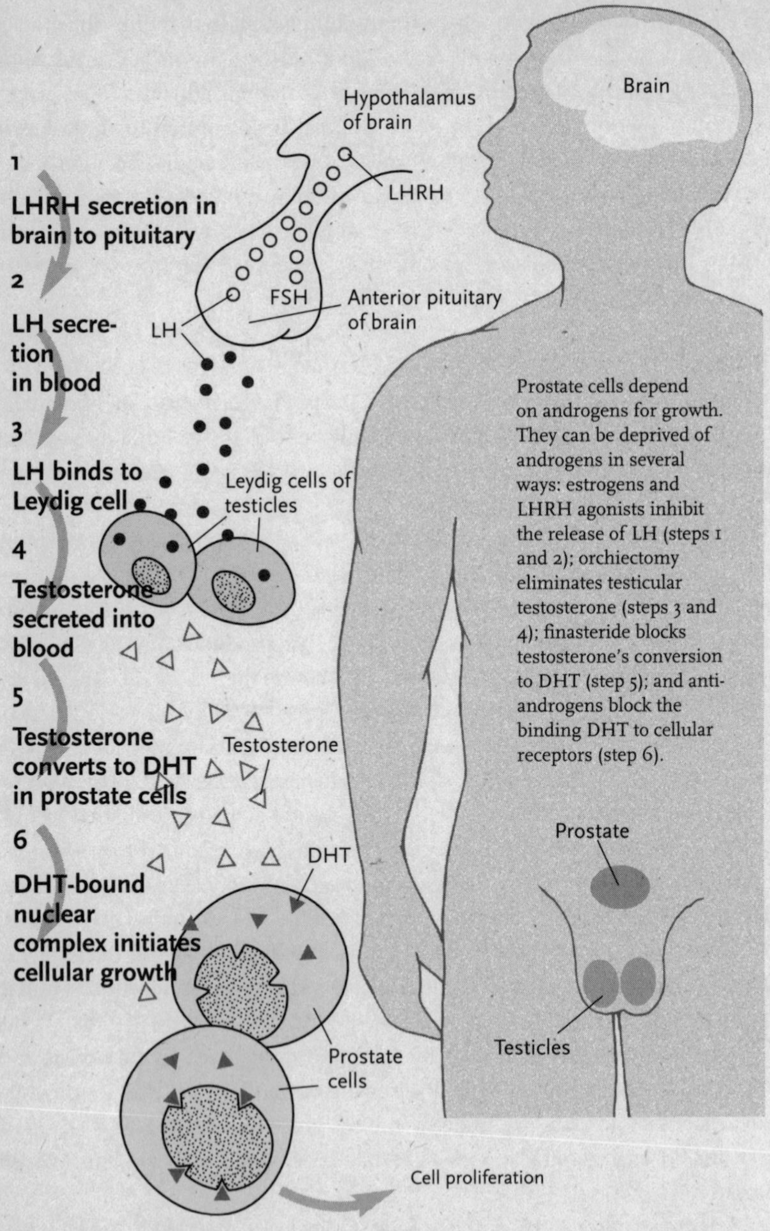

DHT is the final hormone in the long and complex chain that links the brain to the prostate. DHT binds to *androgen receptors* in the prostate cells. The DHT-receptor complex turns on the cells' DNA, stimulating cellular growth.

It is a complex series of events, but it's important to all men. It is what starts the prostate growing in adolescence and what causes the additional enlargement of benign prostatic hyperplasia (BPH) in older men (see Chapter Eleven). And it's what stimulates the growth of malignant cells in men with prostate cancer.

BREAKING THE CHAIN

The doctors who discovered that androgens drive the prostate also learned they could put the brakes on by removing the testicles (*orchiectomy*) or administering *estrogens* (female hormones). The original treatments are still in use, but they have been joined by newer, more popular methods of androgen deprivation. All the methods work in the same way: When prostate cells are deprived of androgens they commit suicide by the process of *apoptosis* or programmed cell death. Androgen deprivation usually succeeds in shrinking prostate cancers and reducing symptoms. Although the improvement is often prolonged, it cannot be expected to produce a permanent cure. That's because a small proportion of the prostate cancer cells do not require androgens to grow. These androgen-insensitive cells continue growing, slowly enlarging enough to produce symptoms that no longer respond to hormonal treatment. And new research suggests that in some patients, prostate cancer cells can undergo mutations of their androgen receptors so they are actually stimulated by anti-androgen medications.

TREATMENT OPTIONS

There are many links in the chain of hormones that stimulate the prostate, and there are many ways to break the chain. Each method has its advantages and its drawbacks. Because studies have not demonstrated the superiority of any method, doctors disagree as to which is best. At present all appear to have similar effectiveness and all share one side effect, the loss of libido and sexual potency. Despite these common features, though, there are important differences in cost and conveniences as well as in certain other side effects. Here is a rundown on the major options.

- *Orchiectomy.* Surgical removal of the testicles is the fastest way to deprive the prostate of androgens. Testosterone levels plummet within hours, and they stay at very low levels permanently. The operation is fast and safe. Side effects include breast enlargement, which is usually mild. Like all forms of androgen deprivation therapy, orchiectomy causes bones to lose calcium, which can lead to osteoporosis. It also leads to hot flashes, which can often be controlled by progestational drugs such as *medroxyprogesterone* (Provera) or *megestrol* (Megace), or by newer treatments such as the antidepressant *venlafaxine* (Effexor), the antiseizure drug *gabapentin* (Neurontin), or a low-dose estrogen patch.

Orchiectomy is a convenient, one-step, inexpensive treatment. Many doctors think it is the best method of androgen deprivation, but most men with advanced cancer opt to take medications instead, no doubt because of psychological reactions to the operation.

- *Estrogens.* In women, natural estrogens help regulate the menstrual cycle by shutting down LHRH. In men, estrogens will also block the release of LHRH, thus reducing testosterone levels (see Figure 12.3).

  Although many estrogens can be used to treat prostate cancer, the standard preparation is *diethylstilbestrol* (DES). In the 1960s, pioneering studies by the Veterans Administration Cooperative Research Group (VACURG) showed that DES worked as well as orchiectomy. But the first VACURG study also gave DES the bad name it retains today, since men treated with DES had an increased risk of death from heart attacks and blood clots. The first VACURG study used 5 milligrams of DES, but a second study found that a 1 milligram dose was as effective clinically, even though it did not produce a full reduction of testosterone. At 1 milligram per day, DES carries a much lower risk of cardiovascular side effects. Estrogens do not cause hot flashes or bone calcium loss, but they do produce breast enlargement. DES is inexpensive. At the 1 milligram dose, DES is a viable option for androgen-deprivation therapy, especially for men with healthy hearts. Viable or not, it is rarely prescribed by American doctors today and the drug is no longer readily available in the United States.

- *LHRH agonists.* These synthetic drugs resemble LHRH, but unlike the real thing, they block the release of FSH and LH by the pituitary, thus reducing testosterone production (see Figure 12.3). LHRH agonists are now the mainstay of androgen-deprivation therapy. They are equivalent to orchiectomy in their ability to reduce testosterone levels and produce a clinical response. Their side effects (loss of libido, hot flashes, breast enlargement) are also similar. The two major preparations are *goserelin* (Zoladex) and *leuprolide* (Lupron). Both can cause a brief flare in symptoms due to a surge in testosterone production that lasts a week or two. After that, testosterone levels remain extremely low. Both drugs are extremely expensive, and both are administered by injections every one to three months.

- *Antiandrogens.* Unlike the other forms of hormonal therapy, antiandrogens do not inhibit testosterone production; instead, they block the action of androgens on the cellular level. Antiandrogens act against testosterone and DHT, and they also block the effects of the weaker androgens produced by the adrenal glands that constitute about 5 percent of the blood's normal androgen activity. Antiandrogens do not usually cause hot flashes and they are less likely to reduce libido and potency than other forms of hormonal therapy. In addition, they do not lead to osteoporosis. However, they may cause breast enlargement, diarrhea, and other side effects. The major preparations include *bicalutamide* (Casodex), *flutamide* (Eulexin), and *nilutamide* (Niladron). All are taken orally and all are expensive.

Doctors are still studying how to best use antiandrogens. Most often, they are prescribed during the first weeks of LHRH agonist therapy to protect against the early rise in testosterone and the temporary symptoms that would otherwise occur. They are sometimes prescribed after orchiectomy or with LHRH agonists to produce *total androgen blockade,* but recent studies cast doubt on the benefit of this approach. Antiandrogens are also being tested for use alone. In a recent trial, castration and bicalutamide produced equally favorable results in 480 men with locally advanced (stages T3 and T4) prostate cancer. After 6.3 years, the overall survival rate was 56 percent. Some men who take antiandrogens alone retain erectile function.

New research suggests that some prostate cancer cells may become paradoxically dependent on antiandrogens. That means that some patients with advanced prostate cancer that has escaped conventional hormonal therapy actually improve after antiandrogens are discontinued. The benefits of the so-called antiandrogen withdrawal syndrome may last a year or even longer.

- *Ketoconazole.* It is a popular antifungal drug that many people use for athlete's foot. In very high doses, though, ketoconazole blocks androgen production, both in the adrenals and the testicles (see Figure 12.3). In these doses, ketoconazole can damage the liver, and it does not appear suitable for long-term use. Because it dramatically reduces androgen levels within twenty-four hours, however, it can be helpful when rapid, if temporary, action is important.

New Prospects

Hormonal therapy can provide important benefits for most men with recurrent or advanced prostate cancer, but many tumors eventually become androgen-insensitive and escape control. To improve the situation, doctors are studying new approaches to hormone therapy. One unresolved issue is whether it is better to start hormonal therapy as soon as recurrent or widespread disease is diagnosed or whether it is better to wait until the tumor grows or symptoms develop. The question is particularly relevant for men who feel well despite having elevated or rising PSAs following prostatectomy or radiotherapy. Another issue is whether androgen-deprivation therapy should be administered continuously or intermittently. Hormonal therapy is also being studied as an adjuvant to radiation therapy for early disease (see page 397); It does not appear successful as an adjunct to surgery, however. Doctors are also investigating various therapeutic combinations and are working to develop new drugs. It is slow work, but it may result in further gains for men with prostate cancer.

Studies in mice are also raising intriguing possibilities for the management of prostate cancers that have become hormone-independent, thus escaping androgen-deprivation therapy. Some research suggests that some of these cells may actually be inhibited by testosterone. Other investigations in mice suggest that a gene called HER-2/neu may be responsible for androgen independence. If so, the drug Herceptin, which is used to treat breast cancer, may help some men with advanced prostate cancer. It is far too early to say if these findings in mice will ever apply to men, but it is an important new avenue of research.

Treating Prostate Cancer: Chemotherapy

It's another frontier in prostate cancer research that is being approached but has not yet been crossed. Far advanced prostate cancer is debilitating and progressive; bone pain, weakness, and weight loss are its major symptoms. At present, it is very difficult to halt the progression of advanced disease, but doctors are testing new chemotherapeutic regimens using drugs such as *vinblastine, suramin, cyclophosphamide,* and *mitoxantrone.* Immunotherapy and gene therapy are also being investigated. Spot radiotherapy can be useful to control symptoms caused by metastatic disease. But even when therapy cannot further extend the length of life, treatment can help improve the quality of life by relieving pain, treating complications, and providing comfort.

Treating Prostate Cancer: Alternative Medicine

As medical care becomes more complex, technological, and expensive, increasing numbers of people are turning to alternative and complementary therapies. According to researchers at the Harvard Medical School, more than 40 percent of all Americans used some form of nontraditional medicine in 1997. Since that represents a 50 percent increase from 1990, the numbers are likely to keep on growing. Even now, Americans spend more than $21 billion each year on unconventional treatments; and they make more visits to nontraditional practitioners (629 million a year) than to primary care physicians (388 million).

Each person who uses alternative medicine has his own reasons for doing so. In many cases, worries about illness and uncertainties about standard medical care came into play. Most men are concerned about prostate cancer, and some men with the disease are confused about conventional treatment. It is understandable, since doctors themselves debate the relative merits of deferred treatment ("watchful waiting"), surgery, radiation, and hormonal therapy. Current studies reveal that 30 to 40 percent of men with prostate cancer experiment with one or more forms of complementary therapy, though few discuss it with their doctors. But is alternative therapy a good idea?

Men with prostate cancer use a broad array of self-selected treatments, ranging from high-dose vitamins or minerals to supplements of lycopene or soy, various herbs, spiritual healing, massage therapy, and chiropractic. But the most widely-promoted alternative therapy is a mix of eight herbs marketed as PC-SPES; the name stands for prostate cancer—hope (in Latin, *spes*). It sounds too good to be true, but studies indicate that it has real activity—and that it has real side effects.

In mice, PC-SPES can retard the growth of experimental prostate cancer. In men with prostate cancer, PC-SPES often reduces PSA levels, sometimes dramatically. Some men also report improvements in pain and fatigue, but at present there is no evidence that PC-SPES prolongs survival.

How does PC-SPES work?

PC-SPES was developed in China and brought to the United States in 1996. In 1998, doctors in New Jersey evaluated a man with recurrent prostate cancer who was treating himself with PC-SPES. After a month, his PSA fell but he developed breast tenderness and loss of libido, suggesting a hormonal effect. To find out if PC-SPES was responsible for these changes, the research team evaluated seven other PC-SPES users. All exhibited similar effects, and one had developed *thrombophlebitis,* a known side effect of estrogen and other female hormones. In addition, all six men who were tested had lower than expected testosterone levels, another bit of evidence suggesting that one or more of the herbs was acting like an estrogen.

Taking their work one step further, the scientists evaluated PC-SPES in the lab. Using two different assay techniques, they found that PC-SPES had potent estrogenic activity.

In 2000 and 2001, three additional studies evaluated PC-SPES therapy in a total of 162 men with advanced prostate cancer. Thirty-three had not received prior hormonal therapy; they responded best, averaging an 80 percent fall in their PSA levels that lasted about thirteen months. Most also improved chemically, but all became impotent and all developed breast tenderness. Their lab results, too, looked just like men taking estrogen. And the men who had failed hormonal treatment before starting PC-SPES also behaved like similar patients given estrogen. About half had a 50 percent drop in their PSA levels, but the response was brief and disease progression resumed in three to four months. In addition to universal impotence and breast tenderness, PC-SPES produced fatigue, nausea, diarrhea, leg cramps, and thrombophlebitis in some men.

PC-SPES, Estrogen, or Neither

Although estrogen is an accepted hormonal treatment for advanced prostate cancer, it has been largely replaced by newer medications. As an estrogen, PC-SPES may actually suppress the growth of some prostate cancers. But it can have serious side effects and it can interfere with prescription treatment for prostate cancer, particularly if a man takes it without his doctor's knowledge.

New trials comparing PC-SPES to estrogen are underway. The results will not be available for several years. Even if a winner emerges, doctors will have to compare it with the androgen-deprivation therapies that are now in use (see page 398).

Like all potent drugs with potential side effects, PC-SPES should be tested carefully before it is made available. In 2002, one set of tests performed by the State of California found that PC-SPES tablets contained *warfarin* (Coumadin), a powerful prescription anticoagulant (blood thinner) that can cause bleeding. Like all powerful drugs, PS-SPES should be monitored for purity and potency, and it should be used only under medical supervision. As a "dietary supplement" PC-SPES is free from these constraints, but in 2002 the FDA issued a warning against its use. And if the warning doesn't get your attention, consider the drug's considerable cost, estimated to be from $162 to $482 a month, which is not covered by most insurance plans. It is up to every man to exercise judgment and restraint on his own, turning to his doctors for treatment of serious diseases instead of purchasing hope in a bottle.

Perspectives

Doctors have learned a great deal about the biology of prostate cancer, and there have been major advances in diagnoses and treatment. Despite this progress, however, much remains to be learned. New research in prevention, diagnosis, and treatment is already underway. It is hard work, and it is frustratingly slow, especially for men who need to make important decisions about tests and treatments. Slow or not, it is the only way to make further progress. And it is the only way to answer the very fundamental questions posed years ago by Dr. Willett F. Whitmore, Jr., the pioneering urologist who died of prostate cancer himself: "Is cure possible in those for whom it is necessary, and is cure necessary in those for whom it is possible?"

CHAPTER THIRTEEN

Disorders of the Kidneys and Bladder

IF MEN THINK OF THEIR URINARY TRACTS at all, they are likely to think first of their prostate glands. It's understandable, since prostate problems are among the most common and troublesome disorders of men. But for all its importance, the prostate is not essential for life, and it is but one small waystation in a complex organ system that is vital indeed.

The Normal Urinary Tract

The kidneys are located deep behind the abdominal organs at the mid-part of the back. As excretory organs, the kidneys have the task of filtering the blood to remove toxic wastes. Blood enters each kidney through a single artery, which divides into small arteries that eventually branch into microscopic vascular tufts called *glomeruli*. Each of a man's 2.5 million glomeruli is a miniature filter. Blood passes through the glomeruli and is returned to the veins, but the waste-containing urine is filtered off into tiny tubules.

The kidney's tubules are more than passive channels that collect urine. In fact, the tubules regulate the composition of urine to meet the body's needs. As urine passes through the tubules, most of the water is reabsorbed into the circulation, preventing dehydration. The kidneys also adjust the concentrations of important minerals, such as sodium, potassium, and calcium, as urine flows through the tubules.

During its passage through the tubules, the urine becomes more and more concentrated. Eventually the tubules join together to form the collecting system at the center of each kidney. Next, the urine flows down long tubes called *ureters*. The ureters do not have any effect on the composition of urine, but they still have an important job. Each ureter is lined by smooth muscle cells that can propel the urine to the bladder, even against the force of gravity.

The bladder stores urine until it is expelled through the final bit of tubing, the *urethra,* which runs down the center of the penis. Like the ureters, the bladder is lined by smooth muscle cells; when these *detrussor* muscles relax, they allow the bladder to fill to its maximum capacity of twelve to sixteen ounces, but when they contract, they forcefully expel urine—providing, of course, that an enlarged prostate does not block the way. Urinary control depends also on a final set of *sphincter* muscles at the bladder neck. The sphincter muscles act like a valve, contracting to retain urine in the bladder, then relaxing to allow it to flow out.

The kidneys are multipurpose organs. They excrete waste products such as urea, creatinine, and acids; if the kidneys fail, these toxins build up in the blood, producing uremic poisoning. The kidneys also regulate the body's fluid balance, retaining water when you are dry, but shedding it when you're overhydrated. A third function is to adjust the blood's mineral content, retaining chemicals such as sodium and potassium if your diet is deficient, but shedding them if you have too much. By converting vitamin D into its active form, the kidneys also have a key role in keeping calcium in balance and preserving bone strength.

And that's not all. The kidneys also produce hormones, including one that regulates blood pressure and another that stimulates the production of red blood cells. That is why people with kidney disease often develop hypertension and anemia.

It is a complex system, and a lot can go wrong. But among the many urinary tract disorders, only a few strike men more frequently than women; the most important of these predominantly male problems are kidney stones and bladder cancer.

Kidney Stones

Can a tiny deposit of minerals, sometimes less than one-tenth of an inch across, produce a medical crisis? It surely can, especially if it lodges in a narrow portion of the urinary tract. Even a small stone can cause excruciating pain, bleeding into the urine, or urinary tract infections, and some stones can even block the flow of urine, eventually damaging the kidney itself. Tiny stones can cause big problems, and since 500,000 stones form in Americans every year, they cause a $2 billion problem for the nation's economy.

Kidney stones have plagued men throughout history. Fortunately, the last few years have witnessed major advances in the diagnosis, treatment, and prevention of this common and painful problem.

Who Gets Kidney Stones?

Men, mostly. Although kidney stones do form in women, they are three-and-a-half times more common in men. In all, one of every eight American men will develop a kidney stone at sometime during his life; the highest risk occurs between the ages of twenty and fifty.

Men with a family history of stone disease are two-and-a-half times more likely to form stones than men without stone-forming relatives. But the people who have the highest risk are those who have already suffered from a stone. That's because stones tend to recur; in fact, if you have had a kidney stone, you have a 50 percent chance of forming additional stones within ten years of your first episode.

What Causes Stones?

Although urine may look like a simple fluid, it is actually a complex liquid that contains hundreds of chemicals, including many minerals. In some circumstances, the minerals can become *supersaturated.* That is when minerals precipitate into crystals that grow into gravel, then stones. Supersaturation and stone formation occur if excessive amounts of a mineral are excreted into the urine or if the volume of fluid is decreased by dehydration.

About 80 percent of the time, the principal mineral in a kidney stone is *calcium,* usually in combination with *oxalate* (60 percent of all stones), but sometimes paired with *phosphate* (20 percent) or other substances. Less often, kidney stones are composed of *uric acid* (10 percent) or *struvite* (7 percent). In rare cases, they contain other chemicals such as *cystine* or even certain medications.

Symptoms

Although most stones form in the kidney, they do not usually cause symptoms until they drop into a narrow part of the kidney or into the ureter, the thin muscular tube that carries urine down to the bladder. Stones that become lodged in a narrow part of the urinary tract can cause three major problems:

Pain. It's called renal colic, and it's one of the most intense of all pains. Renal colic is caused by contractions of the smooth muscle cells in the ureter. The pain often radiates along the path of the urinary tract, beginning high in the back over the kidney and traveling to the lower abdomen, groin, and even into the genitals. The pain begins suddenly, and it quickly becomes unbearable. Renal colic is often accompanied by nausea and vomiting, not because the stomach is involved, but simply because the pain is so severe. People with renal colic are restless, tossing and turning continuously in a futile attempt to find a comfortable position. Restlessness helps doctors distinguish the pain of kidney stones from the pain of intestinal problems such as diverticulitis and appendicitis, which would make you want to lie still. Although it can persist for agonizing hours, renal colic usually ends as abruptly as it begins. Relief comes when the stone moves from a narrow part of the urinary tract into a wider region, such as the bladder.

Bleeding. In about 90 percent of cases, kidney stones cause bleeding into the urine. Although the urine can be bright red in color, more often it looks clear to the naked eye but is found to contain large numbers of red blood cells when it is examined through a microscope. In people who are lucky enough to escape pain, bleeding is the usual clue to the presence of kidney stones.

Blockage. When a stone lodges in the ureter, it blocks the flow of urine. Pressure builds up in the kidney, causing it to swell with fluid, a condition know as *hydronephrosis.* The kidney attempts to protect itself by producing less urine, but permanent damage may occur if the blockage is prolonged. That is uncommon, except if the blockage occurs silently, without the pain or bleeding that usually signal the need for prompt treatment.

DIAGNOSIS

A major technological advance is revolutionizing the diagnosis of kidney stones. Until recently, doctors relied on a plain X-ray of the abdomen, which missed many stones, followed by an *intravenous pyelogram* (IVP), which is accurate but requires an injection of dye that may cause allergic reactions. The next advance was *renal ultrasound.* It is a very good test that does not require injections or medication, but it often misses stones in the lower half of the ureter. The new diagnostic breakthrough is *spiral computed tomography* (spiral CT). It is fast and it does not require dye, though it does use X-rays to produce an image of the urinary tract. That image is extremely detailed; in most cases, it identifies the precise location and size of the stone, and with further refinement it may soon be able to reveal the stone's chemical composition.

High-tech tests are usually expensive, and the spiral CT is no exception.

Because of its speed and accuracy, though, a spiral CT can actually cost less than the combination of tests it is replacing. All in all, the spiral CT is now the best way to diagnose kidney stones.

TREATMENT

The first step is to relieve pain. Although some patients respond to oral medication, many require injections of powerful painkillers, such as narcotics.

The next step is to remove the stone. In most cases, time and fluids will do the job, enabling the stone to pass on its own. But patients with stones larger than 6 millimeters (about the diameter of a pencil eraser) may need help—and a major advance is available here, too. The procedure is called *extracorporeal shock wave lithotripsy* (ESWL). It uses a device that generates high energy sound waves that are beamed through the patient's tissues until they arrive at the stone, where they release their energy. If all goes well, the stone is pulverized into tiny fragments that pass out through the urinary tract.

ESWL requires sedation but it can be performed on an outpatient basis, allowing most people to resume normal activities within a few days. The treatment is successful for up to 90 percent of small stones, but is less useful for stones as large as an inch or more. But even if ESWL cannot be used successfully, other techniques are available. The most common approach is to attack the stone directly, either via a tube inserted through the skin into the kidney (*percutaneous nephroureterolithotomy*) or through a tube passed up into the bladder (*ureteroscopy*). Although both are invasive treatments, they represent a significant advance over open surgery, which is now rarely performed. Needless to say, a urologist will have to decide which treatment is most appropriate for stones that do not pass spontaneously. Retained stones that do not cause pain, bleeding, obstruction, or infection do not need any treatment at all—except, of course, for measures to prevent additional stones from forming.

PREVENTION

Every man who has suffered through a bout of renal colic will be highly motivated to prevent a recurrence; fortunately, most can succeed. Prevention relies on a combination of diet and, sometimes, medication tailored to each type of stone. But one element is essential to prevent all types of stones: fluid.

Although water is a necessary ingredient in every preventive program, specific dietary adjustments and medications depend on the type of stone in question. The first step, then, is to identify the stone's chemical composition. If you are lucky enough to find a stone as it passes, bring it in to your doctor for analysis. If not, you can try filtering your urine through cheesecloth or a coffee filter to trap small bits of gravel. In most cases, though, you will have to collect several twenty-four-hour urine samples for analysis. It's a cumbersome procedure; some doctors request the test after just one stone, while others reserve it for people who have had several episodes. The same goes for blood tests, which sometimes reveal high levels of calcium or uric acid but are usually normal, even in people who form stones recurrently.

Fluids. A high fluid intake will keep the urine dilute, so minerals will not precipitate into crystals and aggregate into stones. The Health Professionals Study determined that nearly any kind of fluid will do; water, coffee, tea, beer, and wine were all protective, but carbonated beverages had a mixed record. In contrast, the Health Professionals Study found that apple and grapefruit juices actually increase risk.

As a rule of thumb, everyone who has had a kidney stone should drink large amounts of fluid, enough to pass at least two quarts of urine each day. That requires drinking at least ten glasses of fluid a day, five of which should be water. It means never passing up a water cooler during the day and it means getting up at least once to urinate at night, and downing a glass of water on the way back to bed. It is a lifestyle that takes getting used to, but it beats being rushed to the emergency ward doubled up with renal colic.

Diet. Most men who have calcium stones excrete excessive amounts of calcium in their urine, sometimes putting out amounts far above the 300 milligrams considered normal for a day. Although this *hypercalcuria* has been recognized for years, its fundamental cause was clarified only recently. In most cases, the fault is not in the kidneys, but in the intestinal tract. Only 2 percent of stone-formers have kidneys that put out too much calcium, but more than 50 percent have an intestinal defect that allows them to absorb excessive amounts of calcium from food. That calcium has to go somewhere, and it does: into the urine.

If excessive calcium absorption is the root cause of calcium stones, the solution seems obvious: reduce dietary calcium. Indeed, that has been the standard approach to prevention. Standard or not, it is wrong. Perhaps the biggest surprise of new research is that dietary calcium restriction does not prevent stones. On the contrary, in fact, a *low* calcium diet seems to make things *worse,* both by increasing the risk of stones and by boosting the risk of *osteoporosis* ("thin bones"). That's because some of the calcium in food normally binds to *oxalate,* preventing the body from absorbing oxalate. If dietary calcium is low, the body absorbs more oxalate, which is excreted in the urine, where it can finally bind to calcium—forming *calcium oxalate* crystals that grow into stones.

The Health Professionals Study revealed a lot about diet and kidney stones. All the 45,619 volunteers provided detailed information on their diets and their medications. None of the men had a history of kidney stones when the study began. During four years of observation, 505 of the men formed stones. When researchers compared dietary calcium with the risk of stones, they discovered that the men who consumed the most calcium from food were actually 44 percent less likely to form stones than the men who had the lowest levels of dietary calcium.

The Harvard study found that dietary calcium was protective, whether it came from milk, cheese, yogurt, oranges, or broccoli. But calcium supplements increased the risk of stones; that's because the calcium in food binds to the oxalate in foods, but the calcium in supplements does not.

The study of male health professionals has been confirmed by other research, including a parallel Harvard investigation of more than 91,000 women in the Nurses' Health Study. In both men and women, other dietary factors were found to influence the risk of kidney stones. As expected, a high fluid intake decreased risk. A high intake of potassium from fruits and vegetables was also helpful. But dietary protein and sodium each increased risk because they increase urinary calcium excretion.

To prevent calcium stones, drink lots of water and other fluids, aiming for about two quarts a day. Eat moderate amounts of calcium-rich foods, but stay away from calcium supplements and from supplements of vitamin D, which increases the intestinal absorption of calcium. Avoid foods with high levels of oxalate; rhubarb, spinach, beets, sweet potatoes, parsley, nuts, instant coffee, tea, and chocolate head the list. Avoid excessive amounts of protein, especially from animal sources such as meat. Reduce your sodium intake, staying below the recommended maximum of 2,400 milligrams per day. Increase your consumption of citrus fruits and juices (except grapefruit juice): in addition to potasium, they provide a second helpful nutrient, *citrate*.

Medication. If diet does not prevent stones, medications can help. *Thiazide diuretics*, such as *hydrochlorothiazide* (Esidrix, HydroDiuril) are particularly beneficial; *potassium citrate* (Urocit-IC) can also be helpful, particularly for the minority of stone-formers who do not have high urinary calcium levels.

Although calcium is a crucial component of most stones, other variants do exist, and they can be just as painful. *Uric acid* stones plague people with gout (see Chapter Fourteen), prevention involves a high fluid intake, a reduction of foods such as shellfish and meat that are rich in *purine,* and medications such as *allopurinol* (Zyloprim) and potassium citrate. Allopurinol can also help prevent calcium stones in people who excrete excessive amounts of uric acid. *Struvite* stones, which are uncommon, require specialized medications.

Do nutritional supplements play a role in kidney stones? Large does of vitamin B_6 are sometimes recommended as a preventive measure, but the Health Professionals Study found no benefit. But the study did provide some good news to men who favor supplements: Contrary to popular belief, vitamin C does not appear to increase the risk of stones, even in large doses.

Bladder Cancer

Kidney stones are a pain, but bladder cancer is a killer.

Bladder cancer is a particular problem for men; in the United States, the disease strikes men about three times more often than women. More than 41,000 American men will be diagnosed with bladder cancer this year, and more than 8,000 will lose their lives to the disease. Although bladder cancer can occasionally affect men in their forties, it becomes progressively more common beyond age fifty. The average age at diagnosis is sixty-nine.

Bladder cancer is the fourth most common internal cancer in American men, and its incidence is rising with each passing year. But early diagnosis can often nip the disease in the bud, and new therapeutic programs are improving the outlook for patients with advanced disease. Best of all, many cases of bladder cancer can be prevented.

Anatomy and Staging

From top to bottom—from the structures that collect urine in the kidneys to the upper two-thirds of the urethra where urine leaves the body—the urinary tract is lined by a special tissue called the *uroepithelium* or *transitional cell epithelium.* In the United States and other industrialized countries, more than 95 percent of bladder cancers arise from the cells of this thin, membranous tissue. The transitional epithelium is only a few cells thick. Cancers that are diagnosed when they are still confined to this superficial layer respond very well to simple treatment, but cancers that penetrate to deeper tissues are much more problematic. Fortunately, about 80 percent of bladder cancers are discovered when they are still superficial.

A membrane called the *lamina propria* lies just beneath the epithelium.

Below that lies the much thicker *muscular layer* that provides the contractile force that empties the bladder. The bladder muscles themselves are divided into superficial and deep zones. The adjacent structures are called *perivesical tissues*. Beyond them lie separate organs such as the prostate, lymph nodes, and bones.

Doctors use the TNM (tumor, node, metastasis) system to stage bladder cancer (see Figure 13.1).

CAUSES

All cancers are caused by varying combinations of environmental and genetic factors (see Chapter Three). In the case of bladder cancer, major environmental triggers have been known for decades, but research is just now identifying the genetic abnormalities that are ultimately responsible.

The most important cause of bladder cancer is cigarette smoking. Many of the toxins that enter the body when smokers inhale are absorbed into the bloodstream, and then excreted by the kidneys into the urine. Because urine dwells in the bladder for hours before it is expelled, the bladder epithelium is exposed to prolonged contact with *carcinogens* (cancer-causing substances). In the United States, tobacco use accounts for about half of all bladder cancers. Cigarette smokers are four times more likely to get bladder cancer than nonsmokers; heavy smokers are at greater risk than light smokers, but the risk gradually diminishes in people who kick the habit, even if they have smoked for many years.

Various industrial toxins can also injure the transitional cells that line the bladder, eventually producing cancer. In the past, workers in the rubber, paint, cable, electric, and textile industries were at substantial risk, but current workplace safety regulations have greatly improved matters. In certain parts of the world, such as the Nile River delta, parasitic infections account for many cases of bladder cancer. Other relatively uncommon causes include prolonged therapy with *cyclophosphamide* (Cytoxan) and overuse of the pain killer *phenacitin*. Although extremely high doses of artificial sweeteners may cause bladder cancer in animals, there is no evidence that they do so in humans. Other dietary factors, however, may play a role (see Prevention, page 420).

Tobacco smoke and other toxins cause bladder cancer by damaging the DNA in the nucleus of transitional cells. Heredity can also produce defects in DNA. The son of a parent with bladder cancer is 35 percent more likely to develop the disease than the son of healthy parents, and a man whose brother was diagnosed with bladder cancer before age thirty-five is seven times more

FIGURE 13.1. STAGING BLADDER CANCER

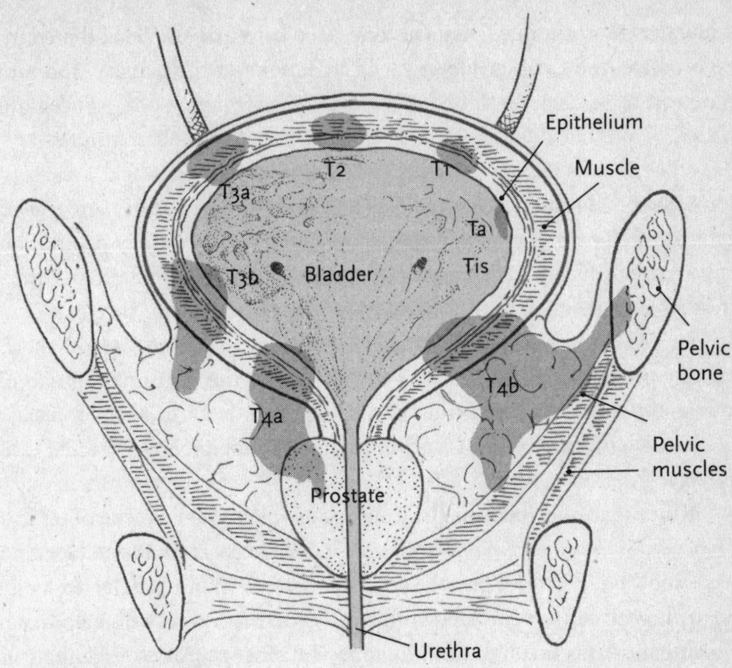

Tumor Location	Tumor Stage
Confined to epithelium	Ta and Tis
Extending just beneath the epithelium	T1
Infiltrating superficial muscles	T2
Infiltrating deep muscle	T3a
Extending just beyond the muscle	T3b
Penetrating adjacent organs (such as the prostate)	T4a
Fixed to the abdomen or pelvis	T4b
Spread to lymph nodes in the pelvis	T (any stage) N+
Spread to distant lymph nodes or organs	T (any stage) N+M+

likely to develop bladder cancer than a man whose family is free of the disease. Genetic abnormalities have been detected on six different chromosomes of malignant transitional cells, and scientists are already using this information to develop new diagnostic tests.

Symptoms

The most common symptom of bladder cancer is *gross hematuria,* blood in the urine that is visible to the naked eye. Although 80 to 90 percent of people with bladder cancer have it as their first symptom, bloody urine is not always a sign of bladder cancer. Indeed, kidney stones (see page 409), BPH and infections of the prostate (see Chapter Eleven), and infections of the urinary tract are even more common causes of blood in the urine. Less often, kidney cancer, trauma, sickle cell anemia, and other conditions can cause gross hematuria.

There is no sure way for a man with hematuria to know if bladder cancer is the cause—but there are some clues. One is the absence of pain or fever. Infections often cause both symptoms, and stones are generally painful, but the typical case of bladder cancer produces bloody urine without other symptoms. Another clue is when the blood appears during urination. In typical cases of bladder cancer, the blood is visible throughout urination, but in men with prostate problems, blood is often concentrated at the beginning or end of urination. But although these clues can be helpful, they can also be misleading. As a result, your doctor should always consider a diagnosis of bladder cancer if you have gross hematuria.

Although bloody urine is the leading sign of bladder cancer, other features can occur. Sometimes the only evidence is *microscopic hematuria,* bleeding that is so scant that it cannot be seen with the naked eye but is detected by testing the urine with a dipstick coated with a chemical that reacts with blood, or by examining the urine through a microscope. But since microscopic hematuria has so many causes, many of which are much more common than bladder cancer, the urinalysis is not a reliable way to screen for the disease; in fact, only 2 percent of people with microscopic hematuria have bladder cancer. Finally, in some cases bladder cancer does not produce any bleeding at all. Some of these patients complain of urinary frequency, urgency, or discomfort caused by bladder irritation, but many have no symptoms at all.

DIAGNOSIS

Two elements are involved in establishing a diagnosis of bladder cancer: ruling out other common causes of gross hematuria and identifying the bladder tumor itself. The first task depends on a urine culture to exclude bladder or kidney infections. A digital rectal exam is used to check for *prostatitis* or BPH (see Chapter Eleven); transrectal ultrasound evaluations are also helpful. CT scans and ultrasound are also helpful in detecting larger bladder cancers, especially if they extend beyond the bladder wall itself.

Until recently, most patients with suspected bladder cancer were asked to have an X-ray test called *intravenous pyelography* (IVP). To perform an IVP, technicians first inject an iodine-containing dye into your bloodstream. Next they obtain a series of X-ray pictures that follow the dye as it appears in your kidneys, ureters, and bladder. Although IVPs remain useful tests for the diagnosis of bladder cancer, spiral CT scans have largely supplanted them in most medical centers, but neither test has challenged the role of cystoscopy.

Most often, cystoscopy is an office procedure that uses a thin, flexible fiber optic tube, the cystoscope. After administering a local anesthetic, the urologist inserts the scope through the urethra into the bladder, allowing him to see and photograph the bladder. But if tumors are found and biopsies are required, cystoscopy is performed in a hospital setting under general anesthesia, which allows the urologist to insert tiny instruments through the scope to obtain biopsies of the bladder wall.

Cystoscopy is the gold standard for the diagnosis of bladder cancer, but it is invasive. As a result, researchers are developing tests to diagnose bladder cancer by checking urine samples. The oldest test is *urine cytology,* the microscopic evaluation of cells in voided urine using a technique similar to the female PAP smear. Unfortunately, while the PAP smear is an excellent way to diagnose cancer of the cervix, urine cytology is much less accurate for the diagnosis of bladder cancer. Newer tests depend on finding tumor markers—abnormal genes or their protein products—in the urine. Three such procedures, the two *bladder tumor antigen* (BTA) tests and the *nuclear matrix protein* (NMP) 22 test, have already been approved by the FDA, and many others are being developed. At present, these tests appear better at keeping track of patients already diagnosed with bladder cancer than at establishing an initial diagnosis.

Follow-up is important because bladder cancers often develop on multiple sites of the uroepithelium and because these tumors tend to recur. Most urologists perform follow-up cystoscopies every three months for the first year after successful treatment of superficial bladder cancer, then every six months for two years, and every year thereafter. It is an effective strategy, but in the future urinary tumor markers may reduce the dependence on cystoscopy.

TREATMENT

Most superficial bladder cancers respond very well to treatment, and in most cases, local treatment will do the trick. The first step is to remove the tumor through cystoscopic surgery (*endoscopic resection*). But even if all the identifiable tumor cells are eliminated, surgery is not enough. That is because bladder cancers often develop in multiple locations and they tend to recur. Fortunately, these problems can be controlled by administering additional therapy within the bladder. Most often, that treatment involves *immunotherapy. Bacillus Calmette-Guerin* (BCG) bacteria, which were developed eighty years ago as a vaccine against tuberculosis, are injected into the bladder, where they boost the body's own tumor-fighting immune cells. An alternative is *intravesical* (within the bladder) *chemotherapy:* A watery solution of a chemotherapy drug is instilled in the bladder. A new, still experimental, approach to the intravesical treatment of superficial bladder cancer is *photodynamic therapy.* At present, most American urologists favor BCG immunotherapy, which appears to have the highest response rate.

Superficial bladder cancers that do not respond to local therapy require more aggressive treatment. The same is true of tumors that have invaded the muscular layers of the bladder wall (Stages T2 and T3). The standard treatment for these tumors is *radical cystectomy,* surgical removal of the entire bladder. In men, the prostate and seminal vesicles are also removed, which produces impotence. Until recently, patients with radical cystectomies required an *ileostomy* to collect urine in a plastic bag worn on the abdominal wall. Although most patients adjusted remarkably well, new surgical techniques can make life even better by using a portion of the patient's intestinal tract to construct a pouch that can be emptied through the skin by periodic self-catheterization. Skilled urologists can even use intestinal tissue to construct an artificial bladder for some men, allowing them to urinate quite naturally. Still, some patients who are unwilling or medically unable to undergo radical cystectomy may also get good results from combination bladder-sparing therapy that involves limited surgical removal of the tumor followed by chemotherapy and radiation. An experienced medical center with a dedicated multidisciplinary team is the key to successful bladder-sparing therapy. Chemotherapy and radiation can help control widespread bladder cancer, and in some cases may even provide a cure.

PREVENTION

Despite important advances in the immunotherapy of superficial bladder cancer and the surgical therapy of invasive disease, prevention is the best treatment of all. Here too, progress is evident.

The first step, of course, is to quit smoking. It is an obvious necessity that will also reduce a smoker's risk of heart attacks, lung cancer, and many other major diseases. But in the case of bladder cancer the benefit accrues slowly, taking ten years or more; ex-smokers should remain particularly alert for warning symptoms during this time.

The second step is to review your work history for possible exposures to cancer-causing chemicals. *Benzene* and various *arylamines* are high on the list. Since bladder cancer develops slowly, usually becoming apparent at least twenty-five years after an exposure, continued vigilance is appropriate long after the exposure itself.

The third step is to improve your diet. Although the details vary, studies from Harvard, the University of Washington, and the University of California agree that a high intake of fruits and vegetables appears to reduce the risk of bladder cancer, while a high fat diet seems to increase risk. The Health Professionals Study singled out cruciferous vegetables, such as broccoli and cabbage, as protective. It also linked a high intake of vitamin E from foods or supplements to a decreased risk and found weaker evidence to a similar effect from vitamin C. The Washington investigation found protection from a dietary pattern rather than specific foods, but it found fried foods particularly harmful. This small study also added the hopeful observation that long-term use of a multivitamin or supplementary vitamin C appeared to reduce the risk of bladder cancer by 40 percent.

The final protective measure is to drink more fluid. It seems intuitive that a high urine volume will dilute toxins in the urine and increase voiding frequency; both should protect the vulnerable bladder cells from carcinogens. Intuitive or not, it took the Health Professionals Study in 1999 to show that dilution is indeed a solution to the bladder cancer conundrum. All 47,909 men in the study were free of cancer when it began in 1986. Over the next ten years, the researchers kept track of each man's consumption of twenty-two different types of beverages as well as the occurrence of bladder cancers. When the results were analyzed, the men who drank the most (averaging about two and one-half quarts a day) were 49 percent less likely to develop bladder cancer than the men who drank the least (averaging less than one and one-quarter quarts per day). Although water was particularly beneficial, all types of beverages contributed to protection, including alcoholic and caffeinated beverages, which had been cited as possible risk factors in some earlier studies. All in all, men can decrease their risk of bladder cancer by 7 percent for each additional eight ounces of fluid they drink each day. In a sense, then, the bladder is like so many other parts of the body: The more it is used, the healthier it stays.

Cancer of the Penis

Cancer of the penis is a rare disease in the United States, where it accounts for less than 1 percent of malignancies in males. In some other parts of the world, however, it is a major problem indeed, accounting for perhaps 10 percent of all cancers in men living in Africa, Asia, and South America. The difference is circumcision and penile hygiene. Cancer of the penis is virtually unknown in males circumcised shortly after birth, and it develops principally in men with phymosis and chronic inflammation of the foreskin and glans (see Chapter Nine). Infection with human papilloma virus (HPV) may also be a risk factor.

Penile cancer usually begins near the tip of the penis in the skin of the glans or foreskin. The earliest symptoms are redness or thickening of the skin, an ulceration, or the appearance of a warty growth, sometimes accompanied by itching or a burning feeling. Without treatment, the tumor grows into a nodule or lump, and then it invades the body of the penis. In more advanced cases, the disease extends to the lymph glands in the groin, finally spreading to various internal organs.

Cancer of the penis can be cured if it is caught early enough, but surgery is required. Doctors can remove small tumors without sacrificing too much normal tissue. To accomplish this, they may operate under a microscope or use laser surgery. In all cases, circumcision is the first step. Radiation therapy may be successful in more advanced cases, but penile amputation is often required. Chemotherapy is used for widespread disease, but cure is difficult.

All in all, penile cancer makes a strong case for prevention. Circumcision or good hygiene will dramatically reduce risk, and self-inspection can help detect the disease in its earliest, most curable stage.

Cancer of the male urethra is rare. Symptoms of pain or urinary obstruction, bloody urine, or a penile discharge usually precede the appearance of a mass in the penis itself. Unfortunately, cancer of the urethra is an aggressive disease that has usually invaded lymph nodes by the time it is diagnosed.

Nighttime Urination

Doctors call it nocturia. Men call it a curse. By any name, nighttime urination is a common problem, particularly for older people.

Until recently, doctors usually blamed nocturia on *benign prostatic hyperplasia* (BPH) and urologists often favored surgery to correct the problem. But many men who underwent technically successful *transurethral resection of the prostate* (TURP) still found themselves stumbling to the bathroom at night (see Chapter Eleven). Now we know why. New research shows that nocturia has many causes, and enlargement of the prostate is actually rather low on the list. It is a rude awakening, but it provides a rational approach to the future treatment of nocturia.

GENDER AND AGE

If nocturia was caused principally by BPH, it should be much more common in men than women. But numerous surveys demonstrate that the problem is equally prevalent in both genders. A survey of 400 American men and 479 women who were healthy and sixty years of age or older tells the tale: 65.2 percent of the men and 62.8 percent of the women reported nocturia. In addition, the number of nighttime trips to the bathroom was similar for men and women; about one-quarter of the subjects reported voiding two or more times in a typical night.

Gender does not account for nocturia, but age does. In both men and women, nighttime urination increases steadily over the years. A twelve-month Austrian study of 1,247 women and 1,221 men illustrates the relationship. Below the age of thirty, 3.1 percent of women and 3.4 percent of men reported nocturia. For age thirty to fifty-nine, 7.2 percent of women and 5.7 percent of men experienced the problem, and at age sixty and beyond the figures were 26.7 percent for women and 32.4 percent for men. In this study, as in others, nocturia was equally bothersome for men and women, with nearly two-thirds of the people reporting that getting up at night has a negative impact on their lives.

Why is nocturia related to age? Many factors contribute, including changes in urine production by the kidneys, changes in the capacity and reactivity of the bladder, changes in the quality of sleep, and the presence of disease in both the urinary tract and the rest of the body.

CAUSES

In many cases, nocturia is explained by an increase in urine production; some people get up at night simply because they have more urine to eliminate. The reason for the high urine volume may be as simple as an excessive fluid intake, particularly late in the day. Patients who take *diuretic* medication in the afternoon or evening will also have to deal with a high urine flow at night. Because alcohol and caffeine are also diuretics that increase urine production, a predinner cocktail or after-dinner espresso can also trigger nocturia.

But even without coffee, alcohol, medications, or lots of liquids, many older people produce excessive amounts of urine at night. Infants and young children produce urine at a steady rate around the clock. But after age seven or so, things change as the body develops ways to protect sleep. Healthy young adults produce urine three times faster during the day than at night. That's because the brain puts out extra amounts of *antidiuretic hormone* (ADH, also known as *vasopressin*) at night. ADH causes the kidneys to reabsorb water, so they produce small volumes of concentrated urine. You will know ADH is at work if you sleep through the night and wake up to void a moderate amount of concentrated, dark yellow urine. But as people age, the *circadian rhythms* that control salt and water excretion (among other things) begin to change. As a result of changes in ADH and other hormones such as *atrial naturetic peptide,* many older people revert to the juvenile pattern of steady around-the-clock urine production. True, they void less during the day, but they pay for that convenience at night.

Changes in the bladder also contribute to nocturia in older adults. With age, the bladder tends to get smaller and stiffer. It also becomes more sensitive to the presence of urine, so it produces the urge to void before it is really full. Inflammation or infections of the bladder make the problem even worse. Though it is no longer considered the primary cause of nocturia, BPH also produces bladder overactivity.

If you pass large volumes of clear urine when you get up at night, you can suspect increased urine production as the cause. If you wake up with the urge to void but pass only a modest amount of yellow, more concentrated urine, your bladder is probably to blame. In many people, though, both problems contribute to nocturia.

SLEEP AND THE NERVOUS SYSTEM

The urge to urinate is the result of a complex series of influences. When its muscles are relaxed, the bladder wall is soft and stretchable. Pressure does not even start to build up until the bladder is half full, and the desire to urinate does not begin until the bladder is three-quarters full. As the bladder gets fuller, it sends nerve impulses to the brain signaling the need to void. But the brain talks back, suppressing the urge to void until it is convenient and socially acceptable or until the bladder is totally full.

When people wake up at night to urinate, they assume that a full bladder wakes them up. In most cases, they are probably right. But as people get older, they often sleep lightly, so instead of suppressing the urge to void until morning, they may sense the urge even before the bladder is three-quarters full. Nocturia may be the effect of disrupted sleep, not its cause.

Surprisingly, perhaps, people are very poor judges of what wakes them up at night. When researchers monitored eighty patients with suspected sleep disorders, they recorded an average of one-and-a-half episodes of nocturnal urination per night. In most cases, the patients said they were awakened by the urge to void, but careful monitoring documented that sleep disturbances were actually responsible for 79 percent of the awakenings. In men, the major cause was *obstructive sleep apnea* (see Chapter Fourteen). Restless leg syndrome, anxiety, and various neurological disorders can also contribute to disturbed sleep and nighttime urination, as can insomnia and simple habit.

OTHER DISEASES

In most cases, nighttime urination is harmless and innocent, even if doctors give it a formidable name like nocturia. But in some situations, nocturia can reflect important diseases outside the urinary tract itself. The two most common examples are *diabetes mellitus* and *congestive heart failure*. In the former, sugar in the urine causes an increase in urine volume, while in the latter, an increased excretion of sodium during recumbency is responsible. Even if these problems are relatively uncommon, they should remind people who have nocturia to discuss the symptoms with their doctors; unfortunately, many do not.

Even if BPH is not the culprit it was once thought to be, it is still an important cause of nocturia. But when BPH is responsible, men experience other symptoms along with nocturia. Urinary urgency, frequency, and hesitancy and incomplete bladder emptying, a slow or narrow urinary stream, and dribbling at the end of urination are typical (see Chapter Eleven). But even when these symptoms suggest that BPH is responsible for nocturia, they do not automatically signal the need for treatment. Instead, men need treatment only if the symptoms are bothersome enough to detract from the quality of life. Men who fall back to sleep after they get up to void and awaken feeling rested in the morning do not need treatment. And even if nocturia produces sleep deprivation, medical treatment with alpha-blockers, finasteride, or even herbs should be considered as alternatives to standard and less invasive surgical therapies (see Chapter Eleven).

PRACTICAL TIPS

Nocturia is a complex phenomenon, but a few simple adjustments can help you manage the problem, whether or not it is caused by BPH. Here are a few tips:

- Do not drink too much. Fluids are important for health, but unless you have kidney stones, urinary tract infections, or certain other medical problems, you do not have to force fluids. Drink enough to quench your thirst and maintain good hydration, but drink as little as possible within four to five hours of bedtime.

- Reduce your intake of alcoholic and caffeinated beverages, particularly late in the day.
- Review your medications. If you are taking a diuretic, ask your doctor if a milder preparation or another type of drug would be as good for you—but do not make changes on your own. And while you are at it, ask your doctor to be sure you do not have diabetes or any other condition that might increase your urine flow.
- Establish good sleeping habits. Do not eat a large meal before you retire. Be sure your bed is comfortable and your bedroom is dark, quiet, and at the right temperature. Particularly if you have a large neck or snore loudly, ask your doctor if a sleep disturbance could be the real reason you are getting up at night (See Chapter Fourteen).
- Protect yourself from falls at night. Be sure your path to the bathroom is not an obstacle course; loose rugs and stray objects can turn nocturia into a broken hip. Use night lights, but try to keep the light bright enough for safety but dim enough to allow you to get back to sleep. Be sure to follow the same rules when you are away from home.

Nighttime urination can result from BPH or a variety of other problems, but even more often, it is a normal consequence of the aging process. With a little planning, most men can minimize the number of times they get up at night and maximize their ability to get back down for a refreshing night's sleep.

Urinary Incontinence

Urinary incontinence is a troublesome problem that can produce enough discomfort, inconvenience, and shame to seriously impair the quality of life. It is usually thought of as a "woman's problem" but men experience it too. Still, the misconception about gender adds to a man's embarrassment; perhaps that's why less than one-third of incontinent men bring the problem to their doctor's attention. The gender bias also explains why so few physicians bother to ask their male patients about bladder control.

While it is true that urinary incontinence is more common in women, it is far from rare in men; the problem affects 15 to 30 percent of older women and

7 to 15 percent of older men. In both sexes, the problem increases with advancing age. A study of 7,763 Swedish men reported incontinence in less than 4 percent of forty-five-year-olds, but the prevalence steadily increased to nearly 30 percent by age ninety. A study of American men reported an even higher rate of incontinence, which peaked at 32 percent for men sixty-one to seventy years of age; 43 percent of incontinent men reported loss of bladder control at least weekly, and 9 percent reported severe loss of control.

CAUSES

In women, urinary incontinence is usually related to childbearing and loss of estrogen after menopause. In men, of course, the causes are entirely different. The leading culprit is the prostate. As men age, the prostate enlarges, stretching the urethra and displacing the bladder neck from its normal position. But three very different problems can produce incontinence in men:

- *Overflow incontinence* results from blockage of the bladder outlet and/or weakness of the *detrussor* muscles that are responsible for emptying the bladder. *Benign prostatic hyperplasia* (BPH) is the usual cause (see Chapter Eleven). Medications can add to the problem. Drugs with *anticholinergic* activity (such as antihistamines, drugs used for intestinal spasms, and tricyclic antidepressants) weaken the contractions of the detrussor muscles, while decongestants (such as pseudoephedrine) tighten the sphincter muscles at the bladder neck, preventing them from relaxing to allow urine to pass freely. Typical symptoms of overflow incontinence include urinary urgency, hesitancy, and a weak, slow stream with starting and stopping that requires the man to strain while voiding. Men with overflow incontinence often void small amounts of urine. They still feel full after urination, and need to void again shortly after they finish. Dribbling is common.
- *Urge incontinence* is technically known as *detrussor instability*, but is commonly called an overactive bladder. By any name, the problem is caused by excessive or inappropriate contraction of the bladder muscles. In many cases, doctors cannot figure out why the muscles are overactive, but in some men they trace the problem to urinary tract infections, bowel problems, or early BPH. Men with urge incontinence typically complain of an irresistible need to void and of frequent uri-

nation; they can also be plagued by large-volume accidents with more than 3 ounces of urinary leakage.

- *Stress incontinence* is common in women, but rare in men—except in men who have had prostate surgery. Because radical prostatectomies remove the entire gland, they deprive the bladder of its usual support; the operation may also injure the nerves that control the bladder sphincter. Stress incontinence is much less common after TURPs, but it can occur. The typical symptom is the loss of small amounts of urine during coughing, straining, lifting, or even just standing up.

EVALUATION

To determine the cause of a man's incontinence, doctors will ask about his surgical history, his medications, his fluid intake, and his use of alcohol and caffeine. A detailed account of symptoms is very important, and the patient may be asked to keep a voiding diary. The doctor will examine his patient's abdomen and will perform a digital rectal exam. If there is any possibility that a neurological disorder is contributing to poor urinary control, a detailed neurologic exam is essential.

The next step in evaluation is quick and simple: it is the cough test, in which a man is asked to cough and strain to see if he has stress incontinence. Routine lab tests include a urinalysis and culture and blood tests to measure kidney function. A PSA test may be indicated as well (see Chapter Twelve).

The most important test is *urine flowmetry,* which measures the rate at which the bladder empties. After receiving instruction and waiting until his bladder feels full, the man simply urinates into a device that uses electronic monitors to record the rate of urine flow. Peak flow rates below 10 ml/minute suggest severe bladder outlet obstruction that can cause overflow incontinence, but slow flows can sometimes reflect very weak detrussor muscles. Another useful test is to determine the amount of urine that remains in the bladder after voiding; the *post-void residual* volume can be measured by catheterizing the bladder or by performing an ultrasound. But if the diagnosis is still unclear after these simple tests, a comprehensive set of urodynamic studies may be needed.

TREATMENT

The treatment of male urinary incontinence depends upon its cause.

Overflow incontinence responds to measures that relieve obstruction.

Men with BPH often improve with medications such as *alpha-blockers* (Hytrin, Cardura, or Flomax) or *finasteride* (Proscar); herbal therapy with *saw palmetto* may also help (see Chapter Eleven). If the symptoms remain bothersome despite medical therapy, surgical treatment may be required. Urge incontinence requires a different strategy. Anticholinergic medications such as *oxybutynin* (Ditropan) or *tolterodine* (Detrol) are the mainstays of treatment. But before men use them, they must be sure that they do not have obstruction in addition to bladder overactivity. Bladder training can also help. This is a behavioral technique that tries to improve control by gradually lengthening the time between voiding until the patient can maintain control for two to four hours without leaking.

Stress incontinence following prostate surgery can be difficult to treat. Mild cases may respond to pelvic muscle exercises or possibly biofeedback, but severe incontinence may require collagen injections or surgical placement of an artificial sphincter.

It is nice to know that tests and treatments can help men with urinary incontinence. Men should put embarrassment aside and discuss the problem with their doctors. And they should also make simple adjustments to help themselves. Pads can provide security and simple measures like restricting fluids and making frequent trips to the bathroom can help a great deal.

CHAPTER FOURTEEN

Other Male Medical Problems

MEN ARE SPECIAL. They have distinctive attributes, characteristic interests, and particular abilities. They also have special illnesses. Thus far, Part III of this Guide has concentrated on genitourinary issues that are truly restricted to men. But there is more to a man than his hormones and reproductive tract, and the rest of a man's body is also subject to disease. This chapter will discuss a metabolic disease (gout), two vascular abnormalities (aortic aneurysms and peripheral arterial disease), two functional difficulties (snoring and sleep apnea), and a hereditary problem (baldness). What do these very different disorders have in common? Just one thing: they are all at least three times more common in men than women.

Gout

Long known as the rich man's disease, modern research reveals that gout has no relationship to social status or wealth and surprisingly little to diet, drink, or corpulence. But gout *is* a man's disease, occurring five to seven times more often in men than women. It is also a common disease, striking an estimated 2.2 million Americans each year. In fact, gout is the most common form of inflammatory arthritis in men over age forty.

What Causes Gout?

Gout is caused by an abnormality in the body's metabolism of *uric acid.* Uric acid has no useful function. In the human body, it is simply a breakdown product of *purines,* a group of chemicals present in all body tissues and many foods. In normal circumstances, the body rids itself of uric acid by excreting it in the urine, keeping blood levels low. But some men have an inherited metabolic glitch that allows blood uric acids to rise; 90 percent of the time it is because the kidneys do not excrete enough uric acid, but sometimes the body just produces too much of the pesky chemical. Certain medications such as *thiazide diuretics* and *niacin* can also increase uric acid levels. Binge drinking, extreme fasting, kidney disease, lead toxicity, and leukemias and lymphomas are much less common causes of high uric acid levels.

High uric acid levels lead to gout, but not right away. In fact, uric acid levels are typically elevated for twenty to thirty years before they cause any trouble, which is why gout usually occurs in middle-aged and older men. Uric acid levels are normally below 7 milligrams per decliliter of blood. The higher the level, the more likely an attack of gout; men with levels above 9 mg/dL have a 22 percent chance of developing gout. But gout can also be triggered by a rapid drop in uric acid levels, which is why up to 30 percent of men with gout have normal uric acid levels at the time of an attack.

An attack of gout occurs when excess uric acid is deposited in a joint. The uric acid forms crystals which irritate the joint lining. White blood cells try to help; they gobble up the crystals but they are not equal to the task. The white blood cells are themselves damaged, releasing chemicals that cause inflammation, swelling, and pain.

SYMPTOMS

Ouch! Gout is painful, very painful.

The most common manifestation of gout is an acute, severe pain in a joint. In most cases, gout strikes just one joint at a time. Half the time, it is the first joint in the large toe; other common sites include the instep, heel, ankle, and knee. Gout is uncommon in the upper body, but it can strike fingers, wrists or elbows. At any site, the attack usually begins abruptly, often at night. Within hours, the joint becomes red, swollen, hot, and painful. The pain and tenderness can be so severe that even the touch of a sheet or blanket can be excruciating. Even though only one small joint is involved, the inflammation can be intense enough to cause fever, muscle aches, and other flu-like symptoms.

Without treatment, gout can also cause long-term arthritis with chronic swelling and permanent joint damage. Uric acid crystals can build up to remarkable levels, producing large, even grotesque, deposits called *tophi* in joints or other tissues. Uric acid crystals may also be deposited in the kidneys and they may precipitate in the urine, forming *kidney stones* (see Chapter Thirteen).

DIAGNOSIS

Gout is easy to recognize when it strikes the big toe, causing the characteristic inflammation called *podogra*. Doctors can often make the diagnosis over the phone, and most men with gout can diagnose themselves, particularly in their second or third attacks of this recurring disease. But in other joints, the diagnosis can be tricky. It is simple to measure the level of uric acid in the blood; a high level supports a diagnosis of gout, but it is not absolutely definitive, since many healthy men have high levels, and some men with gout have normal blood uric acid levels. Other diseases can mimic gout including *rheumatoid arthritis, infections,* and *pseudogout,* which is caused by crystals of another chemical (*calcium pyrophosphate*). If there is doubt about the diagnosis, doctors can remove a small amount of fluid from the inflamed joint. In cases of gout, the fluid contains white blood cells and uric acid crystals, which can be seen through a special polarizing microscope.

TREATMENT

Gout responds very well to *nonsteroidal antiinflammatory drugs* (NSAIDs) if two rules are observed: First, the NSAID should be started as promptly as possible, and second, it should be used at the maximum recommended dosage. Many physicians prescribe *indomethacin* (Indocin) in a dose of 50 milligrams three or four times per day, but the many other NSAIDs are also effective. One exception: Aspirin should not be used for gout because it can affect uric acid levels. After two to three days at full strength, the NSAID dose can be reduced by half, and in most cases treatment can be stopped after just five to seven days.

Some men cannot take NSAIDs because of gastritis, peptic ulcers, or advanced kidney disease. An older medicine, *colchicine,* can be useful in these circumstances, but it has fallen out of favor because it often produces vomiting or diarrhea in the high doses needed to treat acute gout. Fortunately a brief course of *prednisone* or a similar steroid will usually do the job for men who cannot take NSAIDs. Steroids can also be given intravenously to people who cannot take oral medications, and they can be injected directly into the inflamed joint to provide rapid relief.

Joints that are inflamed should be rested, but men can resume normal activities as soon as their gouty attacks settle down.

PREVENTION

For centuries, diet was the mainstay of prevention, but since only about 10 percent of the body's uric acid is derived from dietary sources, it did not work very well. Still, every little bit helps. Men with gout should follow a low-fat, moderate protein diet. They should avoid excess amounts of alcohol, and may wish to cut down on purine-rich foods (see list below). Weight loss may help men who are overweight. A high fluid intake is important to help prevent uric acid kidney stones.

HIGH PURINE FOODS THAT MAY INCREASE THE RISK OF GOUT
All meats, especially organ meats
Meat extracts and gravies
Seafood, especially sardines and anchovies
Yeast and yeast extracts
Beer and other alcoholic beverages
Beans, peas, and lentils
Spinach and asparagus
Cauliflower
Mushrooms

Modified from Emerson, B. T. *The Management of Gout N Engl J Med.* 1966; 334:445.

Although gout usually recurs, months or years can go by between attacks. Men whose attacks are infrequent do not need any preventive medication, but they should have an NSAID on hand for self-treatment at the first sign of another attack. But if gout is a frequent problem—or if very high uric acid levels predict frequent attacks—medications can help. There are three ways to prevent gout:

- *Antiinflammatory Medication.* Taken daily, low doses of NSAIDs (indomethacin 25 milligrams twice a day, for example) or colchicine (0.6 milligrams once or twice a day) can prevent acute attacks.
- *Medication to Promote Uric Acid Excretion. Probenecid* (Benemid) is the traditional choice; the usual dose is 250 to 500 milligrams two or three times a day. Rash and intestinal upset are the most common side effects. Because the drug increases uric acid in the urine, it can predispose to kidney stones and it should be avoided in patients with kidney disease. Because it lowers blood uric acid levels, it can trigger gout early on, so men should always take an antiinflammatory medication during the first two to three months of probenecid therapy. Aspirin, however, blocks the activity of probenecid.

- *Medication to Reduce Uric Acid Production. Allopurinol* (Zyloprim) is the only drug in this category, and it works very well. It is the treatment of choice for men with chronic gouty arthritis or uric acid kidney stones. The typical dose is 300 milligrams per day, but some men need more, others less. The most common side effects are rash and intestinal upset; severe allergic reactions can occur, but are rare. Because allopurinol produces a rapid fall in uric acid that can precipitate gout, men should always take an antiinflammatory medication for the first two to three months of therapy.

Gout is an old disease that has plagued men for centuries. Thomas Sydenham, a great physician of the seventeenth century, wrote that "Gout, unlike any other disease, kills more rich men than poor, more wise men than simple." But the modern era has witnessed major changes in gout. It never kills and it no longer results from errant behavior, if it ever did. Moreover, wise men need not fear the disease. Instead, they can learn to treat and prevent attacks themselves, with just a little help from a physician wise to the ways of gout.

Abdominal Aortic Aneurysms

The *aorta* is the largest artery in the body; it is also the strongest. But size and strength are not enough to protect this crucial blood vessel. In fact, the aorta is one of the body's most vulnerable arteries.

Although many disorders can strike the aorta, the most common is an *aneurysm*. It is an unfamiliar term, but it was wisely selected by the ancient Greeks, who named the disorder with the word that means "to widen."

Any part of the aorta can develop a widening or aneurysm, but most occur in the lower part of the artery as it travels through the abdomen carrying blood to the legs and lower body. *Abdominal aortic aneurysms* (AAA) are common, particularly in older people, and four out of five occur in men. While many are harmless, others can rupture, usually with deadly results. In all, AAAs are responsible for 1 to 2 percent of all deaths in men older than sixty-five, or almost 15,000 deaths in the United States each year, making them the thirteenth leading killer of American men. Fortunately, though, new advances in diagnosis and therapy are dramatically improving the management of this age-old problem.

THE NORMAL AORTA

The aorta is the body's main blood vessel. It receives all the blood pumped out from the *left ventricle* of the heart. Because it lies in the chest, the first part of the artery is called the *thoracic aorta*. After leaving the heart, it ascends toward the neck, and then descends toward the abdomen. When the artery leaves the chest, it becomes known as the abdominal aorta. After traveling along the rear of the abdomen just in front of the spine for about seven inches, the abdominal aorta divides into the two smaller *iliac arteries* that carry blood to the pelvis and legs. In healthy adult men, the top of the aorta is about 3 centimeters (1.2 inches) wide; as it runs through the body and distributes blood to the head and arms, it tapers to a width of about 2 centimeters (.8 of an inch) in the abdomen.

Like all arteries, the aorta's wall has three layers: a thin inner layer lined with *endothelial cells*, a middle layer composed of *smooth muscle cells* and elastic tissue, and an outer layer of supporting tissues. But the middle layer of the aorta distinguishes it from other arteries; it is composed of layer upon layer of elastic tissue, which makes it very thick and strong. It needs that strength to absorb the tremendous force of blood being propelled directly from the heart. And after absorbing the force when the heart pumps blood, the aorta gives some of it back. As the heart relaxes to refill with blood between beats, the elastic fibers in the aorta recoil, pushing the blood along its route to the rest of the body.

The aorta expands with each heartbeat and narrows down again between beats. It is a demanding routine, and over the years it can take quite a toll. In many older people, the elastic tissue in the aorta stiffens, making the artery less flexible; the process contributes to *systolic hypertension* and all its complications (see Chapter Three). And over time, the aorta itself can widen and weaken, developing into an aneurysm.

WHO GETS AN AAA?

Age is the strongest risk factor. AAAs are rare before age fifty, but they become increasingly common thereafter, affecting 4 to 9 percent of men above age sixty-five. It is not surprising that AAA is a disease of aging, since elastic tissue in the artery's wall wears down with time, and the aorta is unable to replenish or repair this vital material. Even so, age alone does not account for the problem, since the aorta remains normal in the majority of senior citizens.

Gender is another important risk factor. AAAs are four times more common in men than women and they tend to occur ten years earlier in males than females. AAAs are also ten times more likely to be fatal in men than women.

Family history contributes to some cases. The impact is greatest in men above sixty who have a sibling with an AAA; up to 18 percent of such men have AAAs themselves.

Another major risk factor is smoking, which triples the chances of developing an AAA. Although the evidence is mixed, most studies agree that high blood pressure is also a contributor. Abnormal cholesterol levels seem to play a role, though to a lesser degree; the same is true for abdominal obesity and the lack of regular exercise. Surprisingly, perhaps, diabetes is not linked to AAAs.

Age, male gender, smoking, hypertension, high cholesterol—it is a familiar recipe for *atherosclerosis*. Indeed, many people with AAAs also have atherosclerosis of smaller arteries, especially those in the heart and legs. It underlines the fact that AAAs are localized manifestations of problems that involve the whole body, and since so many men with AAAs also have heart disease, it also explains why surgery is so tricky in people with AAAs.

SYMPTOMS

Most AAAs are clinically silent, producing no symptoms at all. But as aneurysms enlarge, they can produce pain in the abdomen or back. When such complaints occur, they are usually nonspecific, producing a pulsating sensation or gnawing ache deep in the abdomen or in the mid-back.

Unfortunately, there is no mistaking the tragic event that people worry about most: rupture of an AAA causes severe abdominal pain, a profound fall in blood pressure, and collapse. It is a highly lethal event; 50 percent of victims die before they even get to the operating room, and of the remainder, only about a half make it through surgery.

Doctors often refer to AAAs as time bombs. It is understandable, since they are often entirely silent until they burst with a big bang. But it's now clear that even if AAAs are time bombs, they usually have long fuses—and doctors can now detect them before they explode.

DETECTION

The simplest way for a doctor to detect an AAA is to feel a pulsating swelling in his patient's abdomen, often just to the left of the belly button. As in so much of life, though, the easy way is not the best way; except in very thin people with rather large aneurysms, a doctor's physical exam will miss most AAAs. Since less than a quarter of AAAs have enough calcium in their walls to show up on X-rays, an ordinary X-ray is not much help either.

Fortunately, there is a simple, risk-free way to detect AAAs. Ultrasound will detect more than 95 percent of all AAAs, and it is rare for the test to miss an AAA large enough to cause trouble. Because they are quick, easy, and accurate, ultrasound tests can be repeated to monitor the size of an AAA, thus identifying the ones at risk for rupture. In fact, ultrasound can detect as little as a 3 mm increase in an aneurysm's diameter.

Newer tests, such as computed tomography (CT) and magnetic resonance imaging (MRI), are also very accurate, but they are more expensive and time-consuming than ultrasound. In general, doctors reserve CTs and MRIs for pre-operative evaluations, in which case an injection of dye is often given first (*CT* or *MR angiogram*).

If ultrasound is so accurate and AAAs so worrisome, should everyone have the test as part of an annual physical? It's the 64 dollar question, but doctors do not yet know the answer. At present, most experts advise against routine screening, arguing that the problem is just not common enough to justify the enormous cost of mass testing. But targeted screening is another matter, and abdominal ultrasounds may prove useful in people with AAA risk factors. Men with a family history of the disorder who are sixty or older would fit the bill, as would men with hypertension, high cholesterol levels, clinical evidence of atherosclerosis, or significant smoking histories. Needless to say, any man with symptoms at all suggestive of an AAA should have an ultrasound as promptly as possible.

WHAT TO DO?

Many AAAs are discovered accidentally in the course of abdominal imaging tests performed to evaluate other problems. Some are discovered by physical exams or as a result of routine screenings. What's next?

Using the time bomb analogy, doctors and patients get very nervous about AAAs. It is understandable for a man to want his AAA repaired before it ruptures, but it is not that simple. Far from being a quick fix, surgical repair is difficult and risky, carrying an operative mortality rate of 4 to 8 percent in most hospitals.

It is quite a dilemma, but there is a way out; doctors can now identify the AAAs at highest risk of rupturing. The key determinant is size. As an AAA gets larger, its walls get thinner and weaker, much as a balloon thins out as it is inflated. A 1997 study from Minnesota demonstrates the key role of an AAA's diameter:

SIZE	ANNUAL RISK OF RUPTURE
3–3.9 cm	0
4–4.9 cm	1%
5.0–5.9 cm	11%
6 cm or larger	25%

A recent British study of 1,090 patients with AAAs agrees, setting 5.5 centimeters as the size at which the benefits of surgery outweigh its risks in the average patient.

Although these guidelines are very useful, they are not carved in stone. Some patients with aneurysms smaller than 5 cm may benefit from surgery, particularly if they have few complicating medical problems and access to a top-flight surgical team. On the other hand, older patients with serious illnesses that boost the risk of surgery might do best with conservative management even if they have AAAs larger than 5.5 centimeters. And if these guidelines are not complex enough, new treatment options may soon change the rules.

Even if small AAAs do not warrant repair, they certainly require attention. Ultrasounds should be repeated every six to twelve months. Aneurysms that expand by more than 0.5 centimeter should be considered for repair, as should aneurysms that begin to cause pain. And everyone with an AAA should avoid all forms of tobacco exposure and reduce blood pressure and cholesterol levels that are elevated.

REPAIRING AAAs

AAAs rupture because their walls are thin and weak. To prevent disaster, doctors can place a *prosthetic graft* inside the aneurysm, shoring up its walls.

Conventional surgical repair involves general anesthesia and a large abdominal incision. The surgeon clamps the aorta just above the aneurysm, temporarily halting the flow of blood; since most AAAs are below the *renal arteries,* circulation to the kidneys is preserved. Next, the surgeon opens the aorta and places a Dacron tube within it. After stitching the graft in place, the surgeon closes the aorta, removes the clamp, and sews up the abdomen.

It is an effective procedure but a big operation. Even in the best of hands, a conventional AAA repair has a substantial risk of complications, even death, particularly since the typical patient is an older man with atherosclerosis. But in the past decade, a new option has become available; it's the approach that doctors used to treat Senator Bob Dole's AAA. Like conventional surgery, *endovascular stent grafts* also involve placing a polyester tube inside the aneurysm, but in this case, the graft is threaded up into the aorta through a thin catheter that doctors insert through the skin into a leg (or arm) artery. Doctors take X-rays and monitor the progress of the catheter on a video screen. When the graft is in place, they expand the graft, then withdraw the catheter. Endovascular repair can be performed under epidural or even local anesthesia. Many operative complications can be avoided, and if all goes well, patients recover in a few days.

Endovascular AAA repair is an exciting option, but it is technically demanding and requires a skilled medical team. The procedure can have complications of its own, including bleeding into the space between the graft and the aorta or migration of the graft itself. More research will be needed to compare long-term results of this new treatment with conventional surgical repair.

PERSPECTIVES

AAAs are diagnosed in about 200,000 Americans each year, and about 40,000 surgical repairs are performed annually. In addition, researchers estimate that about 1.5 million Americans have AAAs without knowing it; most are men.

Doctors have made great strides in diagnosing AAAs and in determining which are at risk for rupturing. New treatment options are also very promising. But the incidence of AAAs is increasing steadily; to stem the tide, men should not rely on technology alone. Instead, they should embrace preventive strategies to eliminate smoking and reduce elevated blood pressure and cholesterol levels. It's the way to reduce the risk of AAAs and other manifestations of atherosclerosis. As usual, prevention is the best medicine.

Peripheral Artery Disease

Atherosclerosis is a systemic disease that can affect any artery in the body. Even so, the damage is remarkably local, with plaques damaging one small stretch of an artery while sparing adjacent segments. For unknown reasons, the plaques tend to occur in certain characteristic locations. In the coronary arteries, ather-

FIGURE 14.1. ARTERIAL CIRCULATION OF THE LEGS

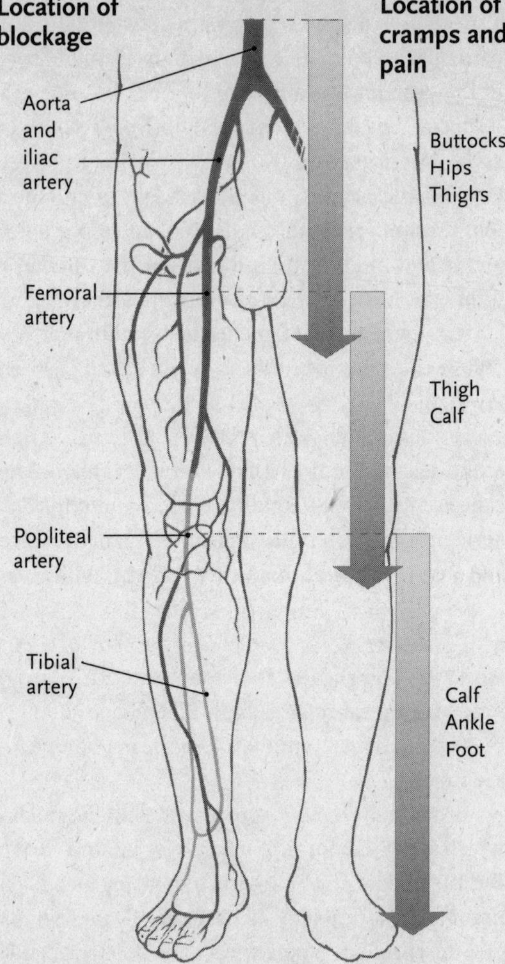

Narrowed arteries do not carry a full supply of oxygen-rich blood to tissues. When muscles exercise, they need more oxygen. Painful cramps develop if blood flow cannot keep up with demand. The location of pain depends on the site of the blockage.

osclerosis causes angina and heart attacks and, in the brain, it causes strokes. In the limbs, atherosclerosis causes *peripheral arterial disease.*

The plaques of peripheral arterial disease are much more common in the legs than the arms. In the legs, the blockages tend to occur in specific locations such as the *aorta* and the *iliac, femoral, popliteal,* and *tibial* arteries (see Figure 14.1). The points of greatest risk are the places where arteries branch into smaller vessels. Many people with symptoms of peripheral artery disease have multiple blockages. In all, about 30 percent have narrowing of the aorta or iliac arteries, 80 percent have disease in the femoral or popliteal arteries, and 40 percent have plaques in the tibial artery.

Peripheral arterial disease gets much less attention than heart disease and stroke, but it is actually a very common problem with very important implications. About 300,000 Americans are diagnosed with peripheral artery disease each year. Rare in people below age fifty, peripheral arterial disease becomes more common with age; about 25 percent of men above seventy-five have the problem, but only a quarter of them have symptoms. Although women get peripheral arterial disease, it is two to five times more common in men.

In most cases, peripheral arterial disease progresses only slowly, and excellent treatment is available. Only about 4 percent of patients develop critical impairments of the blood flow to their legs during the course of a year. But although peripheral arterial disease is typically slow to progress, men with the problem have death rates two to three items higher than men who are free of peripheral artery disease. In all, men with peripheral arterial disease severe enough to cause symptoms have a 15 percent chance of dying within five years and a 50 percent chance of dying within ten years of the initial diagnosis.

If peripheral arterial disease itself is rarely lethal, why do so many patients with the disease die prematurely? About half die from heart attacks, about a quarter from strokes. That is because atherosclerosis truly is a systemic disease, affecting critical arteries in the heart and brain as well as the somewhat less critical arteries in the legs. It's an important message: Patients with peripheral vascular disease must be treated for all the manifestations of atherosclerosis, not just the blockages in their legs.

RISK FACTORS

Peripheral arterial disease is caused by the same problems that produce atherosclerosis in other parts of the circulation. For the legs, diabetes and smoking are the two most potent factors, increasing risk by threefold and twofold, respectively; both are likely to cause more severe, rapidly progressive disease. Close behind are high blood pressure and abnormal cholesterol levels; the Physicians' Health Study recently reported that an elevated ratio of total cholesterol to HDL cholesterol was a particularly strong predictor of risk. Although less carefully studied, other heart disease risk factors such as high levels of *homocysteine* and lack of exercise (see Chapter Three) also play important roles. In addition, the Physicians' Health Study found that elevated levels of C-reactive protein predict a high risk of future peripheral artery disease; it is another indication of the important role of inflammation in vascular disease. Obesity and psychological factors have received less attention, but they may also contribute to peripheral arterial disease, as they do to atherosclerosis in other arteries.

SYMPTOMS

The symptoms of peripheral artery disease occur in three stages: *intermittent claudication, rest pain,* and *critical limb ischemia.*

Intermittent claudication is the earliest and most common symptom. Claudication is derived from the Latin "to limp." It is why the Roman emperor who was born lame was named Claudius. But today the term refers to pain, usually a cramplike discomfort but sometimes experienced as fatigue, weariness, numbness or tingling. Claudication occurs when muscles are not getting all the oxygen they need. Because exercising muscles need oxygen, claudication begins during exercise, particularly walking, and disappears with a few minutes of rest. The intermittent nature of the symptom is reflected in its name. Men with mild blockages can walk substantial distances before claudication sets in, but men with severe arterial narrowing can experience distress in just a few yards.

The location of the discomfort depends on the site of the blockage:

LOCATION OF BLOCKAGE	LOCATION OF PAIN
Tibial artery	Foot
Femoral or popliteal artery	Calf
Aorta or iliac artery	Thigh, hip, or buttock

Because the iliac artery gives rise to the arteries that supply blood to the penis, men with aortoiliac atherosclerosis are also at high risk for impotence (see Chapter Ten).

Although peripheral artery disease is the most common cause of exertion-induced leg pain, other disorders can cause similar symptoms. *Spinal stenosis* is the closest mimic, so close in fact that the pain is called *pseudoclaudication.* Spinal stenosis results from a narrowing of the lower spinal canal that puts pressure on the nerves to the legs, usually caused by degenerative arthritis. It is most common in the same older age groups that are at risk for peripheral artery disease. Like true claudication, pseudoclaudication occurs with exercise; like true claudication, it is relieved by rest, but the relief usually occurs more slowly. Both symptoms are triggered by walking, but people with peripheral artery disease also get leg pain from biking, while those with spinal stenosis do not. That's because people bend forward when they bike, and flexion widens the spinal canal, reducing pressure on the nerves. But even if the symptoms of peripheral artery disease and spinal stenosis overlap, doctors can readily distinguish the two by checking the leg pulses (diminished in arterial disease) and reflexes (decreased after walking in spinal stenosis).

Rest Pain occurs when blockages are so severe that leg muscles cannot get enough oxygen when they are at rest. Foot pain is most common. Initially, it is worse at night, because leg elevation decreases blood flow while gravity improves flow during sitting or standing. As the disorder progresses, the pain becomes severe and persistent. Deprived of oxygen and nutrients, the skin becomes cool, thin, pale, and shiny, then develops ulcers that are difficult to heal and may become infected.

Critical limb ischemia is every bit as bad as it sounds. *Ischemia* means tissue injury caused by lack of blood and oxygen. When severe or prolonged, ischemia results in *necrosis,* or tissue death. In the case of peripheral artery disease, critical ischemia can occur when a plaque closes off an artery, when an artery-blocking clot forms on a plaque, or when a clot breaks off from the heart or large artery and travels downstream to lodge in a narrow artery, where it blocks the flow of blood.

In most cases, the diagnosis of peripheral artery disease is quite straightforward; a doctor will suspect the diagnosis when he hears a man's symptoms, and he will confirm it by feeling the pulses in his legs. For most of their course, the leg arteries are covered by muscle and are too deep to feel, but they can be evaluated in three places (see Figure 14.1); at the ankle (*dorsalis pedis* and *posterior tibial* arteries) at the back of the knee (*popliteal artery*) and in the groin (*femoral artery*). In some cases, the doctor will also use his stethoscope to listen to the blood traveling through the femoral artery; if the artery is narrowed, it may produce a high pitched whooshing sound called a *bruit.*

It is important for the doctor to examine both legs, allowing him to compare the circulation in each. It is also important to check for signs of trouble in the skin. Since impaired blood flow deprives the skin of nutrients, it is often pale, cool, thin, and shiny: in addition, hair growth may be diminished. A few simple maneuvers may also be revealing: elevating the affected leg makes it pale, while dangling it down from the exam table makes it a dusky bluish-red.

Finally, painful, hard-to-heal skin ulcers or infections may be present, particularly in advanced cases.

Detecting peripheral artery disease is one thing, assessing its extent, quite another. Fortunately a simple test, the *ankle-brachial index* (ABI), can give a good estimate of severity, and it can also be used to estimate the risk of coronary artery disease, even in the absence of chest pain or electrocardiographic (EKG) abnormalities.

To understand how the ABI works, just step on a garden hose; the blockage produced by your foot will reduce water pressure at the nozzle. Similarly, a blockage in a leg artery will reduce blood pressure at the ankle.

To measure your ABI, your doctor will first measure your blood pressure in the normal way in both arms at the *brachial arteries.* For the ABI, it is the higher number or *systolic blood pressure* that counts; if your arms differ, the higher pressure will be used for the index. Next, after placing a large blood-pressure cuff around your thigh or calf, your doctor will check the pressure at your ankle, using either the posterior tibial or dorsalis pedis artery. Instead of using a stethoscope, though, he will use a *Doppler probe* to detect the systolic blood pressure at your ankle.

In health, the ankle blood pressure is slightly higher than the brachial blood pressures, but peripheral artery disease usually reduces the ankle pressure without affecting the arm pressure. To calculate the index, your doctor will divide your ankle blood pressure by your arm pressure; to interpret the results he may use the following guide:

ABI	SEVERITY OF BLOCKAGES
0.9 or higher	None or minimal
0.7–0.89	Mild
0.5–0.69	Moderate
Below 0.5	Severe
Below 0.15	Threat of amputation

Doctors can also use the ABI to estimate your risk of having coronary artery disease and stroke. Men with ABIs below 0.9 have twice the risk of heart attack and four times the risk of stroke as compared to men with normal ABIs. Peripheral artery disease is a serious business, often reflecting atherosclerosis in the heart and brain.

In most cases, when a doctor suspects peripheral artery disease, he will order an ultrasound to confirm the diagnosis. Ultrasound can also be used to follow the course of the disease, but more elaborate tests are needed for patients who are candidates for invasive therapy.

Duplex Ultrasound Scanning. This is a direct, noninvasive test that combines ultrasound and Doppler technology. It allows doctors to identify the site of a blockage, to measure the thickness of an artery's wall, and to determine the severity of an artery's narrowing. In general, a narrowing of more than 50 percent is likely to produce symptoms.

Angiography. The gold standard for diagnosis, angiography involves the puncture of an artery and the injection of a dye that allows X-rays to detect the location and extent of blockages. It is a very accurate test but it has risks of its own, including bleeding from the puncture site and allergic reactions or kidney damage from the dye. As a result, angiography is used only as a prelude to revascularization therapy.

Magnetic Resonance Angiography (MRA). MRA is a new approach that may soon replace angiography. MRAs use *gadolinium* instead of dye, and they do not require arterial puncture; as a result, they are safer than angiograms. Because they use magnetic resonance imaging instead of X-rays, MRAs can produce accurate and detailed views of blockages. In some centers, MRAs have already replaced conventional angiograms for preoperative evaluation.

Newer Tests. Still experimental are new tests such as *intravascular ultrasound* and *angioscopy.* Each requires an arterial puncture, which enables doctors to insert an ultrasound probe or fiberoptic tube into the artery, allowing them to visualize the narrowed artery from the inside. A new noninvasive test is the *spiral computed tomographic angiogram;* it is similar to the MRA, but it uses X-rays instead of magnetic resonance images to visualize arteries.

TREATMENT: RISK FACTOR REDUCTION

Because peripheral artery disease is a form of atherosclerosis, everyone who has it should attempt to reduce his atherosclerosis risk factors, and, of course, must avoid tobacco in any form. Abnormal cholesterol levels should be treated with diet, exercise, and weight control. In addition, medications, such as the statin drugs, can be very helpful; in the Scandinavian Simvastatin Survival Study, for example, *simvastatin* (Zocor) therapy reduced the risk of new or worsening intermittent claudication by 38 percent. Although blood-sugar control may not improve peripheral artery disease, it is still important for diabetics to achieve optimal blood sugar levels. Similarly, while blood pressure control may not reduce plaques in leg arteries, it is important to reduce the risk of heart attack and stroke. Because an abrupt or excessive drop in blood pressure can reduce blood flow in a partially blocked artery, however, hypertension must be treated with care in patients with peripheral artery disease.

Can a drink a day keep peripheral artery disease away? Perhaps, according to the Physicians' Health Study, which found that moderate drinking reduces a man's risk of developing peripheral artery disease. After accounting for other risk factors, men who consumed at least one drink a week were 26 percent less likely to develop peripheral artery disease than men who drank less. Since moderate drinking also reduces the risk of coronary artery disease and possibly stroke, the results are logical. But because excessive drinking poses enormous health risks, men who choose to drink must do so with care and moderation, averaging just one to two drinks a day (see Chapter Seven).

TREATMENT: EXERCISE

Although it may seem paradoxical, the most important treatment for intermittent claudication is the very thing that triggers the leg pain: exercise. The most successful regimens begin with supervised exercise training, typically in thirty-to-sixty-minute sessions three times a week. Although walking is the mainstay of treatment, many programs mix in biking, stair climbing, and resistance exercise. In most cases, men who can walk only fifty to one hundred yards before developing pain can walk two or even three times farther at the end of twelve weeks of training, and if they continue exercising on their own, they can expect still more improvement over the next year or so.

Although there is some evidence that exercise may help stabilize or even reduce coronary artery blockages when combined with a strict diet, exercise does not seem to reduce peripheral artery plaques. Instead, the benefit of exercise training depends on its effect on muscles. With training, muscles develop new *capillaries,* the tiny blood vessels that distribute oxygen, and they develop new *enzymes,* proteins that enable them to use oxygen more effectively. Because trained muscles use oxygen more efficiently, they can carry men farther even if their blood supply is limited by peripheral artery disease.

TREATMENT: MEDICATIONS

In general, medications have been only marginally effective in reducing symptoms of peripheral artery disease. The simplest but most useful medication, in fact, does not reduce symptoms at all. Still, low-dose aspirin therapy (81 to 325 milligrams a day) is important to reduce the risk of heart attacks and strokes in patients with atherosclerosis (see Chapter Six), and the Physicians' Health Study found that low-dose aspirin is associated with a 50 percent reduction in the likelihood of needing surgery for peripheral artery disease. *Pentoxifylline* (Trental) is a unique medication that makes red blood cells more flexible. In theory, it should help blood slip past arterial blockages. In practice, it does delay the onset of claudication, allowing patients to walk a bit farther before they have to rest, but the improvement is quite modest. Somewhat better results have been obtained in studies with *cilostazol* (Pletal), but since it is a new drug it does not yet have a long-term track record for safety and efficacy. No one with any degree of congestive heart failure should take cilostazol. *Verapamil* (Calan and other brands) is a calcium-channel blocker that is widely used to treat hypertension; in a recent European trial, it improved walking distance in forty-four patients with intermittent claudication. Among alternative therapies, garlic and Gingko biloba have been reported to help, but the data are sparse and the improvements very modest.

TREATMENT: REVASCULARIZATION

Although doctors have made little progress in the drug therapy of peripheral artery disease, exercise and risk factor reduction can keep the problem under control in more than two-thirds of patients. And when revascularization is needed, doctors have made great strides in developing ways to open blocked arteries with balloons and to bypass blockages with grafts. It is a familiar story, since patients with coronary artery disease benefit from similar treatments.

Before undertaking an *angioplasty,* doctors perform an arteriogram to define the blockages. Next, they thread a catheter through the artery until they reach the blockage. Finally, they inflate a tiny balloon that compresses the plaque, opening the artery. Success rates vary; up to 90 percent of iliac artery blockages improve, but in the femoral and popliteal arteries, initial success rates are only about 65 percent. In either case, about one-third of the blockages redevelop within five years. In an attempt to reduce *restenosis,* doctors are now placing tiny flexible metallic mesh *stents* in the artery after the angioplasty. Stents are very helpful after coronary artery angioplasties, but further research is needed to learn if they are as effective in peripheral artery disease. Antiplatelet medications appear to reduce the risk of recurrent blockages after stent placement.

If less invasive techniques are not successful, surgeons can use grafts to bypass blockages; in general, long or complex blockages require surgery. Synthetic material, such as Dacron, is required for large arteries such as the iliacs, but vein grafts are preferable for the smaller femoral and popliteal arteries in the thigh and knee. Bypass surgery carries risks of its own and should not be undertaken lightly. Still, it can have great benefit for patients with severe pain, and it may be the only way to prevent amputation in cases of severe arterial disease.

TREATING CLOTS

Blood clots can block arteries by forming on cholesterol-laden plaques or surgical grafts (*thrombosis*) or by breaking off from the heart or a large artery and traveling downstream to lodge in a smaller artery (*embolization*). Aspirin and other anticlotting drugs ("blood thinners") can help prevent these events. But when clots block arteries, they can cause immediate, severe damage. *Thrombolytic drugs* ("clot busters") have earned a major role in treating heart attacks, and they appear useful in some types of strokes. Thrombolytic drugs can also help patients with blocked leg arteries, but vascular surgery is an excellent alternative and is more effective in some cases. One way or the other, though, urgent treatment is needed to restore blood flow after acute blockages of peripheral arteries.

NEW HORIZONS, OLD STANDBYS

Researchers are seeking new ways to treat peripheral artery disease; gene therapy is an exciting example. The problems are formidable, but improvements are sure to occur. Still, prevention will always be the best treatment, and in the case of peripheral artery disease and other forms of atherosclerosis, it is very effective indeed. As you stay tuned for new breakthroughs, continue to practice the basics: avoid tobacco; eat a balanced, low-fat diet; keep your weight under control; and get plenty of exercise. Your arteries will thank you for your efforts.

If you have peripheral artery disease, here are some simple but very important ways to avoid further damage:

- Avoid extremes of temperature. Do not use a heating pad on your feet. Do not put your feet in hot water. In cold weather, wear socks to bed at night.

- Keep your feet very clean; wash in lukewarm water at least once a day, and apply lanolin after bathing. Inspect your feet daily.
- Protect your feet at all times. Place lamb's wool between overriding toes. Wear cotton socks, which do not retain moisture, and change them whenever your feet are damp. Wear properly fitting shoes; avoid synthetic materials that do not "breathe." Wear slippers at night and use a night light to avoid stubbing your toes or hitting your shins.
- If your feet ache at night, raise the head of your bed on six-to-ten-inch blocks.
- Avoid exposure to tobacco in all forms (see Chapter Eight).
- Walk to the point of discomfort, then rest and walk again. Try to work up to two miles a day (see Chapter Five).
- Follow a good diet and lose weight if you are obese (see Chapter Four).
- Work with your doctor to control your cholesterol, blood sugar, and blood pressure (see Chapter Three).
- Notify your doctor of any sudden change in symptoms such as increased pain, numbness or tingling, weakness, skin ulcers, or abnormal skin color or temperature.

Disorders of Breathing During Sleep: Snoring and Sleep Apnea

Healthy sleep is quiet and restorative; mind and body slow down, gaining strength for the coming day. Like so many bodily functions, breathing patterns change during normal sleep. Often, however, breathing becomes abnormal at night, with consequences that range from the noise of snoring to the health hazard of sleep apnea. Men are particularly vulnerable to these disorders, but they are usually unaware of the problem because, as Mark Twain observed, "A snorer can't hear himself snore."

Breathing During Sleep

Taking a breath is like expanding a bellows: the chest cage expands and the diaphragm, the large muscle between the chest and the abdomen, contracts. The result is negative pressure that sucks air down into the lungs. For air to reach the lungs, it must first pass through the nose or mouth, then into the back of the throat. The upper airway is narrow, and the tissues at the back of the throat are soft and pliant. The negative pressure of breathing tends to bring these tissues together. If they collapsed inward, they would block the airway, cutting off the flow of air. To prevent this, a special set of muscles in the neck works continuously; these *dilator muscles* spread the tissues apart, keeping the airway open.

All muscles relax during sleep. Because the dilator muscles are less active, the upper airway narrows during sleep. In most people, the airway remains wide enough to permit air to flow smoothly through. But in many men, sleep produces excessive narrowing of the upper airway. The results are nocturnal breathing disorders, which range from mild to very serious indeed.

Snoring

When air flows smoothly, it flows silently; when turbulent, it is noisy. In most cases, snoring results from two problems: excessive inspiratory pressure and excessive narrowing of the upper airway. As a result, airflow is both fast and turbid. The tissues at the back of the throat vibrate and flutter, producing the sound of snoring. Contrary to earlier beliefs, snoring occurs during both inspiration and expiration, and it can occur during mouth breathing or nose breathing.

Sleep Apnea

The term *apnea* is derived from the Greek word for "lack of breath." Sleep apnea is well-named: Breathing stops during sleep. The pause is always temporary, lasting from just a few seconds to a minute or more. Spells of apnea can be rare or frequent, occurring from once or twice a night to more than 500 times a single night. In addition to stopping completely, breathing may become slow, shallow, and ineffectual without halting, a condition called *hypopnea.* To measure the severity of a nocturnal breathing problem the number of apneic and hypopneic spells that last longer than ten seconds are tallied together; scores above 5 per hour are considered significant, those above 15, serious.

There are two major types of sleep apnea. The less common is *central sleep apnea.* Here, the central nervous system is at fault, providing the lungs with too few of the impulses that initiate breathing. Central sleep apnea can be serious, often resulting in congestive heart failure. Patients with central sleep apnea and congestive heart failure benefit from low-flow oxygen therapy at night. New research indicates that an oral medication, *theophylline,* may also help.

When breathing stops during sleep, it is usually caused by *obstructive sleep apnea.* In this condition, the brain signals normally but the lungs cannot respond because the tissues of the upper airway have narrowed to the point of collapse, obstructing the flow of air. In this respect, obstructive sleep apnea has much in common with snoring. Indeed, virtually everyone with sleep apnea snores. Fortunately, however, not all snorers develop sleep apnea.

WHO DEVELOPS NOCTURNAL BREATHING PROBLEMS?

About half of all men snore, and 25 percent snore frequently. Sleep apnea was considered less common, affecting about 4 percent of men, until a 1993 study detected it in 24 percent of healthy middle-aged men. The same type of person tends to be at risk for both snoring and obstructive sleep apnea. About 85 percent of the time, that person is a man, but the reasons for this marked male predominance are obscure. The importance of obesity is far from obscure. The tissues of the upper airway are themselves thickened, and are also subjected to extra pressure from the obese neck. Of course, not all overweight men develop obstructed breathing. Upper body obesity and a large neck (especially size 17 or more) are particular risk factors. Other abnormalities of the upper airway, such as nasal polyps, enlarged tonsils or adenoids, a floppy palate, a large *uvula* (the U-shaped tissue that hangs from the palate), and a short jaw, have also been implicated.

Obstructed breathing during sleep can occur at any age, but it is most common in men between thirty and sixty. Smoking increases the likelihood of obstruction, perhaps because it irritates the tissues of the throat, causing them to swell. Allergies may have a similar effect. Alcohol and sedatives can also increase obstruction because they relax the dilator muscles that must contract strongly to keep the airway open. Much less often, endocrine diseases such as *hypothyroidism* or *acromegaly* are responsible.

WHAT ARE THE CONSEQUENCES?

Although snoring and sleep apnea occur in the same setting, there is a world of difference between the disorders. Snoring is a benign disorder, causing problems for spouses and roommates but not for the snorer himself. But while sleep apnea can also be mild, it can sometimes lead to life-threatening complications.

Sleep apnea thwarts the restorative functions of sleep. When breathing stops, blood oxygen levels fall and carbon dioxide levels rise. Sooner or later, these abnormalities produce *arousal,* activating the resting nervous system. Although the sleeper does not awaken and is unaware of arousal, it can be recognized by a sudden snort or grunt that signals the return of breathing. Arousal prevents suffocation, but it also fragments sleep, preventing it from reaching the deeper stages necessary to refresh mental function. The result is sleep deprivation, which produces daytime sleepiness, headaches, decreased alertness and concentration, and irritability.

Sleep is intended to rest the mind, and it is also meant to rest the heart and circulation. Arousal jolts the circulation. The autonomic nervous system is activated, pouring out adrenaline. The heart rate and blood pressure, normally low during sleep, rise abruptly. In men with heart disease, sleep apnea and arousal can trigger angina, heart attacks, and arrhythmias. In healthy men, repeated nocturnal apnea overloads the circulation, eventually quadrupling the risk of heart attacks and tripling the risk of strokes.

Sleep apnea occurs only at night, but it can affect health all day long.

DIAGNOSIS

Mark Twain was right: More than 80 percent of men with snoring and sleep apnea do not know they have abnormal breathing during sleep. To find out if you have either problem, ask the person sleeping next to you. If you snore loudly, you probably will not even have to ask, since you will have been poked in the ribs during many a night. For sleep apnea, ask if your breathing slows or stops, then resumes with a loud snort or gasp, only to slow or stop again. Restless sleep with jerking and thrashing can also suggest sleep apnea. If you sleep alone, you can tape record your own breathing or simply look for tell-tale signs of restless sleep, such as sheets and blankets that are excessively rumpled or tossed aside.

Although snoring can be a major relationship problem, it is not an important medical concern. But sleep apnea is serious, and it should be detected and treated before it leads to high blood pressure and its complications. If you do not snore, you do not have to worry about sleep apnea. But snoring itself, even it is very loud, does not predict the occurrence of apnea. Even if you cannot hear yourself, you can look for other clues.

The most important is *daytime somnolence.* Men with sleep apnea have fragmented sleep. Instead of being refreshed, they are tired in the morning, often experiencing morning headaches as well as fatigue. The sleepiness persists all day. Diminished concentration, poor work performance, irritability, and mood disorders are quite common, and men with sleep apnea often drift off to sleep during the day. A nap is one thing, falling asleep at the wheel quite another. In fact, motor vehicle accidents are among the most serious consequences of sleep apnea.

Daytime sleepiness is the major clue to sleep apnea, but there are others. In addition to snoring and thrashing, abnormal sleep behaviors can include sleepwalking and frequent night-time urination or even loss of urinary control (see Chapter Thirteen). In addition to sleepiness and morning headaches, daytime abnormalities can include personality changes, episodic disorientation or hallucinations, intellectual decline, and sexual dysfunction. Medical consequences include hypertension and an increased risk of heart disease and stroke.

Because the treatment of sleep apnea is difficult, the diagnosis should always be confirmed medically. Confirmation depends on *polysomnography,* a comprehensive test requiring the patient to spend a night in a specially-equipped sleep lab. Many functions are monitored during sleep, including airflow through the nose to detect apnea, blood pressure and EKG to detect hypertension and cardiac abnormalities, blood oxygen to detect an insufficient air supply, and brain wave and eye motion to detect arousal and fragmented sleep. If that were not enough, some labs also monitor the activity of respiratory muscles and the movements of the limbs during sleep.

Polysomnography is complex, time-consuming, and expensive. Simpler home monitoring devices are also available, but are less reliable. Men should undergo polysomnography before they consider complex medical or surgical treatments, but they can—and should—try lifestyle treatment even before proceeding with elaborate tests.

TREATMENT

Because snoring does not lead to medical complications, it should be treated only to benefit your bed partner. Because sleep apnea can be serious, it should be treated to protect you. The first step is to diagnose and treat any underlying conditions, ranging from simple problems like allergies or nasal polyps to endocrinologic diseases. But most men with snoring or sleep apnea do not have such triggers, and treatment must be directed to the breathing disorders themselves. Both conditions may respond to lifestyle changes, assisted breathing devices, oral appliances, or surgery, but few men will go beyond lifestyle treatment if snoring is their only problem.

Lifestyle Treatment. People who smoke should stop. Men who use sedatives or tranquilizers should omit these medications, particularly late in the day; the same is true for alcohol, which can act like a sedative. Finally, men who are overweight should reduce. It is the most important lifestyle treatment, but it is also the hardest to achieve; diet and exercise are the cornerstones (see Chapters Four and Five).

Airway narrowing during sleep often depends on body position; the usual culprit is sleeping on the back. That's why an elbow to the ribs is the time-tested treatment for snoring. A less traumatic trick is to sew a small pocket on the back of your pajama tops and fill it with a tennis ball when you go to bed. If you sleep at all (and nearly all men manage to), you will not sleep on your back. More elaborate devices to achieve sleep position training include gravity-activated alarms and an indented pillow with a rigid plastic bar at the trough that keeps your head on its side.

If you watch pro football on TV, you have seen some players wearing small plastic strips across their nostrils. These Breathe Right nasal strips pull the nostrils apart, easing air flow through the nose. They were approved for snoring by the Food and Drug Administration (FDA) on the basis of two very small studies involving just twenty-seven people, but newer research casts considerable doubt on their efficacy, both for snoring and for athletic performance. Other simple measures that are worth a try include antihistamines or steroid nose sprays to reduce swelling of the nasal passages in men with allergies.

Breathing Devices. The treatment of sleep apnea has been revolutionized by breathing devices. These machines continuously deliver air under pressure to the patient's nose or mouth during sleep; the positive pressure keeps the airway from collapsing during inspiration. *Continuous positive airway pressure* (CPAP) can be delivered through a nasal mask, nasal prongs, or a mask over the sleeper's mouth and nose; nasal CPAP is most popular (see Figure 14.2).

CPAP is extremely effective, preventing all the complications of sleep apnea. But like all treatments, CPAP works only if it is used properly and regularly. The machine that creates the positive pressure runs on household current, weighs about 5 pounds, and fits easily on most bedside tables. But the system is expensive, generally costing $1,000 or more. The medical benefits of CPAP far outweigh its cost, but many men cannot adjust to the mask; one study found that only 46 percent of patients with CPAP used it properly.

Just a few years after its introduction, CPAP has become the treatment of choice for sleep apnea. Because of its cost and inconvenience, however, it is

FIGURE 14.2. NASAL CPAP

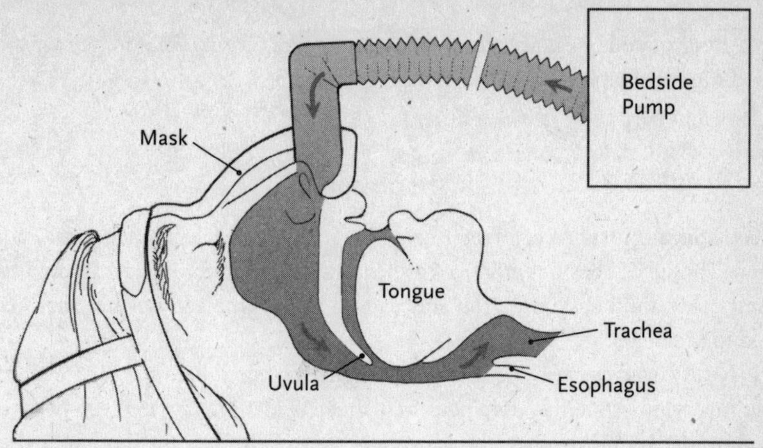

Nasal CPAP pumps air through a mask or prongs into the nose. The pressure opens the airway, allowing air to enter the trachea and lungs.

usually prescribed for men with high apnea-hypopnea scores documented by polysomnography.

Supplementary oxygen can be administered along with CPAP, but it is not necessary if the device is working effectively. Even without CPAP, oxygen may help some men with sleep apnea.

Oral Appliances. A variety of orthodontic devices can be used to reposition the tongue and hold the upper airway open during sleep. Although CPAP is more effective, oral appliances can help, and many men find them more comfortable and convenient.

Surgery. The arrival of CPAP has reduced the need for surgery. It's a good thing, since *tracheostomy* (constructing a breathing hole in the windpipe just below the "Adam's apple") is disfiguring but is the only uniformly effective operation. Many less drastic operations have been proposed; they are most effective for people with anatomic abnormalities of the nose, mouth, or throat, but they should be reserved for men with severe sleep apnea who fail CPAP and oral devices.

Homer described sleep as "the brother of death." Snoring may kill a marriage, but sleep apnea can come close to fulfilling the Greek poet's definition. With dramatic new advances in the diagnosis and management of nocturnal breathing disorders, however, most men should now be able to get a really good night's sleep.

Insomnia

Sleep apnea is just one of many sleep disorders; insomnia is much more common. Though it does not produce cardiovascular complications, it can produce personality and behavioral problems as well as daytime somnolence that may lead to accidents.

Nearly everyone has spent at least one night lying in bed wishing for sleep, and nearly everyone has tried counting sheep, watching late night movies, or sipping warm milk (or something stronger) for relief. All these home remedies may seem to help deal with an occasional sleepless night. Unfortunately, however, it is far more difficult to correct true insomnia.

When specific problems, such as anxiety, depression, nicotine use, excessive use of caffeine or decongestant medications, heart disease, or prostate conditions are responsible for sleep deprivation, the best way to restore sleep is to treat the basic disorder. But people with *primary insomnia* have no underlying conditions. Still, they can get relief by treating the sleep disturbance itself, using behavioral techniques supplemented by medications when necessary.

Behavioral Approaches. You can learn to sleep better. Here are some tips to help:

- Establish a regular sleeping schedule. Respect your body's internal clock by going to bed and getting up at nearly the same time every day, even on weekends. When you begin your schedule, plan to stay in bed for only as long as you sleep on an average night. For example, if you spend eight hours in bed but sleep for only five hours during that time, allot just five to five and a half hours in bed. You may actually lose some sleep at first, but your mild sleep debt will pay off if you go to bed fifteen minutes earlier each week until you are spending your usual amount of time in bed and sleeping for most of it.
- Use your bed only for sleeping or lovemaking, never for reading or watching TV. If you cannot sleep after fifteen to twenty minutes, get out of bed and go into another room. Read quietly with a dim light but do not watch TV, since the full spectrum light emitted by the tube has

an arousing effect. When you feel sleepy, get back into bed, but do not delay your scheduled awaking time to compensate for your lost sleep.

- Do not nap during the day unless it is absolutely necessary. Even then, restrict your nap to fifteen to twenty minutes in the early afternoon.
- Get plenty of exercise. Two 1997 studies show that physical activity during the day promotes sleep at night. In one trial, four weekly sessions of brisk walking or low-impact aerobics added an average of forty-two minutes of nightly sleep to forty-three healthy middle-aged people with insomnia. In the other, three weight-lifting sessions per week improved sleep quality and the overall quality of life in thirty-two elderly people with depression and insomnia. Build up to thirty to forty-five minutes of moderate to brisk exercise nearly every day. Get your workout early in the day, then try some stretching exercises or yoga to relax your muscles and your mind at bedtime.
- Wind down late in the day. Whenever possible, schedule stressful or demanding tasks early and less challenging activities later.
- Eat properly. Avoid caffeine and alcohol, especially after mid-afternoon. Try to avoid all beverages after dinner if you find yourself getting up at night to urinate. If you enjoy a bedtime snack, keep it bland and light.
- Be sure your bed is comfortable and your bedroom is dark and quiet. It should also be well ventilated and kept at a constant, comfortable temperature. Try using a sleep mask, ear plugs, or white noise machine to compensate for problems in your sleeping environment.
- Above all, do not worry about sleep. Watching the clock never helps. Do not keep track of the amount of time you spend trying to sleep; you will probably underestimate your actual sleeping time, and you will deprive yourself of the benefits you can get from resting quietly and peacefully in bed. Try not to lie in bed reviewing your problems and plans. If you really are overloaded, get out of bed and make a list, then return to bed and think of something relaxing and pleasant.
- Learn relaxation techniques such as deep breathing, progressive muscular relaxation, or meditation. If you have trouble relaxing on your own, consider behavioral therapy or counseling.

Medications for Sleep. Sleeping pills are available over-the-counter or by prescription. *Antihistamines* are the active ingredients in most over-the-counter sleeping pills such as Nytol, Tylenol PM, Sominex, and many others. They can promote sleepiness, but most sleep specialists discourage regular use because they may impair sleep quality and hinder daytime alertness. Antihistamines can also produce urinary retention in men with *benign prostate hyperplasia* (BPH) and they should not be used by people with *angle-closure glaucoma.* In addition, *melatonin* and various herbs are sold as dietary supplements to promote sleep, but their efficacy and safety have not been established.

Although many types of prescription medications are available, most physicians recommend a *benzodiazepine,* such as *temazepam* (Restoril), the drug *zolpidem* (Ambien), or an antidepressant, such as *trazodone* (Desyrel). Like all powerful drugs, sleeping pills require careful medical supervision and should be used only when needed. Whether you are treating yourself or using a drug prescribed by your doctor, you should follow several basic guidelines:

- Use medications only as a back-up to behavioral changes.
- Use the lowest dose that is effective.
- Do not take a pill every night. Instead, use medication only when an uninterrupted night's sleep is really important. Even then, restrict yourself to two to four tablets per week.
- Try to stop using medication after three to four weeks.
- Discontinue medication gradually to avoid rebound insomnia.

Baldness

It lacks the pain of gout, the threat of an aortic aneurysm, and the complications of sleep apnea. Still, despite the best efforts of Michael Jordan, millions of men are distressed by hair loss.

Normal Hair Growth

Whether straight or curly, hair grows in a cyclical pattern. The cycle has three phases: growth (called the *anagen* phase by biologists), involution (*catagen*), and rest (*telogen*). In humans, each hair follicle cycles independently of the others; that's why humans do not "shed" each season, as many animals do. In a healthy scalp, more than 90 percent of hair follicles are in the growth phase, less than 1 percent are undergoing involution, and 5 to 10 percent are resting.

At birth, the human body is covered by about 5 million hair follicles, including about 100,000 in the scalp. The number of hair follicles remains constant throughout life, but the activity and productivity of each follicle varies according to the stage of a person's life.

Abnormal Hair Loss

Hair follicles contain living cells; like all cells, they can be damaged. Damaged follicles stop growing hair. If the problem is mild, the follicle recovers and resumes hair growth, but if the damage is severe, it may be permanent.

If it is substantial enough, any stress, physical or emotional, can damage hair follicles, halting hair growth. That's why patients often lose hair two or three months after a major illness or traumatic life event. It is a temporary problem technically known as *telogen effluvium*. It is easy to recognize with a simple pull test: If you can extract more than five or six hairs with a single pull, you are likely to have telogen effluvium, and you are likely to grow back all your hair within a few months, even without therapy.

Medications can damage hair follicles; chemotherapy drugs are the leading examples. Less often, toxic chemicals, radiation, or infection can do the job. Skin diseases that produce scarring can also produce hair loss, which may be permanent. These problems are all uncommon. Contrary to popular belief, common woes like seborrhea and dandruff do not cause hair loss.

Normal Hair Loss

Men with male pattern baldness may not regard it as normal, but it is. Like it or not, loss of scalp hair is part of the human condition. It may cause psychological distress that is important in its own right, but it is not a disease.

Virtually all people, male and female, lose scalp hair as they age. In a sense, male pattern baldness, (known technically as *androgenic alopecia*) is just an exaggerated form of a normal event. It has two prerequisites: a genetic predisposition and the male hormone testosterone.

The genetics of male baldness are complex. Doctors believe one gene is responsible, but several may play a role. In any case, the abnormal gene has *variable penetrance,* which means it is more likely to produce hair loss in some men than others. The abnormal gene can be passed down from a mother or a father, and it can be inherited by boys and girls. But men are much more likely to suffer from the gene's activity because they have the second prerequisite, testosterone.

Testosterone makes the man; it is responsible for the large muscles, strong bones, and deep voice that characterize the gender. The hormone is essential for male genital development during fetal life, for the sexual awakening of adolescence, and for libido and fertility in adulthood. Testosterone acts directly on tissues, to produce all these effects, but it acts on the prostate and on hair follicles indirectly. In these tissues, an enzyme called 5 *alpha-reductase* converts testosterone to *dihydrotestosterone* (DHT), and DHT acts on the tissues.

DHT stimulates the growth of hair follicles in the beard and body, but it has the opposite effect on scalp hair. Hair loss usually starts between age seventeen and forty. By age fifty, about half of all men display some degree of male pattern baldness. It usually begins with a receding hairline over the temples, followed by thinning of the hair at the vertex or top of the scalp. The rate of hair loss is highly variable. Some men go bald in less than five years, but most lose hair gradually over fifteen to twenty-five years. On average, men with androgenic alopecia lose about 5 percent of their scalp hair each year, but the process can slow down or speed up without apparent reason.

Although it's small comfort to balding men, their hair follicles do not actually disappear. Instead, each successive growth phase grows shorter and each resting phase, longer. With a shorter growth phase, the hair becomes shorter and finer; with a longer resting phase, the hairs are less tightly attached to the scalp, so they fall out during washing or combing. In addition, the follicles themselves grow progressively smaller until they are reduced to miniatures that produce only short, fine, unpigmented *vellus hair* that is nearly invisible.

Is Hair Loss Harmful?

Male pattern baldness is not a disease; the only consequences are cosmetic and the only complications are psychological. Although baldness does not cause disease, it may be a marker for cardiac risk. The Physicians' Health Study found that men with bald spots were more likely to develop coronary artery disease than men with full heads of hair; mild vertex baldness was linked to a 23 percent increase, moderate baldness to a 32 percent rise, and severe baldness to a 36 percent increase in risk. The effect was greatest in men with hypertension or high cholesterol levels. Frontal baldness, the receding hairline, was not associated with cardiac risk.

Doctors do not know why baldness and heart disease are linked, but there is no reason to think that hair loss can in any way damage the heart. The only reason to treat hair loss is to improve appearance and self-esteem.

TREATMENT

Doctors may not think male pattern baldness is a serious problem, but millions of men disagree. That is why 33 million Americans spend about $1.5 billion a year to replace or restore lost hair.

Treatment takes many forms, ranging from wigs and toupees to scalp surgery and hair transplants. Many men prefer wigs to surgery; some are worn on top of existing hair, while others are interwoven with a man's own hair. Interwoven wigs have to be adjusted every few weeks as the natural hairs grow, adding to expense and inconvenience.

For generations, a bewildering array of concoctions claiming to regrow hair have been sold to gullible men around the world. In 1989, the FDA issued guidelines that cleared the shelves of many expensive and ineffective products. At present, only two drugs are approved for male pattern baldness.

When sold in tablet form, *minoxidil* is a prescription drug for hypertension. But for more than ten years, it has also been available as Rogaine, a nonprescription lotion for hair loss. Regular Rogaine solution or spray contains 2 percent minoxidil, Extra Strength Rogaine, 5 percent. The drug increases the duration of the hair follicles' growth phase, but it works only on follicles that are still active, and its benefits persist only as long as it is used regularly. Rogaine is more effective for bald spots than receding hairlines, but it is only partially effective at that. In one study, 36 percent of men who had used the product for several years felt it was worth the time and money.

According to the manufacturer, Rogaine should be applied twice daily. Scalp irritation can occur; dizziness and low blood pressure are less common side effects. The drug is expensive.

Finasteride is an oral prescription medication that inhibits 5 alpha-reductase, blocking the conversion of testosterone to DHT. In a 5 milligram tablet, finasteride is sold as Proscar for benign prostatic hyperplasia (see Chapter Eleven). In a 1 milligram tablet it is marketed as Propecia for male baldness. In that low dose, it will not do much for the prostate, but it can affect hair follicles, at least to some degree.

To date, only three studies of Propecia, all funded by the manufacturer, have been reported. Two of the trials involved a total of 1,553 men with mild to moderate male pattern baldness that was most prominent at the top of the scalp. Half the men were given Propecia, the other half a look-alike placebo. After three months, the men who took Propecia were more satisfied with the appearance of their hair. After a year, the men who took the drug had an average of 876 hairs in a one-inch circle on the scalp, while the placebo-treated men had 769 hairs. The third trial evaluated 326 men with mild to moderate frontal hair loss; after a year, 50 percent of the men taking Propecia and 30 percent of the men taking the placebo thought their appearance had improved.

All the 1,879 men in the three trials were between the ages of eighteen and forty-one and none were completely bald. Since Propecia does not regrow hair in older men who are bald, it cannot be expected to revive hair follicles that are inactive. As a result, the drug warrants consideration only by younger men with partial hair loss. Because it must be taken daily to remain beneficial, that means years of therapy will be required to maintain even modest improvements. Propecia is even more expensive than Rogaine. It is well-tolerated, but 1 to 2 percent of men experience diminished libido and potency. Because finasteride can produce genital abnormalities in males exposed before birth, the drug should never be taken by women of childbearing age.

To Treat or Not?

It's a personal decision. From a medical point of view, there is no need to treat normal hair loss. At best, the treatments are only partially effective; although therapy is generally safe, some men may experience side effects. Rogaine is inconvenient, and both it and Propecia require permanent use at considerable expense.

Take a look in the mirror and think it over. But before you make a final decision, try to imagine how Michael Jordan would look with a bit of hair.

EPILOGUE

Preventive Maintenance: Medical Care for Men

ALTHOUGH MUCH HAS CHANGED over two-and-a-half millennia, modern medicine still traces its roots to the ancient Greeks. Those early physicians attributed health to Aesculapius, the god of healing. But Aesculapius, however powerful, did not go it alone. Instead he divided his responsibilities between his two daughters: Hygeia was put in charge of wise living and healthful behavior, while Panacea governed the use of medication.

In this case, as in many others, the Greeks got it right; good health depends on a combination of a healthful lifestyle and effective medical care. Part II of this Guide took a page from Hygeia's book, focusing on the habits that can keep men healthy. But despite our best efforts, illnesses will still strike, and Part III discussed the medical problems of particular importance to men. And now it's time to turn to Panacea's domain to consider the tests and treatments that can help preserve health and prevent illness. Medical treatments can never substitute for wise living, and they are not panaceas; still, preventive maintenance should be part of every man's program for health.

The Health Care System

In case you missed it, here is the secret to our health care system: There is no system. Instead, there are many systems. During the course of the twentieth century, the standard of medical care has shifted from the solo practitioner to the medical group, from the generalist to the specialist, from the private office to the hospital and clinic. Financial responsibility has also evolved, shifting from a fee-for-service model to third-party payers in the form of insurance companies, HMOs, and government programs. As a result of all this, some aspects of care have improved but others have suffered. Even when care has improved, however, confusion and frustration threaten to obscure real gains.

It is a complex situation and it is changing fast. Men should stay informed about new developments so they can help promote reforms that will improve healthcare for all Americans. Above all, men should concentrate on the basics, on the core issues that remain constant in a sea of change: Find a good doctor, get the checkups and tests you should have, and understand how to get help when you need it.

Your Doctor

Your doctor is still the key, but he is not likely to work alone. Instead, your doctor is likely to share responsibility for your care with other physicians and with nurses and assistants.

In this case, more is better, as long as you have a designated individual who is in charge of the team. In most cases, it is a primary care physician; for men, that means an internist or family practitioner.

Picking a physician can be difficult. First, you will need to be sure that your insurance covers his services. Next, check for education, training, and certification; if you are shy about asking, your local medical society will provide the information you need. You can also log on to the American Medical Association's free Physician Select service at www.ama-assn.org/aps, which will allow you to search for any physician in the United States. With a click or two, you can learn the doctor's gender, medical school, year of graduation, residency training, board certification, and specialty. You can also learn if the physician has received special awards or, for that matter, disciplinary actions.

Collecting the information is easy, but evaluating it is not. Not every patient can find a doctor from Harvard or Yale, and even if they could, not every Harvard graduate is a good clinician. Do not be dazzled by fancy diplomas and big name hospitals, but if all things are equal (which they seldom are) go for the name brand, at least until you see if the personal chemistry is right.

Although you are likely to see a variety of doctors over the years, your primary care physician is the linchpin who will handle most of your problems and coordinate specialty referrals. For most men, a doctor who has completed three years of residency training in internal medicine or family practice is best. After completing his residency, a doctor is deemed "board eligible"; if he then passes a rigorous exam in his field he becomes "board-certified." Some internists take two or more additional years of fellowship training to become subspecialists in cardiology, gastroenterology, or other fields; each subspecialty has its own board that administers certifying exams. Long years of training do not always translate into top-notch care, but in general, more training is better.

Be sure to pick a medical team that will be available to answer questions and discuss problems by phone and that will see you in the office on short notice if you are ill. Remember to pick a team that you can reach quickly in an emergency, even during nights and weekends.

Because your doctor is part of a team, you should be comfortable with his colleagues. It is also important to pick a doctor who is associated with a good hospital that offers a broad range of medical and surgical services. If it is available, a university-affiliated medical center is usually a good bet.

Education and affiliations are one thing, personality and style, another. For the best care, chemistry can be as important as intellect. It is not something you can learn about from credentials and diplomas, but you can get helpful leads from friends and relatives who know the doctor. Above all, see for yourself. Give it some time and do your part to establish a trusting, professional relationship. If it does not work out, do not be afraid to make a change.

Sharing Responsibilities

In medicine, at least, autocracy is a thing of the past. The paternalistic model of a physician who tells his patient what to do has been replaced by the concept of a doctor–patient partnership, with both parties working together to solve health-related problems.

Communication is the key. Tell your doctor how much information you want. Do you want your actual test results, a simple "everything's fine," or will you settle for no news is good news. And if bad news comes, how much detail do you want to hear—and how much data, favorable or worrisome, should your doctor share with your family?

Be honest with your doctor and yourself. Not even the best doctor can read your mind. If you have worries or concerns, discuss them. Most men do not, particularly when sensitive issues such as sexuality and emotions are concerned. It's a mistake. Learn to talk frankly—and if your doctor is not a good listener, get a new one.

Be an active, informed health care consumer. Keep lists of your questions and do not hesitate to ask for a clarification if you do not understand an answer. Do not be afraid to ask a "dumb question"—there is no such thing (though there are dumb answers). Do not be surprised if your doctor does not know all the answers; nobody does, and a doctor who thinks he knows it all is a bigger worry than one who will try to learn new things to meet your needs.

Keep your own medical records—not all the details, but the dates of important events, the results of major tests, and the effects of treatments. It is particularly important to keep track of your medications. Know what you are taking and why. Check to be sure that drugs will not interact adversely with each other and find out if they should be taken at a special time of day or if food will affect their absorption. Be sure to inform your doctor and pharmacist about any nonprescription drugs and supplements that you are using. Keep a careful, up-to-date list of allergic reactions and side effects. And take good care of your pills: Store them in their original bottles, in a cool, dry, secure place; do not take them if they look or smell funny; and discard them when they expire or you no longer need them.

Stay informed about new developments in medicine (see the Appendix). Use books, newsletters, newspapers, and magazines. Surf the web and visit your favorite health sites regularly. But do not try to be your own doctor. No consumer health product can convey all the complexities and nuances of medicine and most do not even try. Check the credentials of your sources and discuss what you learn with your doctor before you make any big changes.

A common analogy likens your primary care physician to the quarterback of your health care team. It is an apt description, but it overlooks the fact that you are the owner and general manager. It is okay to let your medical quarterback call the plays, but it is your job to work with him to be sure you are moving in the right direction. And you should never be afraid to ask for a second opinion if you feel your doctor may need a bit of coaching.

In the Office

There are two types of office visits: preventive checkups and problem visits.

The most important checkup is your initial office visit. You should be asked to provide a detailed medical history including your illnesses, operations, medications, immunizations, and allergies. You should also be asked about your family's medical history and your personal health habits such as diet, exercise, tobacco and alcohol use, and safety issues ranging from sex to firearms to seatbelts. You should have a thorough head-to-toe physical, including measurements of your weight and blood pressure. Subsequent visits will depend on your health; they will be less frequent and simpler if your health is fine and you are taking good care of yourself, more frequent if you have problems that need attention. Followup visits will be like miniature versions of your initial visit. You should be asked to update your database and to have another physical exam. Above all, perhaps, you should have ample opportunities to ask questions and discuss your concerns at all visits.

How often should you see your doctor for routine checkups? A healthy man with good health habits can get by with surprisingly few visits, but he will not get to know his doctor and may lose continuity. As a rule of thumb, many physicians recommend checkups every five years for men in their twenties, every three years for men in their thirties, every two years for men in their forties, and every year after age fifty.

If you are ill, of course, you will need more care. It is important for you to know how to reach your doctor to get advice by telephone and how to arrange an unscheduled visit when you need one. You should understand your doctor's coverage system and how to get emergency care when you need a safety net.

In our modern world of high-tech medicine, people expect to have tests when they go to their doctors. In most cases, they will not be disappointed. Tests can be important to screen for diseases before symptoms develop; diabetes and colon cancer are good examples. Tests can also be important to establish baseline values for future comparison; the electrocardiogram (EKG) is an example. But tests must be used wisely. Many are expensive or inconvenient and some can have risks of their own. No test is completely accurate, but some have a higher than average likelihood of providing false reassurance by failing to detect abnormalities, while others may raise false alarms by diagnosing disease when none is present. Doctors describe tests that miss abnormalities as having *low sensitivity* and tests that overdiagnose problems as having *low specificity*. But even if a test is inexpensive and safe with a good sensitivity and specificity, it will be worthwhile only if the results can lead to an intervention that will improve your health.

It is a high standard for a test to meet. Let's see how various tests measure up.

Preventive Services for Men

Prevention is the best medicine. The best prevention depends on your lifestyle (see Part II), not your physician, but your doctor can certainly help. The great Greek physician Galen was among the first to voice the idea when he wrote: "Since, both in importance and time, health precedes disease, so we ought to consider first how health may be preserved, and then how we may best cure disease." Our modern notions of preventive maintenance are much newer, dating from 1900, when Dr. George Gould articulated the concept that periodic medical care could prevent disease. With automobile maintenance as a model, Americans rapidly embraced the idea of preventive care. That's why the preventive checkup is the single most common reason that people see their doctors, accounting for at least 100 million office visits a year.

During the past thirty years, the old concept of preventive maintenance has taken on a new look. Without disputing the importance of prevention, doctors have been reevaluating the value of specific tests and treatments to find out which are really beneficial. The most comprehensive reviews have been performed by the U.S. Preventive Services Task Force and the Canadian Task Force on Preventive Care. In addition, many organizations have issued guidelines of their own. Examples include medical specialty groups such as the American College of Physicians, the American Urological Association, and the American College of Cardiology, and advocacy groups such as the American Cancer Society, the American Heart Association, and the American Diabetes Association.

With so many people at work, disagreements are inevitable. Fortunately, most disputes relate to details, not principles—and even the best guidelines are subject to change as new data accumulate.

Above all, guidelines are suggestions, not commandments. While valuable, they can and should be adapted to meet individual needs. For example, people at higher risk for a particular disease should have more intensive testing than people at low risk.

Here is a set of suggestions for routine tests and immunizations for healthy adult men. They apply to individuals with average risk factors, no symptoms of disease, and normal physical exams. They are based principally on the suggestion of the U.S. Task Force on Preventive Services and the American College of Physicians. Of course, they are subject to modification and change. To check the latest recommendations of the U.S. Task Force, visit the Agency for Healthcare Research and Quality website (www.ahrq.gov).

Table E.1: ROUTINE TESTING FOR HEALTHY MEN

TESTS AND MEASUREMENTS	INTERVAL
Blood pressure	At every physical exam; at least every 1–2 years.
Cholesterol	At the initial checkup, then at least every 5 years.
Complete blood counts	At the initial checkup; then periodically, depending on the physician's practice and the patient's preference.

Urinalysis	At the initial checkup; then periodically.
Fasting blood sugar test	At age 45; then every 3 years.
Electrocardiogram	Baseline at age 40; then periodically.
Chest X-ray	Not recommended for screening.
Eye exam by specialist	Baseline at 50; then every 1–2 years.
Hearing tests	Not recommended for screening.
Dental exam and prophylaxis	At 6–12 month intervals.
Prostate cancer screening	Annual prostate specific antigen (PSA) blood tests and digital rectal exams should be offered to men starting at age 50 (or 40 for African Americans or men with fathers or brothers with prostate cancer). Testing is unlikely to be helpful beyond age 70. See Chapter 12 for the pros and cons of screening.
Colon cancer screening	Strongly recommended starting at age 50. Men at average risk can choose among four options. 1. Annual fecal occult blood testing (FOBT) with colonoscopy for a positive test. 2. FOBT as above plus sigmoidoscopy every 5 years. 3. Colonoscopy every 10 years. 4. Double-contrast barium enema every 5–10 years. Colonoscopy is the most accurate test but is the most arduous (and expensive). Men with higher than average risk should choose colonoscopy; examples include men who have had previous colon polyps and men with colon cancer in a parent or sibling.
Skin cancer screening	Periodic self-examination with physician exams at regular checkup intervals. Exams by specialists for people at high risk.
Testicular cancer screening	Periodic self-examination (see Chapter 9) with physician exams at regular checkups until age 35.
Tetanus diphtheria booster	Every 10 years.
Influenza vaccine	Every fall, starting at age 50.
Pneumococcal pneumonia	At age 65 with boosters every 5–10 years.
Hepatitis A vaccine	Two injections 6 months apart for travelers to high risk areas or men at risk for close contact with infected individuals.
Hepatitis B vaccine	A series of three injections over 6 months for men at risk of exposure to blood or body fluids.
Immunizations for measles, rubella, polio, lyme disease, yellow fever, cholera, typhoid	Individual recommendations for travelers and others at particular risk.

Considering all the tests and treatments that are available for sick people, the list for healthy people is surprisingly short. To keep your own preventive maintenance simple, you will have to take good care of yourself. You will also have to listen to your body. If you detect signs of discord, discuss them with your doctor to see if additional tests may be helpful.

Preventive maintenance is the key to good health. Your doctor can help with advice and exams, tests and recommendations, but the rest is up to you.

Be well!

Sources for More Information

Newsletters

Medical research is producing important new insights into health and disease at a rapid pace. Health newsletters can help you keep up with developments.

Harvard Men's Health Watch is an eight-page monthly newsletter devoted to issues that matter to men most. It is available on the Web at www.health.harvard.edu. You can get more information by calling 1-800-829-3341 or writing to Harvard Health Publications, 10 Shattuck Street, Boston, MA 02115.

Organizations

Many government agencies and independent groups provide excellent consumer health information, typically without charge. Here are some resources of particular interest to men:

Food and Drug Administration
5600 Fishers Ln.
Rockville, MD 20857
(888) INFO-FDA (463-6332)
www.fda.gov

National Cancer Institute
9000 Rockville Pike
Bethesda, MD 20848
(800) 4-CANCER
www.nci.nih.gov

National Center for Complementary and Alternative Medicine
NCCAM Clearinghouse
P.O. Box 7923
Gaithersburg, MD 20898-7923
(888) 644-6226 (toll free)
www.nccam.nih.gov

National Institute of Mental Health
NIMH Public Inquiries
6001 Executive Blvd., Room 8184, MSC 9663
Bethesda, MD 20892-9663
(301) 443-4513
www.nimh.nih.gov

National Heart, Lung, and Blood Institute
National Institutes of Health
NHLBI Information Center
P.O. Box 30105
Bethesda, MD 20824-0105
(301) 592-8573
(800) 575-9355 (Consumer hotline with recorded messages)
www.nhlbi.nih.gov

American Diabetes Association/NCC
1701 North Beauregard St.
Alexandria, VA 22311
(800) 342-2383
www.diabetes.org

American Dietetic Association
216 W. Jackson Blvd.
Suite 800
Chicago, IL 60606
(800) 366-1655
www.eatright.org

American Heart Association
American Stroke Association
7272 Greenville Ave.
Dallas, TX 75231
(800) 242-8721 (AHA)
(888) 478-7653 (ASA)
www.americanheart.org
www.strokeassociation.org

American Cancer Society
1599 Clifton Road NE
Atlanta, GA 30329
(800) 227-2345
www.cancer.org

National Kidney and Urologic Diseases Information Clearinghouse
National Institutes of Health
Building 31, Room 9A04
Center Drive, MSC 2560
Bethesda, MD 20892-2560
(301) 654-4415
www.niddk.nih.gov

WEBSITES

Consumer-friendly health information, reviewed and approved by leading medical and dental experts, is available at www.intelihealth.com.

For a complete bibliography of the Harvard men's health studies cited in this book, please visit www.health.harvard.edu/HMS_mens_health.

Index

Page numbers in *italics* refer to figures and tables.

Illustration Credits

The following illustrations are copyright © Harriet R. Greenfield, West Newton, Massachusetts: Figure 1.2, page 10; Figure 1.3, page 13; Figure 3.1, page 42; Figure 3.2, page 58; Figure 5.2, page 150; Figure 5.3, page 152; Figure 5.4, page 154; Figure 9.1, page 249; Figure 9.2, page 257; Figure 9.3, page 259; Figure 9.4, page 261; Figure 9.5, page 262; Figure 9.6, page 263; Figure 9.7, page 267; Figure 9.8, page 270; Figure 10.1, page 274; Figure 10.2, page 275; Figure 10.4, page 284; Figure 11.1, page 325; Figure 11.2, page 343; Figure 12.1, page 375; Figure 12.2, page 396; Figure 12.3, page 400; Figure 13.1, page 417; Figure 14.1, page 440; Figure 14.2, page 455.

The illustration "Male Karyotype" (Figure 1.1, page 8) is reprinted with permission from WebMD Scientific American Medicine.

The graph "BMI and the Risk of Disease" (Figure 4.1, page 75) is reprinted from "Physical Activity as an Index of Heart Attack Risk in College Alumni" in the September, 1978, issue of the *American Journal of Epidemiology.*

The graph "Benefits of Exercise" (Figure 5.1, page 133) is reprinted from "Body-Mass Index and Mortality in a Prospective Cohort of U.S. Adults" in the October 7, 1999, issue of the *New England Journal of Medicine.*